70

Improving Diabetes Care in the Clinic

Improving Diabetes Care in the Clinic

Editor

Jayendra H Shah MBBS MCPS FACP FACE

Professor of Medicine and Radiology
University of Arizona College of Medicine
Former Chief of Staff, Southern Arizona VA Health Care System, and
Network Research Officer, Veterans Integrated Service Network-18
Tucson, Arizona, USA

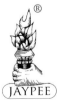

JAYPEE

JAYPEE BROTHERS MEDICAL PUBLISHERS (P) LTD.

New Delhi • London • Philadelphia • Panama

Jaypee Brothers Medical Publishers (P) Ltd

Headquarters

Jaypee Brothers Medical Publishers (P) Ltd
4838/24, Ansari Road, Daryaganj
New Delhi 110 002, India
Phone: +91-11-43574357
Fax: +91-11-43574314
Email: jaypee@jaypeebrothers.com

Overseas Offices

J.P. Medical Ltd
83 Victoria Street, London
SW1H 0HW (UK)
Phone: +44-2031708910
Fax: +02-03-0086180
Email: info@jpmedpub.com

Jaypee Medical Inc
The Bourse
111 South Independence Mall East
Suite 835, Philadelphia, PA 19106, USA
Phone: +1 267-519-9789
Email: joe.rusko@jaypeebrothers.com

Jaypee Brothers Medical Publishers (P) Ltd
Bhotahity, Kathmandu, Nepal
Phone: +977-9741283608
Email: kathmandu@jaypeebrothers.com

Jaypee-Highlights Medical Publishers Inc
City of Knowledge, Bld. 237, Clayton
Panama City, Panama
Phone: +1 507-301-0496
Fax: +1 507-301-0499
Email: cservice@jphmedical.com

Jaypee Brothers Medical Publishers (P) Ltd
17/1-B Babar Road, Block-B, Shaymali
Mohammadpur, Dhaka-1207
Bangladesh
Mobile: +08801912003485
Email: jaypeedhaka@gmail.com

Website: www.jaypeebrothers.com
Website: www.jaypeedigital.com

Improving Diabetes Care in the Clinic

First Edition: **2014**

ISBN 978-93-5090-955-3

Printed at: Samrat Offset Pvt. Ltd.

Dedicated to

Reverend Pandurang Shashtri Athavale (Dadaji), philosopher and modern day sage (Rishi), for teaching the Way of Thinking, Way of Life, and Way of Devotion to humanity through the medium of Swadhyay,
and
My parents, Hiralal and Radhaben Shah, for their constant love and inspiration to excel in all endeavors.

Contents

Contributors

Editor

Jayendra H Shah MBBS MCPS FACP FACE
Professor of Medicine and Radiology
University of Arizona College of Medicine
Former Chief of Staff, Southern Arizona VA Health Care System, and
Network Research Officer, Veterans Integrated Service Network-18
Tucson, Arizona, USA

Contributing Authors

RM Anjana MD Dip Diab (UK)
Joint Managing Director and Consultant
Diabetologist, Madras Diabetes Research
Foundation & Dr. Mohan's Diabetes
Specialities Centre
Chennai, Tamil Nadu, India

David G Armstrong DPM MD PhD
Professor of Surgery and Director,
Southern Arizona Limb Salvage Alliance
Department of Surgery
University of Arizona College of Medicine
Tucson, Arizona, USA

Modassar Awan MD
Southern Arizona Limb Salvage Alliance
Department of Surgery
University of Arizona College of Medicine
Tucson, Arizona, USA

Hemraj B Chandalia MD FACP
Diabetes Endocrine Nutrition
Management and Research Centre &
Jaslok Hospital and Research Center
Formerly, Honorary Professor of Medicine
and Diabetes, Grant Medical College
Mumbai, Maharashtra, India

Michelle Cordoba-Kissee MD
Staff Endocrinologist
Southern Arizona VA Health Care System
Inpatient Endocrinology Consultant
Tucson Medical Center
Assistant Professor of Medicine
University of Arizona College of
Medicine
Tucson, Arizona, USA

Ryan K Crisel MD
Senior Cardiology Fellow
Division of Cardiology
Department of Medicine
Northwestern University Feinberg School
of Medicine
Chicago, Illinois, USA

Joseph Fiorito DPM
Southern Arizona Limb Salvage Alliance
Department of Surgery
University of Arizona College of Medicine
Tucson, Arizona, USA

Alexander A Izad MD
Vitreoretinal Disease and Surgery
Staff Physician, Southern Arizona VA
Health Care System
Assistant Clinical Professor of
Ophthalmology
University of Arizona College of Medicine
Tucson, Arizona, USA

Vikram Kamdar MD
Clinical Professor of Medicine
Department of Medicine
Division of Endocrinology, Metabolism
and Hypertension
David Geffen School of Medicine, UCLA
Los Angeles, California, USA

Shubh P Kaur MD
Chief Resident
Department of Medicine
University of Arizona Medical Center
Tucson, Arizona, USA

Kathleen E Kendle MD FACP
Assistant Chief of Staff
Southern AZ VA Health Care System
Assistant Professor of Medicine
University of Arizona College of Medicine
Tucson, Arizona, USA

Brian Lekyum DPM
Southern Arizona Limb Salvage Alliance
Department of Surgery
University of Arizona College of Medicine
Tucson, Arizona, USA

V Mohan MD FRCP (Lond, Edin, Glasg, Ire) PhD
DSc FNASc DSc (Hon. Causa) FNA
Chairman & Chief Diabetologist, Madras
Diabetes Research Foundation &
Dr. Mohan's Diabetes Specialties Centre
Chennai, Tamil Nadu, India

Glen H Murata MD
Professor of Medicine, University of New
Mexico School of Medicine
Medical Director, Informatics Service
Director, Center for Health Services and
Informatics Research
New Mexico VA Health Care System
Albuquerque, New Mexico, USA

Mordecai M Popovtzer MD FACP FASN
Program Director, Division of Nephrology
Professor of Medicine
Southern Arizona VA Health Care System
and University of Arizona College of
Medicine
Tucson, Arizona USA

R Pradeepa PhD
Senior Scientist and Head
Department of Research Operations
Madras Diabetes Research Foundation &
Dr. Mohan's Diabetes Specialities Centre
Chennai, Tamil Nadu, India

Venkateswara K Rao MD FACP
Professor, Department of Medicine
Division of Nephrology
University of Arizona College of Medicine
Renal Physician, Southern Arizona VA
Health Care System
Tucson, Arizona, USA

Sanjiv J Shah MD
Associate Professor of Medicine
Division of Cardiology
Department of Medicine
Northwestern University Feinberg School
of Medicine
Chicago, Illinois, USA

Craig S Stump MD PhD FACE
Associate Professor of Medicine and
Nutritional Sciences
Chief, Division of Endocrinology,
Diabetes, and Hypertension
Southern Arizona VA Healthcare System
University of Arizona Medical Center
Tucson, Arizona, USA

Stephen P Thomson MD
Director, Endocrinology Fellowship
Program
Staff Endocrinologist
Southern Arizona VA Health Care System
Assistant Professor of Medicine
University of Arizona College of Medicine
Tucson, Arizona, USA

Hussein Yassine MD
Director of Lipid Clinic
Clinical Science Center
University of Southern California
Los Angeles, California, USA

Preface

Globally, diabetes has reached an epidemic proportion. According to United States (US) Center for Disease control and Prevention (CDC), nearly 26 million American have diabetes and 79 million adults (more than one third adults) in US have pre-diabetes. Blood glucose higher than normal, but not high enough to be diagnosed as diabetes defines pre-diabetes, which increases individual's risk for developing type 2 diabetes, heart disease, and stroke. Incidence of diabetes in US is 8.3% in persons of all ages, but 11.3% in persons aged 20 and older. Approximately seven million people (27%) of those with diabetes are unaware that they have diabetes. If this statistical trend continues, CDC has projected that by year 2050, as many as 1 in 3 adults in US may develop diabetes. The International Diabetes Federation has estimated that in 2011, 7% adults (366 million) in the world had diabetes; and further estimated that by 2030, 8.3% (552 million) adults globally will be suffering from diabetes. It is estimated that type 2 diabetes accounts for up to 95% of all individuals with diabetes. In recent years, incidence of type 2 diabetes in youth, 10 to 16 years of age, is also increased. The sedentary lifestyle, ever increasing obesity, and longevity are main causative factors in the increased incidence of type 2 diabetes in adults and youth. The incidence of diabetes is higher in geriatric (individuals above the age of 65) population. It is estimated that in US, over one-fourth of geriatric population suffer from diabetes and nearly half have pre-diabetes. Diabetes affects all organ system in the body and its microvascular complications cause neuropathy, nephropathy, and retinopathy; whereas macrovascular complications cause peripheral vascular, cardiovascular, and cerebrovascular diseases. Diabetes complications are responsible for blindness, amputations, stroke, acute myocardial infarction, heart failure, and chronic renal failure requiring dialysis. This increase burden of diabetes and its complications has profound social and economic implications on the individual patient, family, and society. In US, yearly cost for diabetes is estimated to be $174 billion including $116 billion in direct medical care cost. Indeed, type 2 diabetes is a preventable and manageable disease and a burden of this chronic disease of epidemic proportion is an embarrassment to health care profession.

In providing care to diabetic patients, education to patient and family members is one of the most important aspects of management. The informed decisions about self-monitoring of blood glucose (SMBG), nutrition, exercise, weight control, eye and foot care, use of oral medications and insulin, prevention of micro- and macrovascular complications cannot be effectively managed without knowledge of diabetes. Also, factors such as desire to learn, cognitive abilities, attitudes, depression, family support, barriers to diabetes care, and cultural and ethnic background, influence the learning process. Obviously, physicians and other health care professionals play a pivotal role in providing education and care to patients with this chronic devastating disease. Diabetic patients frequently find that lifestyle changes are overwhelming and for health care providers, managing their diabetes is challenging. The Food Frequency Questionnaires (FFQ) is a tool to quickly identify patients with poor adherence to diet recommendation and poor metabolic control. This can provide information for appropriate intervention, whether for glycemic control or for managing hypertension or hyperlipidemia. FFQ can be easily completed at home by patient with help of spouse or other family members in a non-threatening environment. Health care providers can use information from FFQ in combination with other parameters such as SMBG, HbA1c, weight, blood pressure readings, lipid levels etc. and discuss with the patient attainable realistic goals for diet and overall metabolic control. Frequently, health care providers only focus on glycemic control with pharmacologic agents, while management of hypertension, hyperlipidemia, obesity, and foot hygiene is neglected in diabetic patients. It has been shown that presence of several risk factors in diabetic patients increase mortality to a greater extent at young age than a single factor. Studies have confirmed that treating hyperglycemia, hypertension, and hyperlipidemia decrease mortality. In fact, when hypertension and hyperlipidemia are well controlled in type 2 diabetic patients, the benefit of glycemic control was difficult to ascertain. The pharmacologic treatment should not distract health care providers in dealing with the factors to prevent diabetes and its complications.

In the forthcoming health care reform in USA, emphasis will be placed on prevention, outcomes, quality of care, patient's need, reducing cost, and evidence based guidelines. A new concept in the health care delivery, "Medical Home", for management of chronic disease such as diabetes, which leverages resources and improves the outcomes while holding down the cost, will be utilized for diabetes management. The advent of electronic medical record will aid in processing of complex medical data on individual patient and help the health care provider for care coordination. The electronic data will ease in the formation of patient registries. Diabetes registry can identify which diabetic patient is in need of specific care and it will help health care provider to coordinate SMBG, nutritional, and weight loss tracking; management of hyperglycemia, hypertension, hyperlipidemia, heart failure, and depression; preventing microvascular and macrovascular complications and providing appropriate vaccinations. When most sensitive patient data are used then the diabetes registry will help prevent progression of early diabetes. The diabetes registry can identify patients who can benefit from structured yet parsimonious and cost-effective SMBG to achieve glycemic control and appropriate health care outcomes. The prevention of micro- and macrovascular complications is the arduous task for clinicians caring for diabetic patients. Once the diabetic complications sets in, the health care providers face some of the complex management challenges of diabetic retinopathy leading to blindness, diabetic nephropathy leading to chronic renal failure, dialysis, renal transplantation, diabetic peripheral vascular disease, and neuropathy leading to lower extremity amputations, and diabetic heart disease with or without atherosclerosis leading to coronary artery bypass surgeries and/or onerous treatment task of chronic heart failure. The aforementioned issues are expertly discussed in the exclusive chapters in this book.

Diabetes with its complications has become a multisystem and multifactorial disease. Therefore, it appears that for a physician, knowing diabetes is like knowing internal medicine, sometimes complex and puzzling. There is a vast amount of literature, often confusing and conflicting, is available on multitude of topics concerning diabetes and its complications. To write and publish another such book would be an exercise in futility. However, this book has made a sincere effort to provide new and futuristic information in diabetes management, and it is not overwhelming. The chapters in this book have made an attempt to provide unbiased and evidence-based information in a comprehensive yet concise manner to be a useful guide for practicing primary care physicians, endocrinologists, and other health care providers in their quest of providing excellent care to their diabetic patients. The authors have taken meticulous efforts to provide current practice recommendation. In many chapters, the tables and figures stipulate clear and concise guidance which can be used as ready reference material by busy practitioners. Most of the care of diabetes and steps taken to prevent its complications occurs in the institutional or private practice clinics. I sincerely hope that this book can be used as a diabetes management compendium to improve diabetes care in the clinic.

Jayendra H Shah

Acknowledgments

This book is a concerted effort of many individuals. I am indebted to all contributing authors for their hard work and for making unbiased recommendations in their chapters. They have also tried their utmost to provide an evidence based reviews to make this book unique. Without their contributions, fruition of this book would have been difficult.

I want to express my sincere gratitude to my dear wife, Saroj J Shah, MD for her constant encouragement and support. She has made many sacrifices to support my academic and administrative life and to maintain our family's harmony. She has been a 'sounding board' and constant source of inspiration for me.

I wish to thank Jaypee Brothers Medical Publishers (P) Ltd for publishing this book. I want to extend my special thanks to Dr. Madhu Choudhary, Senior Editor, whose persistent efforts to convince me to write and edit this book paid off. She also provided all the technical help to the contributing authors and I needed to continue writing the chapters.

I am grateful that Veterans Health Administration (VHA) and specifically Southern Arizona VA Health Care System (SAVAHCS) in Tucson, Arizona have provided me the platform to participate in making innovative changes in improving patient care as well as performing clinical research in the field of diabetes. I also wish to thank Lynn Flance MLS and Karen D Douglas MLS, the librarians at SAVAHCS for willingly helping several contributing authors and me in finding appropriate references for the chapters.

Finally, in some of the chapters, I and other authors have used clinical findings emanated from our research which was supported by the VHA and SAVAHCS Research Services.

Diabetes Registries— A Practical Guide to Design, Selection, and Its Use in the Management of Diabetes

Glen H Murata

ABSTRACT

Most major industries—retailing, manufacturing, transportation, financial, hospitality, energy, and natural resources, etc.—rely on information technology to perform a systematic evaluation of operations, identify where processes are suboptimal, and triage those problems to appropriate personnel for corrective action. No one would board an airplane if the pilot not only had to fly the plane but chart the course on paper using a sextant and compass. Moreover, the chances of recovery would be small if the first indication of trouble is a sudden loss in altitude. However, our health care industry has been operating in this mode for decades—without a clear indication of what works and what doesn't, which patients need care and which don't, and which providers are doing well and which are not. Moreover, the first indication of trouble is an adverse patient outcome for which there may be no recovery, exhaustion of resources resulting in withdrawal of care, or poor job satisfaction leading to a decline in the physician workforce. Fortunately, health care systems are now adopting information systems which will bring their enterprises into the modern age. Because they focus on the management of entire populations, registries are the most promising of many tools that will drive much-needed and much-delayed health care reform. As one of the most complicated chronic diseases, diabetes should be the focus of one of the first registries at almost every institution.

INTRODUCTION

Webster's online dictionary defines "disease registry" as a "system of ongoing registration of all cases of a particular disease or health condition in a defined population" (www.websters-online-dictionary.org/definitions/DISEASE+REGISTRY). Although there is a tremendous variation in their functionality, registries share common features including disease focus, specified purpose, targeted population, sponsorship, data sources, data elements, storage format, architecture, data entry, analytical techniques, and reporting services. Each of these domains has undergone a remarkable evolution in recent years. The number of diseases or conditions tracked by disease registries has increased substantially in countries around the world.[1] Registries are now used to track the incidence, prevalence, and risk factors for disease, often to mitigate exposures in populations; to track the natural history of disease; to assemble enough rare cases for systematic study; for research on the association between treatments and outcomes; for quality improvement (QI) through profiling and identifying best practices; for health policy and financial planning; to manage populations by characterizing the needs of and prioritizing services for its members; and to support decision making for individual patients. The targeted population can vary by age, gender, ethnicity, geographic locale, or entitlement. Although registries were first developed by government agencies for epidemiologic purposes, they are now sponsored by professional organizations, health care systems, insurance companies, and pharmaceutical firms. The earliest registries were populated by case reporting from individual clinicians; now, many of the most useful retrieve data automatically from electronic medical records. Data elements range from coded or standardized data to free text and even images. Registries that used to be recorded on paper are now stored in large relational databases residing on institutional computers. Sophisticated software can derive new clinical parameters from raw data and perform sophisticated analyses well beyond the reach of most clinicians. Finally, results can be reported to users through the internet or reporting services of many database software applications.

One of the most common applications for these registries is to help institutions, practices, or individual clinicians deal with chronic diseases. Managing a chronic illness often requires follow-up over years, multiple visits, intensive and repeated testing, many consultants, and care delivered in different settings. Problems may occur with transitions of care from provider to provider, from setting to setting, or from one phase of the disease to another. As a result, their treatment tends to become fragmented, delayed, or incomplete over time resulting in suboptimal outcomes, poor quality of life, and diminished patient satisfaction. Chronic diseases are particularly vulnerable to problems related to access, financing, work force, distribution of services, and legal liabilities. Because most health care systems are struggling with these issues, it is no surprise that there is a surging interest in a technological solution to the problems.

BACKGROUND

The health care crisis in the United States and many other countries represents the confluence of several social trends—poor access to care, dismal health outcomes, unsustainable costs, patient and provider dissatisfaction, and erosion of the primary care base. To a large extent, this "perfect storm" is due to a delivery system based upon the "acute care model". In this paradigm, encounters are initiated by the patient in response to symptoms. This strategy often places the onus for first contact on the person who has the least knowledge about his/her condition or the illness in question. For example, a patient with colonic polyps can miss the next colonoscopy because he or she was unaware of the pathology results, its implications, or recommendations for surveillance. Planning by the physician is done on a case-by-case basis so that it is not possible to anticipate the needs of entire populations or set priorities to maximize collective well-being. Finally, the intervention is reactive, i.e., to ameliorate a condition that has progressed beyond the preclinical phase. The opportunity to treat the condition at an earlier and often more responsive stage is lost.

These problems are compounded by reliance upon the outpatient visit as the principal means of delivering medical services. The "visit-based" approach precludes the neediest patients—those with access barriers who never present for treatment. Progress is tied to the next available appointment, not to the responsiveness of the disease to treatment. For example, insulin titrations often occur every several months even though treatment response can be assessed in just a few days. Despite its disadvantages, administrative processes and financial incentives still favor the acute care, visit-based approach. Examples include the need to identify a "primary diagnosis" for an outpatient encounter and higher reimbursement for an office visit than an equally effective telephone call. The more efficient approach is to track the health status of an entire population, focus attention on the highest priorities, recall patients when services are needed as well as requested, intercede at early rather than late stages of illness, and triage patients to team members with the most appropriate skill level.

Meaningful health care reform, i.e., changes to improve quality while reducing costs, requires a fundamental re-engineering of the nation's health care system. "Population management" provides the overarching conceptual framework in which such reform can occur. Its components include greater emphasis on collective performance, societal impact, and affordability; more realistic expectations of and more active participation by patients; increased accountability of providers for reporting outcomes and justifying expenditure of common resources; prioritization based upon need and likelihood of benefit; optimization based upon correlating processes and outcomes; reducing disparities due to race/ethnicity, geography, or economic status; and setting standards for the delivery of services through health policy. In this new paradigm, health care institutions would develop guidelines that are data driven, evidence based, and individualized to each patient's circumstance; enhance the value of services through performance reviews and cost analyses; provide seamless care through different settings and phases of illness; allocate resources based upon realized and unmet demand for services; assess performance on a 100% sample of cases instead of random audits; and charge QI personnel with interventional as well as analytical responsibilities. Clinicians should also practice in a different way. The emphasis would shift from processes to outcomes; the setting would shift from the office to anything that works; prevention would take precedence over cure; consultations would be prioritized by patient need instead of provider preferences; continuing medical education (CME) would be driven by provider performance instead of interest; practice guidelines would be replaced by individual risk stratification; and equal attention would be given to the psychological, social, and biological determinants of outcomes. All of these needed reforms depend upon gathering comprehensive data on the personal, provider, practice, health system, and national level.

ROLE OF HEALTH INFORMATION TECHNOLOGY

Fortunately, the electronic medical record provides an unprecedented opportunity for promoting these reforms. "Front-end" capabilities include shared access to a comprehensive medical record; practice support as exemplified by automated forms processing, computerized order entry, and treatment advisories; enhanced patient safety through alerts and warnings; and decision-support based upon complex processing of clinical data beyond the reach of a busy clinician. However, it is the "back-end" functionalities that will enable providers, health systems, and government agencies to manage resources in a way that optimize the health status of populations. Systems can now tap into the stream of data populating clinical data repositories. These innovations include cohort tracking in which the work-up of patients is monitored in real time; visit management in which patients are "prepped" for an upcoming visit; prevention management in which services are coordinated at an institutional level on behalf of clinicians; pharmacy management in which indications, safety, cost, effectiveness, and adherence are concurrently monitored; and consult management in which appropriate cases are referred to specialists even if they are "missed" by their primary care providers (PCPs). Registries are the most influential of these back-end functionalities. They can track the status of an entire population with a given condition and stratify its members by risk, need, severity, or complexity. Identifying patients at high risk allows providers to focus behavioral modification and preventive services on the group most likely to benefit. Some patients may have greater need for services than others because they are less able to afford such care on their own, more likely to respond, suffer greater consequences of unmanaged illness, or are more overdue. Those with more severe disease should be given higher levels of care than milder cases. Finally, case management and care coordination would be reserved for complex cases involving multiple specialties.

DIABETES REGISTRIES

Diabetes is one of the most common diseases for which care coordination is critical. Patients must adhere to a healthy diet, exercise regularly, watch their weight, take (and even adjust) their medications regularly, monitor their own blood sugars, and care for their feet. Clinicians must provide eye screening and foot care; give vaccinations; offer counseling on diet, exercise, and weight loss; manage hyperglycemia to reduce the risk of microvascular complications; treat hypertension and hypercholesterolemia to decrease the incidence of macrovascular events; manage devastating complications such as blindness, end-stage renal disease, myocardial infarction, or stroke; and even deal with the psychological and social consequences of the illness. The latter include depression, loss of employment, economic deprivation, and family discord related to the need for care giving or change in eating habits for the entire family. It is not surprising that diabetes was the focus of the earliest disease registries.[2-4]

It is beyond the scope of this chapter to describe existing diabetes registries in detail. Besides, many are proprietary and their functionalities are offered only to members who subscribe. Suffice it to say that long-standing registries have been sponsored by municipalities (New York City), academic health centers (Penn State Milton S Hershey Medical Center), specialty care centers (Joslin Diabetes Clinic), integrated health systems (Kaiser Permanente), programs in foreign countries (National Diabetes Surveillance System in Canada), and international collaborations (DIABCARE Q-NET in Europe).

IMPACT ON THE QUALITY OF CARE

Several studies have analyzed the impact of diabetes registries on the quality of patient care.[5-10] Although a variety of approaches has been used, most have demonstrated a favorable effect. Studies of this type can be very difficult to design, conduct, and analyze. Registries can identify patients who need critical services, but an improvement in outcomes requires an effective action plan for the findings. This plan can fail because of "clinical inertia", resistance to change, hostility over fault finding or loss of autonomy, confusion about roles and responsibilities, and suspicions about the quality of the data. Even if clinicians are motivated, corrective actions may require additional personnel, staff training, assigning new tasks, changing the practice's priorities, and finding the time and expertise for managing the data. Perhaps the most important impediment is that registry-driven care may not generate revenue and is therefore given lower priority than activities that do. Thus, the benefits of a registry may depend more upon the practice's action plan than on the quality of information presented. In addition, their full impact may not be realized until reimbursement is aligned with patient outcomes instead of the workload generated by conventional activities.

Another problem is that the "gold standard" for efficacy—the randomized clinical trial (RCT) is not feasible for diabetes registries. The RCT is considered the best test of an intervention because it is the only method that handles measured and unmeasured patient covariates, i.e., patient attributes that affect the study's end-point other than the groups to which subjects have been assigned. Randomization balances the prognostic factors across the intervention and control groups whether they are measured or not, while statistical methods can only handle those that are measured. Many patient attributes (such as motivation, family support, or commitments to a job or school) are important determinants of diabetes outcomes but not measurable. RCTs are difficult to apply to diabetes registries for practical and ethical reasons. Patients might object to being randomly assigned to practices with or without registries. On the other hand, it is unreasonable to expect practitioners to consult a registry for intervention patients but not for controls when information is available for both. Finally, trials are ethical only if there is "equipoise" or legitimate uncertainty about the risks and benefits of the two treatment arms. It would be difficult to argue that knowing about a critical deficiency in patient care can either be better or worse than not knowing about it.

As a result, most studies testing the benefits of diabetes registries resorted to less rigorous study designs—the pre/post study, the cohort study, and the group-randomized trial. A pre/post study compares outcomes before and after the implementation of a registry. For example, Pollard et al.[6] studied processes and outcomes of diabetes care in 661 subjects at six federally-qualified health care centers in West Virginia. Data pre- and post-registry were compared for three levels of registry utilization. The registry significantly improved 12 of 13 process and three of six outcomes measures for patients exposed to at least medium levels of registry utilization. Likewise, Ciemens and associates[9] analyzed metabolic status and preventive services in 495 adult diabetic patients through a baseline and two intervention phases. The latter consisted of a "low-dose" phase emphasizing provider and patient education and a "high-dose" phase based upon the registry and workflow changes. Significant improvements were noted in blood pressure, glycosylated hemoglobin, low-density lipoprotein, and the proportion of patients receiving recommended eye, foot, and renal evaluations.

Pre/post studies should be interpreted with caution if there is temporal drift in the study's end-points, co-interventions have been introduced, efforts to measure end-points in the "pre" phase are not robust, and outcomes are sensitive to patient or provider motivation. Temporal changes in the study's outcome may offset the benefits of registries—giving the impression that they are ineffective. For example, suppose that the prevalence of childhood obesity is steadily increasing in a community. A registry that tracks patient status and guides interventions may stabilize the incidence. However, a pre/post analysis would show no changes. On the other hand, a spontaneous decline in the rate could be attributed to the registry when, in fact, it had no effect. Co-interventions are those introduced into practice while a study is underway. One example is the patient-centered medical home. If the co-intervention is adopted during the "post" phase, it would not be possible to separate its effect from the use of a registry. In many pre/post studies, outcomes during the "pre" phase are measured by routine procedures, while in the "post" phase, they are evaluated in a prospective and robust manner. For end-points that are silent or have atypical presentations, there can be an apparent change from "pre" to "post" that represents a measurement artifact. For example, myocardial infarction can be "silent" among diabetic patients. In the "pre" phase they might be missed, while in the "post" phase they might be picked up by electrocardiogram (EKG) surveillance. Finally, because so many diabetes outcomes depend upon patient or provider motivation, a spurious benefit of registries might arise from the "Hawthorne" effect. This effect is a change in a study's outcome due to participants' knowledge that they are being observed. Improvement might be attributed to registries when it actually represents a more conscientious effort by providers or greater adherence to recommendations by patients. Thus, study designs using parallel controls tend to yield more convincing evidence of efficacy than pre/post studies.

A cohort study compares two or more groups that differ by an important attribute. However, the groups are assembled without specific techniques (such as randomization, matching, or stratification) to assure that they are similar. This design is exemplified by the study of Coppell and coworkers.[7] These investigators compared 3,646 patients enrolled to the Otago Diabetes Registry in New Zealand with 1,103 who were not. Enrolled patients were more likely to receive recommended process measures as well as angiotensin-converting enzyme (ACE) inhibitors, other antihypertensive medications, and lipid-lowering agents. However, because randomization was not used, the groups could have been imbalanced with respect to patient characteristics affecting completion of recommended tasks. Moreover, because the practices were not randomized to registry-driven versus routine care, the apparent benefit of registries could have been due to differences in office policies or procedures other than the registry. This bias is possible because practices that adopt registries are likely to use other measures to assure high quality of care.

Randomizing practices to the two study arms is a better approach than a cohort design because it addresses such differences. This approach is known as a group-randomized trial. The terminology refers to the fact that patients belonging to each practice are assigned en bloc to the arm to which the practice has been randomized. As noted above, the principal advantage is that covariates arising from the practice level are balanced. Nevertheless, special statistical procedures are needed to adjust for differences in patient attributes as well as cluster effects. The latter result from the fact that the data are "nested" (i.e., patients are grouped under practices). It is beyond the scope of this chapter to discuss the implications of this data structure other than to note that the power of the study is reduced if there is significant variation in outcomes across the practices. Fischer et al.[8] used a sophisticated design to test whether patient and provider report cards generated from a computerized diabetes registry had an effect on glycemic, lipid, and blood pressure outcomes. Randomization for mailed patient report cards was done at the patient level. However, a 2 x 2 factorial design was used to evaluate the effectiveness of point-of-care patient report cards and provider report cards containing patient-specific data. The four arms in this design were: patient + provider report cards, provider report cards alone, patient report cards alone, and neither. One large and one small practice were randomized to each of these four arms. Neither the mailed nor point-of-care patient report cards had a beneficial effect.

Patients of providers receiving report cards were more likely to achieve their targets for glycemic control than those of control providers (6.4% versus 3.8%, respectively; P < 0.001). This study represents the most rigorous evaluation of registry-generated reports to date, although the benefits were modest at best. Unfortunately, treatment plans were not standardized, and it was not clear that the practices had resources to act upon the information.

In summary, most studies have shown that diabetes registries improve the quality of care, although the issue is by no means settled.[11,12] The evidence supporting this conclusion is modest because of limitations in study design or in the plans for corrective actions. Finally, as pointed out by Trief and Ellison,[12] diabetes registries are not without risk. Harm could arise from the intrusion of a third party (the registry developers) into an otherwise confidential patient-provider relationship as well as loss of protected health information.

Like others,[13,14] we will focus our remaining discussion on developing population management tools at the New Mexico Veterans Affairs Health Care System (NMVAHCS). The objective is to review the features of registries that the reader may wish to consider when selecting or designing one for his or her own situation.

IDENTIFYING THE DIABETIC POPULATION

The first functionality of a diabetes registry is to identify appropriate patients. Many factors will affect case identification including its sensitivity and specificity, data sources, search criteria, data validity, search period, sampling biases, and the number of criteria required.

Sensitivity and Specificity

Registries that are highly sensitive capture most patients who have diabetes at the expense of misidentifying some who do not. On the other hand, those that are specific will correctly classify cases that are retrieved but miss cases with marginal criteria. There are no optimal criteria that serve every purpose. For example, if the purpose of the registry is to prevent the progression of early diabetes, then highly sensitive criteria should be used. However, if the purpose is to recruit patients with advanced disease to a clinical trial of experimental treatment, then highly specific criteria are more appropriate. At the NMVAHCS, we build the most highly sensitive and comprehensive registries possible. Our reasoning is that subsets can then be selected by querying the master registry. This approach is more efficient than building a different registry for every purpose.

Data Sources

Diabetes can be identified from five conventional data sources: (1) hospitalization records, (2) outpatient encounters, (3) problem lists, (4) laboratory tests, and

TABLE 1: Data Sources and Case Identification (n = 13,999)			
Source	Cases identified	First criterion met	Single criterion*
Hospitalizations	3,498 (25.0%)	553 (4.0%)	216 (6.9%)
HbA1c ≥6.5%	10,134 (72.4%)	5,146 (36.8%)	1,070 (34.4%)
Medications	8,647 (61.8%)	1,382 (9.9%)	80 (2.6%)
Problem lists	11,165 (79.8%)	4,095 (29.3%)	908 (29.2%)
Visits	10,780 (77.0%)	2,823 (20.2%)	839 (27.0%)

*3,113 were diagnosed by only one criterion; the number in parentheses is the proportion of these cases detected by each of the five criteria.

(5) medications. On occasion, other files can be interrogated as well. For example, procedure files can be searched for laser photocoagulation—an intervention most commonly used for diabetic patients with proliferative retinopathy. Likewise, pathology files might be used to identify patients with nodular glomerulosclerosis (Kimmelstiel-Wilson disease). However, caution should be exercised when using these unconventional data sources because the etiology might not be specified. For example, neither laser treatment nor Kimmelstiel-Wilson disease is entirely specific for diabetes. Table 1 shows the data sources used to identify 13,999 patients at NMVAHCS in 2011.

Note that there are marked differences in the proportion of cases identified depending upon the source. Problem lists capture the greatest proportion of patients followed by outpatient encounters and hemoglobin A1c (HbA1c). However, HbA1c is most frequently the first criterion met and is the most common finding in 22% of patients with a single criterion.

Search Criteria

The search for cases is greatly facilitated if data are coded or expressed in standard terminology. Commonly used coding systems include the International Classification of Diseases (ICD), e.g., ICD-9 for diagnoses, Systematized Nomenclature of Medicine-Clinical Terms (SNOMED-CT) for pathology specimens, Current Procedural Terminology (CPT), e.g., CPT-4 for interventions, and Logical Observation Identifiers Names and Codes (LOINC) for laboratory tests. Many of these codes have several dimensions so that the search can be highly refined. For example, LOINC has six parts: (1) name, standardization, and type of challenge (if any); (2) the physical property; (3) the timing of measurements; (4) the organ system source and type of specimen; (5) the scale of measurement; and (6) the analytical method. Searching for nonstandard terms is a challenge because clinicians may describe a disease in a wide variety of ways. For example, a radiologist may use the terms "pneumonia", "pneumonitis", "infiltrate", "alveolar filling pattern", "consolidation", "haziness", or "air bronchograms" to describe the same abnormality on a chest X-ray. The problem is amplified if the term of interest is not placed in a dedicated field but rather buried in free text. Not only must the term be found, but the user must deal with qualifiers such as "probable", "possible", "consistent with", "not likely to be", or "rule out". While extremely valuable, free-text searching adds a whole new level of complexity to searching. For this reason, our diabetes registry is built only on coded data and standardized terminology.

Discharge diagnoses, outpatient encounters, and problem lists are usually coded using ICD-9 or ICD-10. The Appendix lists the ICD-9 codes used for diabetes at NMVAHCS. Note that, because our philosophy is to use highly sensitive criteria, the Appendix includes gestational and neonatal diabetes, diabetes complications (e.g., ICD-9 code 364.42: rubeosis iridis), laboratory abnormalities [ICD-9 code 790.22: impaired glucose tolerance test (oral)], and even adverse side effects or poisoning by diabetic agents (ICD-9 codes 962.3 and 932.3). Including terms used by specialists is important for tertiary facilities. Many PCPs in the community might use the facility only for consultative purposes. In that case, terms most commonly used for diabetes (e.g., ICD-9 code 250.00: diabetes mellitus without mention of complication, type II or unspecified type, not stated as controlled) will not be found in outpatient encounters or problem lists. Including symptoms, signs, and laboratory tests may capture patients for whom the diagnosis is likely but not firmly established. The rationale for including adverse drug effects or overdoses is that they are more likely to occur in patients prescribed the medication than those who are not.

A consistent approach is required even for searching for standardized terms. The best starting point is to get a complete ICD list in an electronic, searchable format. We create a "match list" by using principles employed in free-text searching and taking advantage of the hierarchical structure of the coding system. In addition to convention terms (like diabetes), we search for root syllables ("*diab*"), abbreviations ("DM"), synonyms, and acronyms ("AODM") in the diagnosis and description fields. The asterisk in the search for root syllables represents a "wild card", i.e., any combination of characters preceding or following the text of interest. We then edit the "hits" to include only the relevant terms and resort by ICD-9 code. Finally, we examine the neighboring entries to the "hits" to find related entries that might otherwise be missed. Our list of diabetes ICD-9 codes was generated using this strategy. It is stored as a table in a relational data base so that a comprehensive search can be done simply by joining a source file (e.g., problem list) to the reference table by ICD-9 code.

Searching laboratory files for diagnostic test results must also be done carefully. Standard test names are often not used, assays may not be standardized; results are expressed as text to accommodate comments ("cancelled"); many results are outside a reportable range; assays and reference values change with time and vary across sites; and there can be disagreement over what constitutes a "positive" test. We focus on abnormal HbA1c because the conditions under which glucose values are drawn are often unknown. For example, even nondiabetic patients can develop glucose intolerance when given large volumes of dextrose-containing intravenous fluids or re-fed after prolonged starvation. The first step is to tabulate the test names and then search for characteristic patterns ("*a1c*"), root syllables ("*hem*" for hemoglobin and "*gly*" for glyco-, glycated, or glycosylated), and abbreviations. Records containing the relevant test names are then pulled from the source file. After replacing the comments, we search for the leading characters "<" or ">" in the results field, replace them with a null string, and then convert the text entries to numeric. Failure to follow this procedure will result in a null entry for results outside of the reportable range and a loss of patients with the most abnormal results. If results from different assays have to be compared, it is necessary to express the raw values as a percent of the upper limit of normal. The results can then be reparameterized to a common scale by multiplying the percent by the upper limit for the assay currently used. Fortunately, both the American Diabetes Association and the World Health Organization have settled upon the same value of HbA1c ($\geq 6.5\%$) as diagnostic of diabetes.

The same issues must be addressed while searching for diabetes drugs in prescription records. Preparations may be described by their generic name, brand name, or an abbreviation; formats for tablet strength may vary ("2 mg" or "2_mg" or "2.0 mg"); the dosage form ("tablet" or "capsule") may or may not be included; and the formulations may differ ("vial" versus "prefilled") for the same medication. Each variation in terminology creates a separate entry even for preparations that are pharmacologically identical. The search is greatly facilitated if each prescription has been assigned to a drug class or can be linked to a standard entry in a drug reference. For example, Veterans Affairs (VA) uses the drug class HS500 for exenitide, HS501 for insulins, HS502 for oral hypoglycemic agents (OHA), and HS509 for pramlintide. Searching for these four classes achieves the same results as searching for dozens of diabetes medications.

Data Validity

The validity of data can vary widely depending upon the source. Discharge diagnoses are usually accurate because they are made by clinicians who have taken care of the patient over days if not weeks. At the NMVAHCS, only PCPs may enter problems onto the problem list, presumably after careful review of the evidence and a determination that the condition is long term and of sufficient priority to be tracked from visit to visit. Quality control is used to assure that prescription and laboratory data are accurate. On the other hand, encounter diagnoses may be entered by administrative personnel; data entry may not be standardized; results are rarely audited; diagnoses may be provisional; or they may be made after an encounter lasting only few minutes or by a clinician unfamiliar with the case. Nevertheless, external review organizations often use a small sample of outpatient encounters to assess the quality of care. By using all data sources and 100% sampling, registries may provide a much more valid assessment of an institution's processes and outcomes.

The most sophisticated electronic medical records also contain features that minimize entry errors such as logic checking, range checking, validation rules, error messages, and input masks. Logic checking compares data in two or more fields to determine if the results are compatible. For example, a high value for prostate specific antigen should not be found in a woman. Range checking consists of comparing the result to a range of plausible values. For example, an HbA1c of 20% is not possible if the reportable range for the assay is 4–18.7%. Validation rules often determine whether an entry is acceptable depending upon whether a Boolean statement evaluates to true or false. In each case, the error may be relayed to the user through error messages. An input mask presents the desired format to the user so that there is never any ambiguity about what should be entered. They are commonly used for social security numbers (XXX-XX-XXXX) or telephone numbers [(XXX) XXX-XXXX]. The user is only responsible for entering the "X's" and not the formatting characters. There is usually an option to store the entire sequence or only the characters entered. Registries are more likely to be valid if there are mechanisms to reduce entry errors at the clinical interface. Surprisingly, even advanced applications like VA's computerized patient record system (CPRS) do not have these functionalities.

Search Period

At NMVAHCS, we search for cases as far back as the system will permit. There are several reasons for this approach. Patients who have successfully managed their diabetes with diet and exercise will not have a high HbA1c, be on medications, have an outpatient encounter where diabetes is addressed, or be hospitalized for a diabetes-related condition. Moreover, this situation may persist for years. A search of recent records may miss these patients even though they are most likely to benefit from intensified preventive care. Table 2 illustrates the effect of search period on the proportion of 13,999 diabetic patients identified by the NMVAHCS registry in 2011.

TABLE 2: Impact of Search Period on Case Identification (n = 13,999)	
Start date	Cases identified
FY 1997*	13,978 (99.8%)
FY 1999	13,872 (99.1%)
FY 2001	13,661 (97.6%)
FY 2003	13,408 (95.8%)
FY 2005	13,057 (93.3%)
FY 2007	12,548 (89.6%)
FY 2009	11,308 (80.8%)

FY, fiscal year.
*Fiscal year October 1996 to September 1997.

TABLE 3: Diagnosis Cohort and Current HbA1c (n = 13,999)		
Cohort	Cases (%)	HbA1c (mean ± SD)
1995–1996	966 (6.9%)	7.77 ± 1.49%
1997–1998	924 (6.6%)	7.41 ± 1.51%
1999–2000	1,089 (7.8%)	7.26 ± 1.51%
2001–2002	1,677 (12.0%)	7.32 ± 1.46%
2003–2004	1,710 (12.2%)	7.18 ± 1.51%
2005–2006	1,984 (14.2%)	6.87 ± 1.29%
2007–2008	2,613 (18.7%)	6.66 ± 1.20%
2009–2010	3,036 (21.7%)	6.69 ± 1.15%

Note that a search period of 8 years is required to identify greater than 95% of current patients previously diagnosed with diabetes.

Another reason for an extended search is to identify the date of diagnosis and assign the patient to an "inception cohort". The VA Diabetes Trial has shown that diabetes of more than 20 years duration is an independent risk factor for cardiovascular event.[15] Moreover, because type 2 diabetes is a progressive illness, it is reasonable to anticipate a gradual increase in HbA1c over time. This phenomenon is shown in table 3. Note that patients belonging to the 1995–1996 cohort have much higher values for HbA1c than those diagnosed in the past 2 years. This finding has major implications for provider profiling. Because established providers may have had closed panels for many years, their patients will have had diabetes much longer than recently diagnosed patients assigned to new staff. Accordingly, it is unfair to set the same standards for glycemic control for providers in two groups.

Finally, a comprehensive search of old laboratory records provides information about long-term glycemic control and the subsequent risk of microvascular complications (see Section "Advanced Functionalities").

Sampling Bias

A sampling bias is a systematic error in the description of a population that arises from the data sources chosen for the search. Discharge diagnoses are biased toward patients with advanced complications. An elevated HbA1c misses patients who are well controlled. The medication file does not contain patients managed by diet and exercise alone. Outpatient encounters identify patients who not only have active diabetes but also have the resources to seek medical treatment. At NMVAHCS, problem lists are managed by PCPs and do not capture patients referred only for tertiary care. Thus, single sources of data not only miss certain cases but also produce results that are biased toward the ends of the severity spectrum. This phenomenon is shown in table 4.

TABLE 4: Data Sources and Quality Metrics (n = 13,999)			
Criterion	Cases	HbA1c not done*	HbA1c (mean ± SD)**
Hospitalizations	3,498	466 (13.3%)	7.43 ± 1.59%
HbA1c ≥6.5%	10,134	781 (7.7%)	7.35 ± 1.40%
Medications	8,647	581 (6.7%)	7.40 ± 1.48%
Problem lists	11,165	862 (7.7%)	7.12 ± 1.42%
Visits	10,780	975 (9.0%)	7.15 ± 1.44%

*Within the preceding 24 months.
**Latest value for those obtaining HbA1c in the preceding 24 months.

As expected, HbA1c is highest for cases detected through hospital records and lowest for those with a problem list entry. This observation reinforces our policy of using all five conventional data sources for the NMVAHCS diabetes registry. This strategy increases the sensitivity of the search and produces the least biased results.

Criteria Table

The NMVAHCS diabetes registry contains the first qualifying discharge date, diagnosis, and ICD-9 code; the first qualifying visit date, diagnosis, and ICD-9 code; the first qualifying problem list diagnosis, ICD-9 code, and entry date; the date and value of the first HbA1c greater than or equal to 6.5%; and the prescription type and date for the first diabetes medication. Users can search on individual criterion, the total number of criteria, or specific combinations. This option can be used to confirm diagnoses based on less reliable sources. Also, this feature facilitates the identification of patients for special initiatives (e.g., an early prevention program).

DATA ELEMENTS

Certain data elements should be incorporated into every diabetes registry including patient identifiers, contact information, and the names of the PCP, team, and practice site. Other items may be included depending upon the purpose of the registry. For example, a registry focusing on prevention, screening, and lifestyle intervention might include:
- Body mass index (BMI)
- Date of the last nutritional and exercise counseling
- Vaccination dates for influenza, pneumonia, and tetanus
- Date and results of the last foot examination
- Date of the last eye referral.

If the registry will be used to support intensive treatment of hyperglycemia, it might contain:
- Most recent HbA1c
- Prior HbA1c

- Magnitude and rate of change
- Most recent serum creatinine, estimated glomerular filtration rate (GFR), and urine albumin/creatinine ratio
- Type and dose of OHA
- Type, dose and timing of insulin injections.

If the registry will be used for macrovascular risk management, it should contain:

- Recent tobacco history
- Most recent blood pressure
- Most recent low-density lipoprotein (LDL) cholesterol measurement and liver function tests
- Current dose of aspirin, statin, and blood pressure medication.

Note that this arrangement allows the user to identify individuals who have not received appropriate testing; have not been seen for an abnormal value; or have failed to reach metabolic targets. This assessment allows the user to stratify the entire population by risk, severity, or need for services. Resources can then be managed to achieve optimal results for the entire population.

The contents of a diabetes registry should be aligned with the duties of the user. For example, if cardiovascular risk reduction is the responsibility of the diabetes team, it should contain information on LDL and lipid-lowering agents. However, if a separate team is assigned the responsibility for cardiovascular risk management for all patients, then those fields can be eliminated from the diabetes registry.

ADVANCED FUNCTIONALITIES

The primary purpose of diabetes registries is to improve patient outcomes. However, they are more likely to be adopted if there are benefits for clinicians as well. These benefits include identifying lapses in care and reducing malpractice exposure, reducing workload, saving time, off-loading tasks to other members of the team, providing information otherwise difficult to retrieve, triaging cases to specialty and support services, and performing complex but highly relevant calculations that clinicians are unable to do. Examples include identifying serious drug interactions that otherwise would have gone unnoticed, registry-based vaccination programs, automated referral of OHA dose titrations to the advanced practice nurse, deriving the rate of change in estimated GFR, referring cases who have repeatedly failed primary care management for a psychosocial evaluation, and estimating long-term glycemic burden from routine laboratory tests.

Poorly designed registries could significantly increase provider workload and frustration while providing minimal benefits. One example is displaying a provider's abnormal HbA1c results in a "dashboard" without determining whether they are "actionable". "Actionable" means that the notification will ordinarily result in some remedial action on the part of the recipient. There are many reasons why an elevated HbA1c might not be actionable:

- It was drawn from a patient for whom treatment intensification is inappropriate (e.g., terminal cancer)
- The result represents a significant decline from a previous value indicating that the patient is already on effective treatment
- The abnormality has already been treated
- The abnormality has already been seen by the PCP
- The HbA1c was drawn too soon after the last treatment change to assess the patient's response; recall that it takes several weeks for HbA1c to equilibrate
- The same result has been observed for years suggesting that the case is a refractory treatment failure.

We used the 2011 diabetes registry of 13,999 cases at the NMVAHCS to assess the extent to which HbA1c's are "actionable" in a primary care population. The analysis was done for three cut points: ≥9.0%, ≥8.0%, and ≥7.0%. In table 5, note that only 20% of values greater than or equal to 9% were drawn at a time appropriate to evaluate a previous action. This finding suggests that those ordering the tests do not consistently review records to determine whether the results will be interpretable. In fact, HbA1c's are drawn on admission to certain units at our medical center as a matter of policy. Reviewing charts for results that are actionable would require a tremendous effort by our primary care staff. To detect the 214 actionable values ≥9, our providers would have had to review over 1,000 charts. While the yield is better for HbA1c greater than or equal to 8% or 7%, we estimate that our providers would have to review 3–4 charts to find one value that warrants intervention. Note that this requirement penalizes practices that are highly efficient in following up their laboratory tests because the number of untreated abnormalities would be small. Thus, diabetes registries should do more than retrieve data—they should process them. Advanced functionalities can be assigned to three areas:

1. Automated triage or prioritization of cases: Triage is defined as the process of routing patients to the most appropriate level of treatment. Prioritization refers to setting the order in which cases are handled. Health systems can markedly improve their operational efficiency through registries that automatically screen, triage, and prioritize cases. These programs can be installed on the institutional servers, interrogate the data streaming into repositories from electronic medical records, and be set to update at a frequency determined by the user. The ultimate objective is to identify the health system's highest priorities at any given time and to refer those cases to the appropriate level of care. For example, registries can generate

TABLE 5: Proportion of HbA1c That is Actionable			
	≥9.0%	≥8.0%	≥7.0%
Total patients	1,049	2,129	4,559
≥70 days after last medication change	214 (20.4%)	510 (24.0%)	1,429 (31.3%)

daily task lists for each member of a diabetes team. The administrative assistant may get a list for patients due for HbA1c testing or needing an appointment. The advanced practice nurse may get another for patients needing uptitration of an OHA, while the physician may get a third for patients needing conversion to insulin. The certified diabetes educator (CDE) may get yet another for patients failing multi-injection insulin treatment to be sure that they know how to use carbohydrate counting to adjust their rapidly-acting preparations.

Registries are most effective when the application replicates the decisions that a clinician would make for an individual patient except that the program would perform the designated task for every patient every day. The first step is to develop a consensus among the clinicians about how a specific problem would be solved. Not only does this approach foster a spirit of collaboration between clinicians and informaticists, but it also increases the likelihood that the application would be used. The clinical process is then reduced to a decision algorithm (Figure 1) characterized by a branching sequence of decision notes. Because each decision is based on a patient attribute, the algorithm defines the data elements that should be incorporated into the registry. It then becomes a simple matter to separate the entire population into groups each of which requires a specific intervention. Each path through the algorithm represents a specific pattern of data. Queries can be written to identify patients with each specific pattern and consequently the task (if any) that should be accomplished. This approach can eliminate a large number of unnecessary chart reviews while preserving the ability to find "missed cases". The accompanying diagram illustrates the decision algorithm used to triage elevated HbA1c's at NMVAHCS. Note that the decision notes are the boxes containing questions, while the required tasks are shown in the boxes on the right. Thus, the application prioritizes the entire diabetes population into those needing an immediate adjustment in treatment, those for whom additional testing is needed, and those for whom no action is necessary.

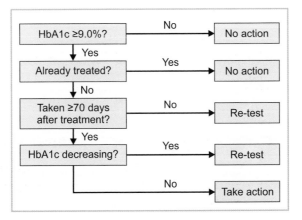

FIGURE 1 An algorithm for triaging elevated HbA1c's.

Although the computer program retrieves the appropriate data from regional servers, some of the questions cannot be answered by the raw data. In fact, the application uses sophisticated methodology to derive the answers for some of the nodes. Date mapping refers to placing events along a timeline to determine their sequence and intervals. At our facility, the last HbA1c is actionable if it is greater than 10 weeks after the last change in medications but not if it antedates the last change or the interval is less than or equal to 10 weeks. Registries can also be programmed to do trend analysis. For example, no action may be appropriate if the HbA1c is decreasing rapidly. The rate can be determined by "self-joining" each value to the preceding one, calculating the difference between the two readings, determining the testing interval, and dividing the former by the latter. Clinicians often find trends in data to be far more useful than the absolute values.

Our system triages cases to members of the diabetes team using an algorithm based upon the natural history of type 2 diabetes. Most patients are initially treated with diet and exercise. When lifestyle intervention fails, OHAs are started and gradually uptitrated. When that fails, patients are started on basal insulin. Eventually, patients wind up on complicated multi-injection regimens the most sophisticated of which require carbohydrate counting. Starting a new OHA requires an assessment of indications, drug interactions, side-effects, patient acceptance, and health literacy as well as a considerable amount of education and emotional support. Because this task is complex, our software assigns this task to the PCP. On the other hand, uptitrating an existing OHA requires only an evaluation of its effectiveness and tolerance—a task assigned to the advanced practice nurse. Pharmacists might be assigned to patients on combination insulin regimens focusing on basal (e.g., premeal and bedtime) hyperglycemia. However, CDEs are assigned cases treated with lispro, glulisine, or aspart. The reason is that CDEs are the only team members at our facility skilled in carbohydrate counting used to adjust doses before meals. This triage to team members is shown in figure 2.

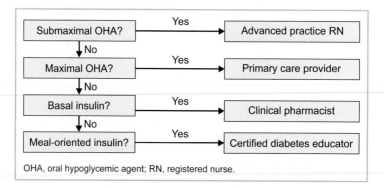

OHA, oral hypoglycemic agent; RN, registered nurse.

FIGURE 2 An algorithm for triaging patients to members of a diabetes team.

Note that, as long as the PCP approves the protocol and writes standing orders for his/her cases, the system can triage cases automatically to the most appropriate team member. This approach avoids the "bottleneck" created by having the PCP evaluate every HbA1c on every patient. The system is also designed to make sure that all team members are operating at the highest level of their abilities.

2. Advanced clinical parameters: Computer programs can perform cutting-edge analyses of large volumes of clinical data going back many years. These analyses result in highly relevant patient assessments that have not previously been possible. For example, our diabetes registry can be linked to a chronic kidney disease registry that tracks temporal changes in estimated GFR for the entire NMVAHCS population. It also estimates the aggregate dose of nonsteroidal anti-inflammatory drugs (NSAIDs) prescribed by NMVAHCS providers over the past 15 years. The amount dispensed through each prescription is converted to an "ibuprofen equivalent" through propriety methodology, and the total is then derived from all prescriptions in the drug class. High aggregate NSAID doses have been implicated in the pathogenesis of chronic kidney and cardiovascular disease. Our diabetes registry can also be joined to a pain/narcotics registry at NMVAHCS that tracks pain scores and narcotic use. One useful feature of the latter registry is its ability to detect aberrant behaviors such as repeated early refills and prescriptions from multiple providers. The application keeps a running tabulation of the proportion of narcotics dispensed through early refills so that there is never any ambiguity about whether patients are taking their medications as prescribed. This information is highly useful to monitor narcotic use by patients with painful neuropathy.

Perhaps the most useful of the advanced clinical parameters is an estimation of long-term glycemic burden. Basic research has shown that protein glycation (and, therefore, microvascular injury) is a function of glucose level and exposure time. It would be very useful to have a measure of long-term glycemic burden, but there is no laboratory test that spans the many years over which such injury occurs. Our application solves this problem by integrating the area under the HbA1c versus time curve using all available values in the patient's medical record. There are several uses for this information. Patients with a large glycemic burden should be assessed for subclinical microvascular injury even if they are not yet symptomatic. Unsuccessful treatment of hyperglycemia over years suggests that the primary care approach has repeatedly failed. These patients may benefit from a detailed analysis of the psychological, behavioral, or social barriers to treatment intensification before such treatment is again attempted. Finally, this feature of our software allows managers to determine if practice variation in glycemic control is correlated with microvascular complications over periods much longer than are feasible in clinical trials. In fact, this type of analysis should be the driving force for QI activities because it uncovers the relationship of local variations with local outcomes. Quality improvement activities that rely on published guidelines may fail because the trials that generated the "evidence" may focus on procedures or populations not relevant at the local level.

3. Rigorous statistical treatment of the data: Computerized disease registries can perform meaningful statistical analyses of the data not previously possible. One example is to derive time-weighted averages of clinical parameters to assess clinical severity. Time-weighting is an important strategy to avoid serious biases in summary statistics that arise from the fact that measurements are taken more frequently when they are abnormal. For example, suppose that a patient is hospitalized for hyperglycemia. On the first day, six measurements of 1,000 mg/dL are obtained while treatment is initiated. On the second day, when treatment has taken effect, a single value of 100 mg/dL is obtained before the patient is discharged. The unweighted average over the seven readings for two days is $[(6 \times 1000) + 100]/7 = 871$ mg/dL. However, a more reasonable estimate would be 550 mg/dL because each of the 1,000 mg/dL readings on the first day represented only 4 hours, while the single reading on the second represented 24. The correct approach is to time-weight each reading by the amount of time that it represents. Another statistical procedure is to perform transformations of skewed data so that z-scores can be interpreted as markers for "outliers". For example, our application can be linked to a pharmacy registry that identifies drug utilization and costs for all preparations, patients, and providers in the region. The distribution of patient costs is positively-skewed, i.e., there is a long tail toward the right that drags the mean away from the median toward higher values. Calculating a standard deviation in cost for each patient is not useful because the resulting "z-score" cannot be interpreted with respect to percentile ranking. The pharmacy registry solves this problem by normalizing the cost distribution through a logarithmic transformation of raw values before calculating z-scores. Thus, a person with costs two standard deviations above the transformed mean is within the highest 2.5% of the population as a whole.

REPORTING FORMATS, VALIDATION, AND USER UPTAKE

We have discussed the importance of clinician participation in the design of diabetes registries. Getting a much larger group of health care providers to use the application for routine care represents a formidable challenge. As a group, physicians have resisted the change from paper to electronic records despite the evidence that the latter improve patient outcomes. Moreover, some practices may be too stressed and overburdened to allow the implementation of novel approaches even if they improve workflow and efficiency. Although health policy and financial incentives may require the adoption of information technology, the benefits of diabetes registries will be realized only if they are embraced by the community of practitioners. How, when, or if this transition occurs is beyond the scope of this chapter.

The same aversion for information technology may make it difficult to deliver useful information to clinicians. The options include paper reports, spreadsheets (like Microsoft Excel) familiar to many casual users, desktop relational database applications (such as Microsoft Access), the reporting services of mainframe programs (like Microsoft SQL Server) or customized applications on the internet that are integrated with diabetes registries residing on institutional servers. We use the Microsoft products as examples because the company is the principal software vendor for the Department of Veterans Affairs, but many other options are available. In general, there is a trade-off between user friendliness and functionality. Early in the transition, it is reasonable to place the emphasis on the former and gradually increase the functionality of the products as clinicians become technically more sophisticated.

BusinessDictionary.com defines beta-testing as a "second level, external pilot test of a product (usually a software) before 'commercial quantity production'. At the beta-test stage, the product has already passed through internal validation (alpha testing) and glaring defects have been removed. But since the product may still have some minor problems that require user input, it is released to selected customers for testing under everyday conditions to spot the remaining flaws". Another reason is to refine its aesthetic features or improve its functionalities. However, at the beta-test phase, extensive reprogramming of the application is usually not feasible. It is reasonable to perform beta-testing on a diabetes registry before it is released for use under ordinary circumstances.

Adoption will be enhanced if there are validation studies that not only demonstrate that the registry delivers accurate information but that its use also improves the efficiency or outcomes of care. Comparing the effectiveness of two care-delivery systems is the objective of comparative effectiveness research—an area that has recently been given the highest priority for research sponsored by federal agencies. Clinical trials should be done comparing registry-driven versus conventional medical care for improving prevention, treating hyperglycemia, and managing cardiovascular risk in diabetic patients. Because this intervention represents a change to the health system infrastructure, trials randomized at the patient level are probably not feasible. However, group randomization (e.g., by practice site) may be used to balance covariates at higher levels, particularly when coupled with matching or stratification for the major confounders. Differences in outcomes between registry-based and usual care can then be statistically adjusted for differences in patient attributes. It should also be remembered that patient-centric outcomes are extremely important for a chronic, potentially-disabling disease like diabetes. These outcomes include psychological, physical, or social functioning; quality of life; preservation of the activities of daily living; satisfaction with care; more informed decision making; perception of and satisfaction with health; and improved patient-provider communication. Diabetes registries have the potential for improving these patient-oriented as well as disease-specific outcomes. Again, the federal government has placed renewed emphasis on this type of research through the Patient Centered Outcomes Research Institute (PCORI).

However, the success of diabetes registries will ultimately be achieved when they alert a clinician to serious problems that otherwise would be missed, increase the practice's efficiency, or improve the practitioner's outcomes, revenue, or satisfaction. At that point, the benefits change from theoretical and general to actual and personal. A diabetes registry will then become an integral part of a sustainable business model where the additional burdens of information technology are more than offset by tangible gains. This goal may be achieved only by keeping the ultimate "clients" in mind—the individual patient and his/her practitioner.

OTHER USES FOR THE DIABETES REGISTRY

Practice Profiling

Because the registry contains all diabetic patients and their current assignments to clinicians, group practices, or sites, it is a simple matter to calculate "panel-wide" statistics for the processes and outcomes of treatment, determine average values across the institution, and identify those whose performance is significantly above or below the norm. Moreover, it is possible to stratify this analysis by or adjust for differences in patient variables (e.g., diabetes duration), physiology (e.g., BMI), or treatment (OHA versus insulin) to make the comparisons meaningful. This approach is far superior to auditing a small number of charts per provider and applying external (and perhaps irrelevant) standards without adjusting for panel characteristics.

Continuing Medical Education

Although providers choose their CME activities on the basis of interest, the new paradigm may require that providers take courses based upon their performance. Registries can be used to identify patients for case presentations, providers whose performance is suboptimal, or topics for general education. Thus, registries have the potential for aligning educational requirements with the needs of providers so that there is collective improvement in the health status of the entire population.

Meaningful Quality Improvement

Scientific evidence is only the starting point for determining how diabetic patients should be managed. Basic research and clinical trials are done under contrived conditions where psychological, behavioral, social, and financial barriers to treatment are minimized. On the other hand, practitioners must deal with these practical issues every day and often develop solutions on their own. Effective QI requires identifying practices with optimal outcomes, ascertaining the reasons, replicating successful solutions across the institution, and re-evaluating performance. Registries can play a central role in this iterative process.

Practice Support

We have already discussed how registries can be used to manage preventive services. Visit management consists of preparing a patient so that the encounter is not wasted for lack of data. The last testing dates for HbA1c and LDL in the registry can be reviewed to determine if they are current. If not, patients can be instructed to obtain them prior to their next visits so that the time can be spent making therapeutic decisions rather than ordering labs. Pharmacy management consists of a systematic review of drug use by the population so that pre-emptive actions can be taken. The most useful aspects of such management relate to drug safety or interactions and patient adherence. For example, the registry can be queried for patients with progressive renal insufficiency so that they can be switched from agents cleared by renal mechanisms (e.g., glyburide) to those that are not (glipizide). Medication adherence can be ascertained from prescription records. The medical possession ratio (MPR) is defined as the proportion of days for which a patient has enough medication to take the prescribed dose. It is derived by dividing the number of days supplied by the interval between the last and prior fill dates. Registries can be designed so that the MPR can be calculated for all diabetic drugs for the entire population. Counseling should then be directed at those with low levels of adherence.

Research

An ancillary benefit of a diabetes registry is that it can serve as a sampling frame for clinical and basic research. It can be designed to evaluate the entire population for a study's inclusion and exclusion criteria so that every patient can undergo a rigorous screening process with minimal effort. A search of computerized records usually requires a waiver of informed consent and Health Insurance Portability and Accountability Act (HIPAA) authorization. A waiver is usually justified if it creates an unbiased sampling frame to maximize validity, assures equal representation of women and minorities, and is associated with minimal risk because of rigorous security precautions. At the NMVAHCS, an "honest broker" with no vested interest in the research is responsible for searching files, obtaining the approval of PCPs, and sending solicitation letters to patients. The broker is "honest" because he/she receives no benefit from the study and therefore can represent the interests of patients and the institution without a conflict of interest. Basic research can be supported by creating a sampling frame across a phenotypic spectrum. For example, the registry can be examined for "super-responders" and "nonresponders" in LDL to a given dose of a statin. Proteomics or genomics research can be done to identify the mechanisms for this phenotypic variation.

CONCLUSION

Most major industries—retailing, manufacturing, transportation, financial, hospitality, energy and natural resources, etc.—rely on information technology to perform a systematic evaluation of operations, identify where processes are suboptimal, and triage those problems to appropriate personnel for corrective action. No one would board an airplane if the pilot not only had to fly the plane but chart the course on paper using a sextant and compass. Moreover, the chances of recovery would be small if the first indication of trouble is a sudden loss in altitude. However, the US health care industry has been operating in this mode for decades—without a clear indication of what works and what does not, which patients need care and which do not, and which providers are doing well and which are not. Moreover, the first indication of trouble is often an adverse patient outcome for which there may be no recovery, exhaustion of resources resulting in withdrawal of care, or poor job satisfaction leading to a decline in the physician workforce. Fortunately, health care systems are now adopting information systems which will bring their enterprises into the modern age. Because they focus on the management of entire populations, registries are the most promising of many tools that will drive much-needed and much-delayed health care reform. As one of the most complicated chronic diseases, diabetes should be the focus of one of the first registries at almost every institution.

REFERENCES

1. Larsson S, Lawyer P, Garellick G, Lindahl B, Lundström M. Use of 13 disease registries in 5 countries demonstrates the potential to use outcome data to improve health care's value. *Health Aff.* 2012;31(1):220-7.
2. Young RJ, Khong CK, Vaughan NJ, New J, Roxburgh M. The evolution of diabetes information systems. *Diabet Med.* 2002;19(suppl 4):6-12.
3. Zai A, Grant R, Andrews C, Yee R, Chueh H. Improving diabetes population management efficiency with an informatics solution. *AMIA Annu Symp Proc.* 2007:1168.
4. Khan L, Mincemoyer S, Gabbay RA. Diabetes registries: where we are and where are we headed? *Diabetes Technol Ther.* 2009;11(4):255-62.
5. Russell KG, Rosenzweig J. Improving outcomes for patients with diabetes using Joslin Diabetes Center's Registry and risk stratification system. *J Healthc Inf Manag.* 2007;21(2):26-33.
6. Pollard C, Bailey KA, Petitte T, Baus A, Swim M, Hendryx M. Electronic patient registries improve diabetes care and clinical outcomes in rural community health centers. *J Rural Health.* 2009;25(1):77-84.
7. Coppell KJ, Anderson K, Williams SM, Lamb C, Farmer VL, Mann JI. The quality of diabetes care: a comparison between patients enrolled and not enrolled to a regional diabetes register. *Prim Care Diabetes.* 2011;5(2):131-7.
8. Fischer HH, Eisert SL, Durfee MJ, Moore SL, Steele AW, McCullen K, et al. The impact of tailored diabetes registry report cards on measures of disease control: a nested randomized trial. *BMC Med Inform Decis Mak.* 2011;11:12.

9. Ciemins EL, Coon PJ, Fowles JB, Min SJ. Beyond health information technology: critical factors necessary for effective diabetes disease management. *J Diabetes Sci Technol.* 2009;3(3):452-60.

10. Harris MF, Priddin D, Ruscoe W, Infante FA, O'Toole BI. Quality of care provided by general practitioners using or not using division-based diabetes registers. *Med J Aust.* 2002;177(5):250-2.

11. Littenberg B, MacLean CD. Mandated diabetes registries will benefit persons with diabetes. *Arch Intern Med.* 2008;168(8):797-9.

12. Trief PM, Ellison RA. Mandated diabetes registries will not benefit persons with diabetes. *Arch Intern Med.* 2008;168(8):799-802.

13. Gabbay RA, Khan L, Peterson KL. Critical features for a successful implementation of a diabetes registry. *Diabetes Technol Ther.* 2005;7(6):958-67.

14. Campion FX, Tully GL, Barrett JA, Andre P, Sweeney A. Improving quality of care using a diabetes registry and disease management services in an integrated delivery network. *Dis Manag.* 2005;8(4):245-52.

15. Duckworth W, Abraira C, Moritz T, Reda D, Emanuele N, Reaven PD, et al. Glucose control and vascular complications in Veterans with type 2 diabetes. *N Engl J Med.* 2009;360:129-39.

Appendix

ICD-9 codes for diabetes at the New Mexico Veterans Affairs Health Care System (NMVAHCS)		
Code	Diagnosis	Description
249.00	SEC DM WO CMP NT ST UNCN	Secondary diabetes mellitus without mention of complication, not stated as uncontrolled, or unspecified
249.01	SEC DM WO COMP UNCONTRLD	Secondary diabetes mellitus without mention of complication, uncontrolled
249.10	SEC DM KETO NT ST UNCNTR	Secondary diabetes mellitus with ketoacidosis, not stated as uncontrolled, or unspecified
249.11	SEC DM KETOACD UNCNTRLD	Secondary diabetes mellitus with ketoacidosis, uncontrolled
249.20	SEC DM HPROS NT ST UNCNR	Secondary diabetes mellitus with hyperosmolarity, not stated as uncontrolled, or unspecified
249.21	SEC DM HPROSMLR UNCNTRLD	Secondary diabetes mellitus with hyperosmolarity, uncontrolled
249.30	SEC DM OT CMA NT ST UNCN	Secondary diabetes mellitus with other coma, not stated as uncontrolled, or unspecified
249.31	SEC DM OTH COMA UNCNTRLD	Secondary diabetes mellitus with other coma, uncontrolled
249.40	SEC DM RENL NT ST UNCNTR	Secondary diabetes mellitus with renal manifestations, not stated as uncontrolled, or unspecified
249.41	SEC DM RENAL UNCONTRLD	Secondary diabetes mellitus with renal manifestations, uncontrolled
249.50	SEC DM OPHTH NT ST UNCN	Secondary diabetes mellitus with ophthalmic manifestations, not stated as uncontrolled, or unspecified
249.51	SEC DM OPHTH UNCONTRLD	Secondary diabetes mellitus with ophthalmic manifestations, uncontrolled
249.60	SEC DM NEURO NT ST UNCN	Secondary diabetes mellitus with neurological manifestations, not stated as uncontrolled, or unspecified
249.61	SEC DM NEURO UNCONTRLD	Secondary diabetes mellitus with neurological manifestations, uncontrolled
249.70	SEC DM CIRC NT ST UNCNTR	Secondary diabetes mellitus with peripheral circulatory disorders, not stated as uncontrolled, or unspecified
249.71	SEC DM CIRC UNCONTRLD	Secondary diabetes mellitus with peripheral circulatory disorders, uncontrolled
249.80	SEC DM OTH NT ST UNCONTR	Secondary diabetes mellitus with other specified manifestations, not stated as uncontrolled, or unspecified
249.81	SEC DM OTHER UNCONTRLD	Secondary diabetes mellitus with other specified manifestations, uncontrolled
249.90	SEC DM UNSP NT ST UNCON	Secondary diabetes mellitus with unspecified complication, not stated as uncontrolled, or unspecified

Contd...

Contd...

ICD-9 codes for diabetes at the New Mexico Veterans Affairs Health Care System (NMVAHCS)		
Code	**Diagnosis**	**Description**
249.91	SEC DM UNSP UNCONTROLD	Secondary diabetes mellitus with unspecified complication, uncontrolled
250.00	DMII WO CMP NT ST UNCNTR	Diabetes mellitus without mention of complication, type II or unspecified type, not stated as uncontrolled
250.01	DMI WO CMP NT ST UNCNTRL	Diabetes mellitus without mention of complication, type I [juvenile type], not stated as uncontrolled
250.02	DMII WO CMP UNCNTRLD	Diabetes mellitus without mention of complication, type II or unspecified type, uncontrolled
250.03	DMI WO CMP UNCNTRLD	Diabetes mellitus without mention of complication, type I [juvenile type], uncontrolled
250.10	DMII KETO NT ST UNCNTRLD	Diabetes with ketoacidosis, type II or unspecified type, not stated as uncontrolled
250.11	DMI KETO NT ST UNCNTRLD	Diabetes with ketoacidosis, type I [juvenile type], not stated as uncontrolled
250.12	DMII KETOACD UNCONTROLD	Diabetes with ketoacidosis, type II or unspecified type, uncontrolled
250.13	DMI KETOACD UNCONTROLD	Diabetes with ketoacidosis, type I [juvenile type], uncontrolled
250.20	DMII HPRSM NT ST UNCNTRL	Diabetes with hyperosmolarity, type II or unspecified type, not stated as uncontrolled
250.21	DMI HPRSM NT ST UNCNTRLD	Diabetes with hyperosmolarity, type I [juvenile type], not stated as uncontrolled
250.22	DMII HPROSMLR UNCONTROLD	Diabetes with hyperosmolarity, type II or unspecified type, uncontrolled
250.23	DMI HPROSMLR UNCONTROLD	Diabetes with hyperosmolarity, type I [juvenile type], uncontrolled
250.30	DMII O CM NT ST UNCNTRLD	Diabetes with other coma, type II or unspecified type, not stated as uncontrolled
250.31	DMI O CM NT ST UNCNTRLD	Diabetes with other coma, type I [juvenile type], not stated as uncontrolled
250.32	DMII OTH COMA UNCONTROLD	Diabetes with other coma, type II or unspecified type, uncontrolled
250.33	DMI OTH COMA UNCONTROLD	Diabetes with other coma, type I [juvenile type], uncontrolled
250.40	DMII RENL NT ST UNCNTRLD	Diabetes with renal manifestations, type II or unspecified type, not stated as uncontrolled
250.41	DMI RENL NT ST UNCNTRLD	Diabetes with renal manifestations, type I [juvenile type], not stated as uncontrolled

Contd...

Contd...

ICD-9 codes for diabetes at the New Mexico Veterans Affairs Health Care System (NMVAHCS)		
Code	Diagnosis	Description
250.42	DMII RENAL UNCNTRLD	Diabetes with renal manifestations, type II or unspecified type, uncontrolled
250.43	DMI RENAL UNCNTRLD	Diabetes with renal manifestations, type I [juvenile type], uncontrolled
250.50	DMII OPHTH NT ST UNCNTRL	Diabetes with ophthalmic manifestations, type II or unspecified type, not stated as uncontrolled
250.51	DMI OPHTH NT ST UNCNTRLD	Diabetes with ophthalmic manifestations, type I [juvenile type], not stated as uncontrolled
250.52	DMII OPHTH UNCNTRLD	Diabetes with ophthalmic manifestations, type II or unspecified type, uncontrolled
250.53	DMI OPHTH UNCNTRLD	Diabetes with ophthalmic manifestations, type I [juvenile type], uncontrolled
250.60	DMII NEURO NT ST UNCNTRL	Diabetes with neurological manifestations, type II or unspecified type, not stated as uncontrolled
250.61	DMI NEURO NT ST UNCNTRLD	Diabetes with neurological manifestations, type I [juvenile type], not stated as uncontrolled
250.62	DMII NEURO UNCNTRLD	Diabetes with neurological manifestations, type II or unspecified type, uncontrolled
250.63	DMI NEURO UNCNTRLD	Diabetes with neurological manifestations, type I [juvenile type], uncontrolled
250.70	DMII CIRC NT ST UNCNTRLD	Diabetes with peripheral circulatory disorders, type II or unspecified type, not stated as uncontrolled
250.71	DMI CIRC NT ST UNCNTRLD	Diabetes with peripheral circulatory disorders, type I [juvenile type], not stated as uncontrolled
250.72	DMII CIRC UNCNTRLD	Diabetes with peripheral circulatory disorders, type II or unspecified type, uncontrolled
250.73	DMI CIRC UNCNTRLD	Diabetes with peripheral circulatory disorders, type I [juvenile type], uncontrolled
250.80	DMII OTH NT ST UNCNTRLD	Diabetes with other specified manifestations, type II or unspecified type, not stated as uncontrolled
250.81	DMI OTH NT ST UNCNTRLD	Diabetes with other specified manifestations, type I [juvenile type], not stated as uncontrolled
250.82	DMII OTH UNCNTRLD	Diabetes with other specified manifestations, type II or unspecified type, uncontrolled
250.83	DMI OTH UNCNTRLD	Diabetes with other specified manifestations, type I [juvenile type], uncontrolled
250.90	DMII UNSPF NT ST UNCNTRL	Diabetes with unspecified complication, type II or unspecified type, not stated as uncontrolled

Contd...

Contd...

ICD-9 codes for diabetes at the New Mexico Veterans Affairs Health Care System (NMVAHCS)		
Code	Diagnosis	Description
250.91	DMI UNSPF NT ST UNCNTRLD	Diabetes with unspecified complication, type I [juvenile type], not stated as uncontrolled
250.92	DMII UNSPF UNCNTRLD	Diabetes with unspecified complication, type II or unspecified type, uncontrolled
250.93	DMI UNSPF UNCNTRLD	Diabetes with unspecified complication, type II [juvenile type], uncontrolled
357.2	NEUROPATHY IN DIABETES	Polyneuropathy in diabetes
362.01	DIABETIC RETINOPATHY NOS	Background diabetic retinopathy
362.02	PROLIF DIAB RETINOPATHY	Proliferative diabetic retinopathy
362.03	NONPROLF DB RETNOPH NOS	Nonproliferative diabetic retinopathy NOS
362.04	MILD NONPROLF DB RETNOPH	Mild nonproliferative diabetic retinopathy
362.05	MOD NONPROLF DB RETINOPH	Moderate nonproliferative diabetic retinopathy
362.06	SEV NONPROLF DB RETINOPH	Severe nonproliferative diabetic retinopathy
362.07	DIABETIC MACULAR EDEMA	Diabetic macular edema
362.10	BACKGRND RETINOPATHY NOS	Background retinopathy, unspecified
362.14	RETINA MICROANEURYSM NOS	Retinal microaneurysms NOS
362.16	RETINAL NEOVASCULAR NOS	Retinal neovascularization NOS
362.29	PROLIF RETINOPATHY NEC	Other nondiabetic proliferative retinopathy
364.42	RUBEOSIS IRIDIS	Rubeosis iridis
366.41	DIABETIC CATARACT	Diabetic cataract
648.00	DIABETES IN PREG-UNSPEC	Diabetes mellitus of mother, complicating pregnancy, childbirth, or the puerperium, unspecified as to episode of care or not applicable

Contd...

Contd...

ICD-9 codes for diabetes at the New Mexico Veterans Affairs Health Care System (NMVAHCS)		
Code	Diagnosis	Description
648.01	DIABETES-DELIVERED	Diabetes mellitus of mother, with delivery
648.02	DIABETES-DELIVERED W P/P	Diabetes mellitus of mother, with delivery, with mention of postpartum complication
648.03	DIABETES-ANTEPARTUM	Antepartum diabetes mellitus
648.04	DIABETES-POSTPARTUM	Postpartum diabetes mellitus
648.80	ABN GLUCOSE IN PREG-UNSP	Abnormal glucose tolerance of mother, complicating pregnancy, childbirth, or the puerperium, unspecified as to episode of care or not applicable
648.81	ABN GLUCOSE TOLER-DELIV	Abnormal glucose tolerance of mother, with delivery
648.82	ABN GLUCOSE-DELIV W P/P	Abnormal glucose tolerance of mother, with delivery, with mention of postpartum complication
648.83	ABN GLUCOSE-ANTEPARTUM	Abnormal glucose tolerance of mother, antepartum
648.84	ABN GLUCOSE-POSTPARTUM	Abnormal glucose tolerance of mother, postpartum
775.0	INFANT DIABET MOTHER SYN	Syndrome of infant of a diabetic mother
775.1	NEONAT DIABETES MELLITUS	Neonatal diabetes mellitus
790.2	ABN GLUCOSE TOLERAN TEST	Abnormal glucose tolerance test
790.21	IMPAIRED FASTING GLUCOSE	Impaired fasting glucose
790.22	IMPAIRED ORAL GLUCSE TOL	Impaired glucose tolerance test (oral)
790.29	ABNORMAL GLUCOSE NEC	Other abnormal glucose
962.3	POISON-INSULIN/ANTIDIAB	Poisoning by insulins and antidiabetic agents
E932.3	ADV EFF INSULIN/ANTIDIAB	Insulins and antidiabetic agents causing adverse effects in therapeutic use

Epidemiology and Its Application to Clinical Care in Diabetes

2

V Mohan, R Pradeepa, RM Anjana

ABSTRACT

Epidemiologic studies published between 1950s and 1970s began to have an important clinical impact and led to an increasing appreciation of the value of epidemiology as a scientific basis for clinical and public health practice. The Framingham study and Bogalusa Heart Study are examples of studies that laid the foundation for knowledge of cardiovascular disease risk factors in humans. The prospective studies conducted by Doll and Hill and the American Cancer Society also formed the basis for the now well-known relationship of cigarette smoking with lung cancer and pulmonary airway disease. The term "clinical epidemiology," which was first proposed by John Paul in 1938, is now used to characterize the application of epidemiology in clinical settings. He defined it as "a marriage between quantitative concepts used by epidemiologists to study disease in populations and decision making in the individual case which is the daily fare of clinical medicine". Clinicians can use the facts derived from epidemiological studies before deciding on the management aspects. In the context of diabetes such information, can be used to guide how we define, diagnose, and screen for diabetes, to describe the present and future burden of diabetes, and to highlight opportunities for intervention. This chapter reviews the available literature on how knowledge of epidemiology in the field of diabetes can be applied to the clinical care of diabetes. Thus, application of clinical epidemiology of diabetes to the care of individual patients termed as evidence based medicine will help clinicians to formulate specific clinical questions and find the best available research evidence to improve patient care and also influence medical decision.

INTRODUCTION

The term epidemiology originally meant the scientific study of epidemics, with particular reference to communicable diseases. Last et al.[1] in 1988 defined epidemiology as "the study of the distributions and determinants of health-related states or events in specified populations, and applications of this study to control health problems. The word epidemiology is derived from the Greek word epidemic which means "upon the people" (Greek: epi means upon, among; demos means people, district). Though not specifically termed as "epidemiology", several studies and ideas resembling epidemiological work have been done over the centuries. John Snow's work "On the mode of communication of cholera" in 1855 is considered a classic in the field of epidemic investigation.[2]

Epidemiologic studies published between 1950s and 1970s[3-6] began to have an important clinical impact and led to an increasing appreciation of the value of epidemiology as a scientific basis for clinical and public health practice. The Framingham study[3] and Bogalusa Heart Study[4] are examples of studies that laid the foundation for knowledge of cardiovascular disease (CVD) risk factors in humans. The prospective studies conducted by Doll and Hill[5] and the American Cancer Society[6] also formed the basis for the now well-known relationship of cigarette smoking with lung cancer and pulmonary airway disease. The term "clinical epidemiology", which was first proposed by John Paul in 1938,[7] is now used to characterize the application of epidemiology in clinical settings. He defined it as "a marriage between quantitative concepts used by epidemiologists to study disease in populations and decision making in the individual case which is the daily fare of clinical medicine".[7] Clinicians can use the facts derived from epidemiological studies before deciding on the management aspects. In the context of diabetes, such information can be used to guide how we define, diagnose, and screen for diabetes, to describe the present and future burden of diabetes, and to highlight opportunities for intervention.[8] In this chapter, we will attempt to review the available literature on how knowledge of epidemiology in the field of diabetes can be applied to the clinical care of diabetes.

BURDEN OF DIABETES

Diabetes, a potentially life-threatening disorder, is considered as "an apparent epidemic which is strongly related to lifestyle and economic change" according to the World Health Organization (WHO).[9] This devastating disorder can affect nearly every organ system in the body. It can cause blindness, lead to end-stage renal disease, lower-extremity amputations and increase the risk for stroke, ischemic heart disease, peripheral vascular disease (PVD), and neuropathy. Diabetes creates an economic burden not only as a costly disease requiring expensive treatment, but also in terms of man hours lost due to the debilitating effect the disease has on an individual.[10] The explosion of diabetes increases the risk of developing diabetes-related complications.[11] It causes profound alterations in both the micro- and macrovascular tree affecting almost every organ in the body leading to increased morbidity and mortality. The increasing burden of diabetes and its complications has led to interest in epidemiological studies relating to diabetes mellitus. Epidemiologic data can be used to define the present and future burden of diabetes and its complications and also to plan therapeutic measures.

Epidemiology of Diabetes and its Complications

The rising prevalence of diabetes with its concomitant complications has become a global concern. Diabetes currently affects 5–10% of most populations and has become the most frequently encountered metabolic disorder in the world. Epidemiological studies of diabetes have an extensive history. To do a comparative analysis on the epidemiology of prevalence of diabetes in the first half of 20th century is difficult as there were no standard criteria for diagnosing diabetes. Most of the earlier studies conducted in the early and mid-20th century were based on hospital and clinic records and used glycosuria as the diagnostic criteria. In the early 1980s, descriptive epidemiology of type 1 and type 2 diabetes were obtained and projections of the future burden of diabetes were made.[12] The WHO and International Diabetes Federation (IDF) have utilized methods that combine available country data at regular intervals and extrapolated estimates for remaining countries without data.

The WHO first published the prevalence of diabetes and the number of adults with diabetes in all countries of the world for three points in time, i.e., the years 1995, 2000, and 2025.[13,14] According to the WHO, the prevalence of diabetes in adults worldwide was estimated to be 4% in 1995 and to rise to 5.4% by the year 2025 and the number of adults with diabetes in the world would rise from 135 million in 1995 to 300 million in the year 2025. Wild et al.[15] in 2004 estimated the prevalence of diabetes for all age groups worldwide to be 2.8% in 2000 and 4.4% in 2030. The total number of people with diabetes was projected to rise from 171 million in 2000 to 366 million in 2030. Table 1 presents the IDF regional estimates and projections for diabetes (20–79 years age group) using epidemiological studies conducted from the year 2000 to 2011.[16-20] According to recent estimates by IDF, approximately 366 million adults worldwide (7%) had diabetes in 2011 and by 2030, 552 million people of the adult population (8.3%) are expected to have diabetes.[20] In addition, according to the Global Burden of Disease study, systematic analysis of all available national health surveys and published estimates, gathering data from 2.7 million participants and 370 country-years, estimated that diabetes affects 347 million adults worldwide.[21]

Data from different regions have largely confirmed these prevalences and projections. The recently conducted large national study in India, called the Indian Council of Medical Research-INdia DIABetes (ICMR-INDIAB) study, conducted in three states and one union territory of India,[22,23] reported the prevalence of diabetes (both known and newly diagnosed) to be 10.4% in Tamil Nadu, 8.4% in Maharashtra, 5.3% in Jharkhand, and 13.6% in Chandigarh. The overall number of people with diabetes in India in 2011 was estimated to be 62.4 million[23] and this was similar to the IDF projection for India, which gave a figure of 61.3 million people with diabetes in India in the age group of 20–79 years.[20] A study from China published in 2010 reported age-standardized prevalence of diabetes to be 9.7%,[24] which is comparable to the 9.0% prevalence given by IDF in 2011.[20]

From table 1, it can be observed that the largest increases will take place in the regions dominated by developing economies. While this burden of greater absolute

TABLE 1: International Diabetes Federation Regional Estimates and Projections for Diabetes (20-79 Years Age Group) Using Epidemiological Studies – 2000 to 2011[16-20]

Regions	Year and corresponding projections								
	2000[16] n* (%)	2003[17] n* (%)	2025[17] n* (%)	2007[18] n* (%)	2025[18] n* (%)	2010[19] n* (%)	2030[19] n* (%)	2011[20] n* (%)	2030[20] n* (%)
Africa	2.5 (1.2)	7.1 (2.4)	15.0 (2.8)	10.4 (3.6)	18.7 (4.5)	12.1 (3.8)	23.9 (4.7)	14.7 (4.5)	28.0 (4.9)
Eastern Mediterranean and Middle East	17.0 (7.7)	19.2 (7.2)	39.4 (8.0)	24.5 (9.2)#	44.5 (10.4)	26.6 (9.3)	51.7 (10.8)	32.6 (11.0)	29.7 (11.3)
Europe	22.5 (4.9)	48.4 (7.8)	58.6 (9.1)	53.2 (6.6)	64.1 (7.8)	55.2 (6.9)	66.5 (8.1)	52.8 (6.7)	64.0 (6.9)
North America	21.4 (7.8)	23.0 (7.9)	36.2 (9.7)	28.3 (8.4)$	40.5 (9.7)	37.4 (10.2)	53.2 (12.1)	37.7 (10.7)	51.2 (11.2)
South and Central America	8.5 (3.7)	14.2 (5.6)	26.2 (7.2)	16.2 (6.3)	32.7 (9.3)	18.0 (6.6)	29.6 (7.8)	25.1 (9.2)	39.9 (9.4)
South-East Asia	34.8 (5.3)	39.3 (5.6)	81.6 (7.5)	46.5 (6.5)	80.3 (8.0)	58.7 (7.6)	101.0 (9.1)	71.4 (9.2)	120.9 (10.0)
Western Pacific	44.1 (3.6)	43.0 (3.1)	75.8 (4.3)	67.0 (4.4)	99.4 (5.1)	76.7 (4.7)	112.8 (5.7)	131.9 (8.3)	187.9 (8.5)

*In millions.
#Middle East and North Africa from 2007.
$North America and Caribbean from 2007.

numbers of diabetes may be partially explained by larger population size in these regions, the rates at which diabetes is increasing in the developing countries amid rapid epidemiological and nutritional transition are much steeper when compared to those in more developed affluent countries. This is substantiated by the Global Burden of Disease study, which noted that the absolute growth in number of people with diabetes was primarily driven by population growth and aging in the world's largest countries (e.g., India and China).[21] It is observed that, in terms of population size, Asians living in the Asia-Pacific region and their diaspora cumulatively account for ~4 billion out of the world's 6.95 billion inhabitants.[25]

Globally, several epidemiological studies have been conducted to assess the prevalence and incidence of diabetic complications—both macrovascular diseases (CVD, which comprises coronary heart disease and cerebrovascular disease, and PVD) and microvascular diseases (retinopathy, nephropathy, and neuropathy). However, due to nonavailability of internationally agreed standards for diagnosing and assessing complications associated with diabetes, comparison between different populations and obtaining estimates for the same is difficult.

To assess the prevalence of diabetic retinopathy (DR), the Wisconsin Epidemiologic Study of Diabetic Retinopathy (WESDR) was initiated in Southern Wisconsin, USA in 1979[26]], which was followed by landmark epidemiological studies including the Barbados Eye Study (West Indies),[27] Beaver Dam Eye Study (USA),[28] Blue Mountains Eye Study (Australia),[29] Liverpool Diabetic Eye Study (UK),[30] Los Angeles Latino Eye study (USA),[31] Chennai Urban Rural Epidemiology study (CURES) Eye Study (India),[32] Aravind Comprehensive Eye Survey (India),[33] Multi-Ethnic Study of Atherosclerosis (MESA),[34] Singapore Malay Eye Study,[35] and several others.[36] Epidemiological studies on the prevalence of DR in different populations show prevalence rates varying from 17.6% in the CURES Eye Study[32] to 50.3% in the WESDR.[26] A recent meta-analysis of population-based studies around the world reported that there are approximately 93 million people with DR, 17 million with proliferative DR, and 21 million with diabetic macular edema worldwide.[36] However, there are few limitations as the data pooled are from studies at different time points, with different methodologies and population characteristics. Similarly population-based studies have been done on the PVD, CVD, neuropathy and nephropathy.[37-42]

Data on diabetic complications in India from the CURES and the Chennai Urban Population Study (CUPS) have reported interesting differences in the patterns of complications seen in Asian Indians. For example, the prevalence of DR,[32] nephropathy,[43] and PVD appear to be lower,[44] while that of neuropathy appears to be similar to prevalence rates reported in the West.[45] The prevalence of CVD, however, was higher[46] than that reported in the West. Figure 1 shows the prevalence of the most common diabetes complications among people with type 2 diabetes in urban South Indian population.[32,43-46] The Diabcare Africa project, which was conducted across six sub-Saharan African countries reported that DR (18%) and cataract (14%) were the most common eye complications; 48% had neuropathy while macrovascular disease was rare in that population.[47]

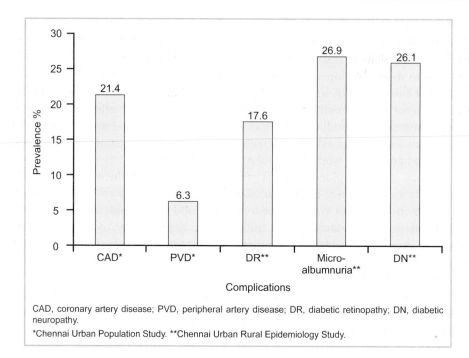

CAD, coronary artery disease; PVD, peripheral artery disease; DR, diabetic retinopathy; DN, diabetic neuropathy.
*Chennai Urban Population Study. **Chennai Urban Rural Epidemiology Study.

FIGURE 1 Prevalence of diabetic complications in Asian Indian population.[32,43-46]

Factors Implicated in the Causation

Diabetes has now reached epidemic proportions and a number of common predisposing factors can be found with regard to patterns of diabetes and rising prevalence rates globally. Identifying the pathophysiological mechanism and causative factors that lead to diabetes is essential to understand the etiology of the disorder and for the development of sound policies, including prevention and treatment strategies for improved health. The reasons for the escalation in diabetes include genetic factors, ethnic susceptibility, aging, family history of diabetes, stress, and environmental factors particularly associated with urbanization (obesity, diet, and physical inactivity). A number of investigators have explored the relationship between the various risk factors and the development of type 2 diabetes.[48,49]

Studies have consistently demonstrated that insulin resistance and hyper-insulinemia[50-52] are strong predictors of type 2 diabetes. A 5-year prospective study of insulin resistance in Pima Indians demonstrated that low insulin response and increased insulin resistance are both predictors of type 2 diabetes, and each variable acts as an independent risk factor.[50] There is extensive evidence from a number of epidemiological studies that certain ethnic groups, particularly Mexican Americans and African-Americans, have an increased risk of developing of type 2 diabetes when compared with the US population as a whole.[53,54]

Age is known to be an important determinant of diabetes largely due to increases in insulin resistance related to obesity and physical inactivity.[55,56] As age increases, β-cells fatigue occurs due to the increased insulin secretion needed to compensate for increasing levels of insulin resistance. Unlike the West, where elderly people are affected, in developing countries the trend in age of onset of diabetes is shifting from middle-aged adults to a younger age in the recent years.[57,58] The onset of diabetes at younger ages may be attributed to an earlier decline in metabolic homeostasis and/or a shorter latency to disease development.

Family history of diabetes is a strong and independent risk factor for diabetes. It represents expression of genetic determinants of diabetes and also interactions between the environment, behaviors, and genes in previous generations.[59,60] Studies of parental transmission of diabetes is useful as it may give insight into the relative contributions of underlying maternal and paternal influences. Genes play an important role in the development of diabetes. Putative susceptibility genes could be the key to the development of diabetes. A combination of genetic and environmental factors is most likely the cause of type 1 diabetes. However, type 2 diabetes is a polygenic disorder with multiple genes located on different chromosomes contributing to its susceptibility.[61] Genome-wide association (GWA) studies have focused on European populations and few gene variants have been investigated in Asians. A GWA study[62] conducted in type 2 diabetic individuals of South Asian ancestry from London, Pakistan and Singapore identified six new loci that are associated with diabetes (GRB14, ST6GAL1, VPS26A, AP3S2, HMG20A, and HNF4A). The findings from various genetic studies provide additional insight into mechanisms underlying type 2 diabetes. However, all the genes still together only explain around 10% of the diabetes disease burden.

The primary driver of the epidemic of diabetes is the rapid epidemiological transition associated obesity, unhealthy dietary practices, and sedentary lifestyle, all of which are lifestyle related. A number of studies have shown a higher risk of diabetes in association with greater general/abdominal obesity.[63-66] Data from the Obesity in Asia Collaboration, comprising 21 cross-sectional studies in the Asia-Pacific region with information on more than 263,000 individuals, indicate that measures of central obesity, in particular, waist circumference (WC), are better discriminators of prevalent diabetes in Asians and Caucasians, and are more strongly associated with prevalent diabetes as compared with body mass index (BMI).[63] A cross-sectional population-based study of 4,136 Chinese, Malays, and Asian Indians residing in Singapore reported that general adiposity explained the difference in insulin resistance between Chinese and Malays, whereas abdominal fat distribution, inflammation, and other unexplained factors contributed to excess insulin resistance in Asian Indians as compared with Chinese and Malays.[65]

There is strong evidence to show that physical inactivity increases the risk of type 2 diabetes.[67,68] Lee et al.[67] estimated that physical inactivity causes 7% (ranging from 3.9% in southeast Asia to 9.6% in the eastern Mediterranean region) of type 2 diabetes. Twenty percent of type 2 diabetes was attributable to physical inactivity. A recent study showed that Korean men with overweight, obese I, and obese II classifications had 1.47, 2.05, and 3.69 times higher risk of type 2 diabetes, respectively, as compared with normal weight men after adjustment for physical activity. In addition, men with low, medium, and high activity had 5%, 10%, and 9% lower risk of type 2 diabetes, respectively, as compared with inactive men after adjustment for body mass index.[69] It has been demonstrated that physical activity decreases concentrations of fatty acid metabolites, which decreases the risk of fatty acid-induced insulin resistance[70] and stimulates the translocation of glucose transporter type 4 to the plasma membrane, thereby improving glucose uptake.[71] In a recent study, Grontved et al.[72] reported that weight training was associated with a significantly lower risk of type 2 diabetes, independent of aerobic exercise, and combined weight training and aerobic exercise conferred a greater benefit.

Both the quantity and the quality of dietary components impact risk for diabetes. Excessive caloric intake increases weight and over time degrades hepatic glucose control and metabolic homeostasis. Unhealthy diet such as low intake of dietary fiber, low glycemic carbohydrates, or whole-grain cereals, high intakes of saturated fatty acids and trans fat increases the risk of developing diabetes.[73,74] In China between 1992 and 2002, the proportion of energy intake from animal foods increased from 9.3% to 13.7% and that from fats from 22% to 29.8%.[75] Substantial increases in animal fat intake have also been reported in India, Japan and Thailand.[76-78] Higher intake of *trans* fatty acids has been associated with weight gain and insulin resistance.[79] In the CURES study conducted in South India, a high intake of foods with a high glycemic load was associated with a fourfold increased risk of type 2 diabetes.[73] Similar findings have been reported in China[80] and Japan.[81] The CURES study has also reported that higher intake of refined grains (predominantly white rice) was associated with insulin resistance and metabolic syndrome in the Chennai population who habitually consume high-carbohydrate diets.[82] The same study demonstrated that the diet of the urban South Indian population consisted mainly of refined cereals with low intake of fish, fruit and vegetables, and all of these could possibly contribute to the increased risk of noncommunicable diseases like diabetes.[83]

APPLYING EPIDEMIOLOGY IN CLINICAL CARE OF DIABETES

The main purpose of clinical epidemiology is to foster methods of clinical observations and interpretations that lead to valid conclusions and better patient care. Over the last few years, considerable attention has been paid on the capacity for epidemiology to contribute to diagnosis, prognosis, treatment, and prevention for the individual with diabetes.

Diagnosis and Screening for Diabetes

For decades, the diagnosis of diabetes has been based on glucose criteria, either the fasting plasma glucose (FPG) or 75 g oral glucose tolerance test (OGTT). The criteria proposed by Fajans and Conn in 1954[84] did not use a fasting glucose criterion but relied on 1-, 1.5-, and 2-hour post glucose load values and recommended a 2-hour cut point of 140 mg/dL. In 1964, the US Public Health Service[85] criteria for the diagnosis of diabetes included a FPG of 125 mg/dL and a 2-hour value of 140 mg/dL. National Diabetes Data Group in 1979[86] and WHO in 1985[87] recommended a FPG of 140 mg/dL and a 2-hour value of 200 mg/dL. The American Diabetes Association (ADA) Expert Committee on the diagnosis and classification of diabetes mellitus[88] revised the diagnostic criteria, using data from three cross-sectional epidemiologic studies (Pima Indians in the US,[89] among Egyptians,[90] and in the Third National Health and Nutrition Examination Survey (NHANES III) in the US[91]) based on the association between FPG levels and presence of retinopathy as the key factor with which to identify threshold glucose level. The data from the epidemiological studies helped to inform a new diagnostic cut point of greater than or equal to 126 mg/dL (7.0 mmol/L) for FPG from the earlier value of greater than or equal to 140 mg/dL and confirmed the long-standing diagnostic 2-hour plasma glucose value of greater than or equal to 200 mg/dL (11.1 mmol/L).

There are recent recommendations to use glycated hemoglobin (HbA1c) greater than or equal to 6.5% as a diagnostic tool to detect type 2 diabetes based on the International Expert Committee (IEC),[92] ADA,[93] and WHO.[94] Nevertheless, there are concerns about using HbA1c for diagnosis or at the selected threshold.[95] Analyses of NHANES data indicate that, assuming universal screening of the undiagnosed, the A1c cut point of greater than or equal to 6.5% identifies one-third fewer cases of undiagnosed diabetes than a FPG cut point of greater than or equal to 126 mg/dL (7.0 mmol/L).[96] In Asian Indians,[97] the A1c cut points of 6.1% and 6.4% defined diabetes by 2-hour post load plasma glucose or FPG criteria, respectively, and in China, the screening model using both FPG greater than or equal to 6.1 mmol/L and HbA1c greater than or equal to 6.1% had specificity of 96.3% and sensitivity of 96.5% for detecting undiagnosed diabetes.[98] Mustafa et al.[99] in a population-based and an at-risk multi-ethnic cohort compared the test performance for detecting diabetes on OGTT using either HbA1c greater than or equal to 6.5% or two HbA1c thresholds where the first cut-point "rules out" and the second "rules in" diabetes, and showed that HbA1c greater than or equal to 6.5% produced sensitivity of 62.1% for detecting diabetes in white Europeans and 78.9% in South Asians. Using two selected thresholds, HbA1c less than or equal to 5.8% (rule in, 40 mmol/mol) and HbA1c greater than or equal to 6.8% (rule out, 51 mmol/mol) produced high sensitivity/specificity (> 91.0%) for detecting diabetes; however, 28.8% of the cohort with HbA1c 5.9–6.7% required a subsequent glucose test.

One of the unfortunate aspects about diabetes is that more than 50% of the people with diabetes are unaware of their disorder. The rate of undiagnosed diabetes is high in most developing countries. In the ICMR-INDIAB study conducted in four states of India, the prevalence of undiagnosed diabetes among urban residents of Tamil Nadu, Maharashtra, Jharkhand and Chandigarh were 5·2%, 7·2%, 5·1%, and

7·6% and that among rural residents 3·8%, 4·9%, 2·3%, and 5·2%, respectively.[22] In the Screening India's Twin Epidemic (SITE) Study conducted across diabetes center in 10 Indian states, 7.2% had undiagnosed diabetes.[100] Detecting people with undiagnosed type 2 diabetes is important for both public health policy and everyday clinical practice. Because of the rapidly increasing prevalence of type 2 diabetes, early screening of individuals at high risk of having diabetes is recommended and several risk score questionnaires have been developed to detect this high-risk group using a combination of demographic, clinical, and sometimes biochemical information derived from epidemiology studies conducted in different populations (Table 2).[101-113] Studies have shown that all perform equally well, with a sensitivity of 65–84% and a specificity of 40–96%.

Prognosis

Diabetes exerts a significant burden globally resulting in escalation of burdens in the form of morbidity, mortality, decreased life expectancy, reduced quality of life, loss of human and social capital, as well as individual and national income losses. Epidemiological evidence indicates that type 2 diabetes is an independent risk factor for macro and microvascular complications, which subsequently become the cause of mortality. Diabetic microvascular complications together may contribute to serious morbidity and mortality.[114] It has been demonstrated that along with the presence of external risk factors, some associations have also been noted between diabetic microvascular complications themselves.[114,115] In addition, studies have shown that the presence of DR may reveal patients at risk of diabetic nephropathy[116] and neuropathy.[117] The CURES study reported on all microvascular complications of diabetes and revealed that the association between DR and nephropathy was stronger than that with neuropathy.[115]

It is well established that subjects with type 2 diabetes are at two to fourfold increased risk of CVD as compared to people without diabetes.[118] This risk persists even after accounting for traditional cardiovascular risk factors such as smoking, hypertension and dyslipidemia. In the Australian Diabetes, Obesity, and Lifestyle Study (AusDiab), known diabetes [hazards ratio (HR): 2.6] was an independent predictor for CVD mortality after adjustment for age, sex, and other traditional cardiovascular risk factors.[119] Earlier studies have reported associations of DR with risks of CVDs, such as stroke and coronary heart disease.[120,121] In a population-based cohort of diabetic persons free of clinical heart disease, even after controlling for age, gender, race, smoking, diabetes duration, insulin use, blood pressure, lipid profile, and other risk factors, participants with retinopathy had more than 2.5 fold higher risk of developing heart failure than those without retinopathy (HR: 2.71).[122] These findings suggest that this increased risk for vascular disease could be attributed directly or indirectly to elevated glucose levels. Apart from hyperglycemia, severe hypoglycemia has also been shown to be strongly related to the incidence of major macrovascular

TABLE 2: Risk Scores for Diabetes Developed Using Data From Population Based Studies

Author/year	Population	Risk score derived from	Risk factors	Sensitivity (%)	Specificity (%)	AUC (%)
Griffin et al. 2000[101]	UK	Community in Cambridgeshire	Age, sex, BMI, HTN, steroids, smoking, FH	77	72	80
Tabaei et al. 2002[102]	Egyptian	Diabetes in Egypt project	Age, sex, BMI, RPG, PP time	65	96	88
Lindstrom and Tuomilehto 2003[103]	Finnish	National Population Register	Age, BMI, WC, history of antihypertensive drug treatment and high blood glucose, PA and daily consumption of fruits, berries, or vegetables	78	77	85
Glumer et al. 2004[104]	Danish	Inter99 study	Age, sex, BMI, HTN, PA at leisure time, and FH	73	74	80
Colagiuri et al. 2004[105]	Australian	Australian Diabetes Obesity, and Lifestyle Study	Age, BMI, CVD, FH, GDM, HTN, IGT or IFG, obese women with PCO and race	80	80	–
Mohan et al. 2005[106]	Indian	Chennai Urban Rural Epidemiology Study	Age, WC, FH and PA	73	60	70
Ramachandran et al. 2005[107]	Indian	National Urban Diabetes Survey	Age, BMI, WC, PA and FH	77	60	73
Aekplakorn et al. 2006[108]	Thai	Cohort of employees from Electric Generation Authority	Age, BMI, WC, HTN and history of diabetes in parents or siblings	77	60	74
Al-Lawati and Tuomilehto 2007[109]	Oman	Oman's National Diabetes Survey	Age, WC, BMI, FH and HTN	79	63	83
Bang et al. 2009[110]	US	National Health and Nutrition Examination Survey	Age, sex, FH, HTN, obesity and PA	79	67	83
Gao et al. 2010[111]	Chinese	Urban community in Qingdao	Age, WC and FH	84	40	67
Doi et al. 2012[112]	Japanese	Population of Hisayama	Age, sex, FH, WC, BMI, HTN, regular PA and current smoking			70
Lee et al. 2012[113]	Korean	Korean National Health and Nutrition Examination Survey	Age, FH, HTN, WC, smoking and alcohol intake	81	54	73

AUC, area under the curve; BMI, body mass index; HTN, hypertension; FH, family history of diabetes; RPG, random plasma glucose; PP, postprandial; WC, waist circumference; PA, physical activity; CVD, cardiovascular disease; GDM, gestational diabetes mellitus; IGT, impaired glucose tolerance; IFG, impaired fasting glucose; PCO, polycystic ovary events (HR: 2.9), major microvascular events (HR: 1.8), death from cardiovascular causes (HR: 2.7) and all-cause mortality (HR: 2.7) in a retrospective analysis of the Action in Diabetes and Vascular Disease—Preterax and Diamicron Modified Release Controlled Evaluation ADVANCE study.[123,124]

Although diabetes is often not recorded as a cause of death, it is already the fifth leading cause of mortality globally (4 million deaths annually), outnumbering global deaths from human immunodeficiency virus/acquired immunodeficiency syndrome (HIV/AIDS); 80% of this mortality occurs in low- and middle-income countries.[125] Even though the prevalence of diabetes is low in low-income countries as compared to high-income countries, there are nearly equal numbers of deaths due to diabetes in low-income countries (492,000) as in high-income countries (544,000).[20]

The majority of deaths among diabetic individuals is due to cardiovascular and cerebrovascular diseases and end-stage renal diseases.[126,127] The CUPS study conducted in South India provided some evidence on the effect of type 2 diabetes on mortality rates in a population.[128] The overall mortality rates were nearly threefold higher in diabetic subjects as compared to nondiabetic individuals (18.9 vs 5.3 per 1,000 person-years). The HR for all-cause mortality for diabetes was found to be 3.6 as compared to nondiabetic subjects. The study also showed that the leading cause of mortality in diabetic subjects was cardiovascular (52.9%) and renal (23.5%) diseases. In another study done by Zargar et al.,[129] of the 234,776 admissions to their tertiary care hospital, 16,690 (7.11%) died, of whom 741 had diabetes mellitus as mentioned in the death certificate. The causes contributing to death were infections (40.9%), chronic renal failure (33.6%), coronary artery disease (16.9%), cerebrovascular disease (13.2%), chronic obstructive pulmonary disease (6.9%), acute renal failure (6.2%), malignancy (4.2%), hypoglycemia (3.5%), and diabetic ketoacidosis (3.4%).

MANAGEMENT

Aggressive management of type 2 diabetes is essential to achieve glycemic and nonglycemic treatment goals. Attainment of treatment goals is associated with a decreased risk of diabetes-related complications, costs, and health care utilization. The relationship between metabolic control of patients with diabetes and the development of micro and macrovascualr complications has always been the primary concern of clinicians, but has also been a much debated issue in the literature over the years.[130,131] The Diabetes Control and Complications Trial (DCCT) carried out in individuals with type 1 diabetes was the first large clinical trial which focused on this issue. The mean HbA1c levels during the 9-year study were 7.2% for intensively-treated subjects and 9.1% in conventionally-treated subjects. The study clearly demonstrated that improved glycemic control reduced the risk of development and progression of diabetic complications in type 1 diabetic individuals (~60% reduction).[132-134]

The United Kingdom Prospective Diabetes Study (UKPDS) carried out on type 2 diabetes demonstrated a 25% reduction in the risk of microvascular endpoints in patients with type 2 diabetes who were treated using an intensive glucose-lowering strategy as compared with a conventional approach.[135] Subsequent observational analyses from the UKPDS study showed that a 1% decrease in HbA1c was associated with 12% reduction in incidence of stroke, 14% in myocardial infarction, 16% in heart failure, 37% microvascular disease and 43% lower extremity amputation or fatal PVD.[136]

After the completion of the landmark DCCT, the study subjects were requested to take part in an epidemiologic follow-up study, the Epidemiology of Diabetes Interventions and Complications (EDIC) study, to determine whether the effect of improved blood glucose control will result in a decrease in the occurrence of circulatory complications and advanced stages of kidney disease. Differences in HbA1c levels between intensively- and conventionally-treated subjects at the end of the DCCT were lost well before the end of the 11-year observational period of the EDIC study which was completed in 2005. Despite this loss of glycemic separation, cardiovascular events were reduced by 57% at the end of the observational period.[137,138] These landmark studies have shown that optimal glycemic control is vital to manage diabetes and its complications. However, estimates in the US indicate that only 57% of type 2 diabetes patients reach the ADA glycemic target of A1c less than 7%, and 33% achieve the American Association of Clinical Endocrinologists (AACE) glycemic target of A1c less than or equal to 6.5%.[139]

The results of major randomized clinical trials on the benefits of intensive versus standard glucose control are, however, controversial.[140-142] In the Action to Control Cardiovascular Risk in Diabetes (ACCORD) study, an intensive glucose-lowering regimen was associated with increased mortality (HR: 1.22).[140] A significant reduction in the rate of microvascular and renal events after intensive glycemic control (median HbA1c was lowered to 6.3% as compared with standard glycemic control achieving an HbA1c of 7.0%) was shown in ADVANCE trial.[141] However, the Veterans Affairs Diabetes Trial (VADT)[142] reported that microvascular complications were same in both the intensive therapy and the control groups. Skyler et al.[143] state that the lack of significant reduction in CVD events with intensive glycemic control in ACCORD, ADVANCE, and VADT should not lead clinicians to abandon good control of diabetes. Indeed the target of HbA1c less than 7.0% is now universally accepted for most patients. The recent ADA-EASD guidelines rightly emphasize the need for individualized glycemic target for people with diabetes depending on their level of morbidity and comorbid conditions.[144]

PREVENTION

In addition, although observational data are imperative to identify risk factors for a disease and their possible role in the natural history of a disease, randomized clinical trials of risk factor intervention are mandatory in the prevention of diabetes. Also, pharmacological agents may be used to prevent diabetes, and the evidence again has to come from controlled clinical trials. In early 1980s, descriptive epidemiology of diabetes was assessed and the areas where interventions, if systematically applied, could impact health status were reported. It was predicted that lifestyle modification through diet and exercise could prevent up to 50% of type 2 diabetes or almost 300,000 cases of diabetes per year.[145] Several large trials from Finland [Finnish Diabetes Prevention Study (FDPS)],[146] China [DA Qing impaired glucose tolerance (IGT) and Diabetes Study],[147] USA [diabetes prevention program (DPP), STOP-NIDDM trial, ACT NOW, Diabetes REduction Assessment with ramipril and rosiglitazone Medication Trial (DREAM)],[148-152] India [(Indian Diabetes Prevention Program (IDPP)],[153] and Japan[154] have demonstrated the ability of lifestyle changes/pharmacotherapy to prevent diabetes in high-risk individuals (Figure 2). These findings may enhance efforts in the development of targeted primary prevention programs for type 2 diabetes.

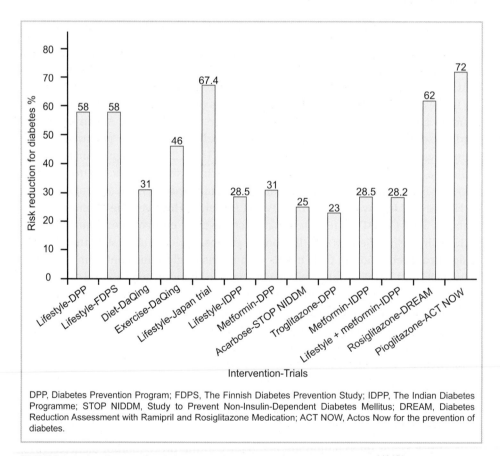

DPP, Diabetes Prevention Program; FDPS, The Finnish Diabetes Prevention Study; IDPP, The Indian Diabetes Programme; STOP NIDDM, Study to Prevent Non-Insulin-Dependent Diabetes Mellitus; DREAM, Diabetes Reduction Assessment with Ramipril and Rosiglitazone Medication; ACT NOW, Actos Now for the prevention of diabetes.

FIGURE 2 Risk reduction for diabetes with various intervention strategies.[146-154]

CONCLUSION

Epidemiological studies of diabetes worldwide indicate that diabetes is a major and growing public health issue globally. The findings from the epidemiological studies emphasize the need for such data for clinicians to better understand the consequences of diabetes, to understand the pathophysiology and risk factor profile (both biomedical and behavioral), to explore the interaction of genetics and environment as determinants of diabetes risk and also identify the effective tools (lifestyle/pharmacological interventions) for diabetes prevention in high-risk population. Thus, application of clinical epidemiology to the care of individual patients termed as evidence-based medicine will help clinicians to formulate specific clinical questions and find the best available research evidence to improve patient care and also influence medical decision.

REFERENCES

1. Last JM. A Dictionary of Epidemiology. 2nd edition. New York, NY: Oxford University Press; 1988.
2. Snow J. On the mode of communication of cholera 1855. *Salud Publica Mex.* 1991;33: 194-201.
3. Dawber TR, Meadors GF, Moore FE Jr. Epidemiological approaches to heart disease: the Framingham Study. *Am J Public Health Nations Health.* 1951;41:279-81.
4. Berenson GS, Wattigney WA, Bao W, Srinivasan SR, Radhakrishnamurthy B. Rationale to study the early natural history of heart disease: the Bogalusa Heart Study. *Am J Med Sci.* 1995;310(suppl 1):S22-8.
5. Doll R, Hill AB. Smoking and carcinoma of the lung: preliminary report. *Br Med J.* 1950;2:739-48.
6. Hammond EC, Horn D. Smoking and death rates; report on forty-four months of follow-up of 187,783 men. I. Total mortality. *J Am Med Assoc.* 1958;166:1159-72.
7. Paul JR. President's Address Clinical Epidemiology. *J Clin Invest.* 1938;17:539-41.
8. Herman WH. Diabetes epidemiology: guiding clinical and public health practice: Kelly West Award Lecture, 2006. *Diabetes Care.* 2007;30:1912-9.
9. King H, Rewers M. Diabetes in adults is now a Third World problem. World Health Organization Ad Hoc Diabetes Reporting Group. *Ethn Dis.* 1993;3 Suppl:S67-74.
10. Songer TJ, Zimmet P. Epidemiology of Type 2 diabetes: an international prospective. Pharmacoeconomics. 1995;Supl 1:1-11.
11. Donnelly R, Emslie-Smith AM, Gardner ID, Morris AD. ABC of arterial and venous disease: vascular complications of diabetes. *BMJ.* 2000;320:1062-6.
12. Herman WH, Sinnock P, Brenner E, Brimberry JL, Langford D, Nakashima A, et al. An epidemiologic model for diabetes mellitus: incidence, prevalence, and mortality. *Diabetes Care.* 1984;7:367-71.
13. King H, Rewers M. Global estimates for prevalence of diabetes mellitus and impaired glucose tolerance in adults. WHO Ad Hoc Diabetes Reporting Group. *Diabetes Care.* 1993;16:157-77.
14. King H, Aubert RE, Herman WH. Global burden of diabetes, 1995–2025: prevalence, numerical estimates, and projections. *Diabetes Care.* 1998;21:1414-31.

15. Wild S, Roglic G, Green A, Sicree R, King H. Global prevalence of diabetes: estimates for the year 2000 and projections for 2030. *Diabetes Care*. 2004;27:1047-53.

16. International Diabetes Federation: Diabetes Atlas 2000. Brussels: International Diabetes Federation; 2000.

17. Allgot B, Gan D, King H, Lefèbvre P, Mbanya JC, Silink M, et al. (Eds). Diabetes Atlas, 2nd edition. Brussels: International Diabetes Federation; 2003.

18. Sicree R, Shaw J, Zimmet P. Diabetes and impaired glucose tolerance. In: Gan D (Ed). Diabetes Atlas. International Diabetes Federation, 3rd edition. Belgium: International Diabetes Federation; 2006. pp. 15-103.

19. Unwin N, Whiting D, Gan D, Jacqmain O, Ghyoot G (Eds). International Diabetes Federation, Diabetes Atlas, 4th edition, Brussels, Belgium: International Diabetes Federation; 2009. pp. 1-27.

20. Unwin N, Whiting D, Guariguata L, Ghyoot G, Gan D (Eds). International Diabetes Federation, Diabetes Atlas, 5th edition. Brussels, Belgium: International Diabetes Federation; 2011. pp. 11-74.

21. Danaei G, Finucane MM, Lu Y, Singh GM, Cowan MJ, Paciorek CJ, et al. National, regional, and global trends in fasting plasma glucose and diabetes prevalence since 1980: systematic analysis of health examination surveys and epidemiological studies with 370 country-years and 2.7 million participants. *Lancet*. 2011;378:31-40.

22. Anjana RM, Pradeepa R, Deepa M, Datta M, Sudha V, Unnikrishnan R, et al. The Indian Council of Medical Research-India Diabetes (ICMR-INDIAB) study: methodological details. *J Diabetes Sci Technol*. 2011;5:906-14.

23. Anjana RM, Pradeepa R, Deepa M, Datta M, Sudha V, Unnikrishnan R, et al. ICMR–INDIAB Collaborative Study Group. Prevalence of diabetes and prediabetes (impaired fasting glucose and/or impaired glucose tolerance) in urban and rural India: phase I results of the Indian Council of Medical Research-INdia DIABetes (ICMR-INDIAB) study. *Diabetologia*. 2011;54:3022-7.

24. Yang W, Lu J, Weng J, Jia W, Ji L, Xiao J, et al.; China National Diabetes and Metabolic Disorders Study Group. Prevalence of diabetes among men and women in China. *N Engl J Med*. 2010;362:1090-101.

25. Gholap N, Davies M, Patel K, Sattar N, Khunti K. Type 2 diabetes and cardiovascular disease in South Asians. *Prim Care Diabetes*. 2011;5:45-56.

26. Klein R, Klein BE, Moss SE, Davis MD, DeMets DL. The Wisconsin epidemiologic study of diabetic retinopathy. III. Prevalence and risk of diabetic retinopathy when age at diagnosis is 30 or more years. *Arch Ophthalmol*. 1984;102:527-32.

27. Leske MC, Wu SY, Hyman L, Li X, Hennis A, Connell AM, et al. Diabetic retinopathy in a black population: the Barbados Eye Study. *Ophthalmology*. 1999;106:1893-9.

28. Klein R, Klein BE, Moss SE, Linton KL. The Beaver Dam Eye Study. Retinopathy in adults with newly discovered and previously diagnosed diabetes mellitus. *Ophthalmology*. 1992;99:58-62.

29. Mitchell P, Smith W, Wang JJ, Attebo K. Prevalence of diabetic retinopathy in an older community. The Blue Mountains Eye Study. *Ophthalmology*. 1998;105:406-11.

30. Varma R, Torres M, Pena F, Klein R, Azen SP; Los Angeles Latino Eye Study Group. Prevalence of diabetic retinopathy in adult Latinos: the Los Angeles Latino eye study. *Ophthalmology*. 2004;111:1298-306.

31. Broadbent DM, Scott JA, Vora JP, Harding SP. Prevalence of diabetic eye disease in an inner city population: the Liverpool Diabetic Eye Study. *Eye (Lond)*. 1999;13:160-5.

32. Rema M, Premkumar S, Anitha B, Deepa R, Pradeepa R, Mohan V. Prevalence of diabetic retinopathy in urban India: the Chennai Urban Rural Epidemiology Study (CURES) eye study, I. *Invest Ophthalmol Vis Sci.* 2005;46:2328-33.

33. Nirmalan PK, Katz J, Robin AL, Tielsch JM, Namperumalsamy P, Kim R, et al. Prevalence of vitreoretinal disorders in a rural population of southern India: the Aravind Comprehensive Eye Study. *Arch Ophthalmol.* 2004;122:581-6.

34. Wong TY, Klein R, Islam FM, Cotch MF, Folsom AR, Klein BE, et al. Diabetic retinopathy in a multi-ethnic cohort in the United States. *Am J Ophthalmol.* 2006;141:446-55.

35. Ding J, Cheng CY, Haaland BA, Saw SM, Venketasubramanian N, Chen CP, et al. Visual impairment, age-related eye diseases, and cognitive function: the Singapore Malay eye study. *Arch Ophthalmol.* 2012;130:895-900.

36. Yau JW, Rogers SL, Kawasaki R, Lamoureux EL, Kowalski JW, Bek T, et al.; Meta-Analysis for Eye Disease (META-EYE) Study Group. Global prevalence and major risk factors of diabetic retinopathy. *Diabetes Care.* 2012;35:556-64.

37. Tapp RJ, Shaw JE, de Courten MP, Dunstan DW, Welborn TA, Zimmet PZ; AusDiab Study Group. Foot complications in Type 2 diabetes: an Australian population-based study. *Diabet Med.* 2003;20:105-13.

38. Klein R, Sharrett AR, Klein BE, Moss SE, Folsom AR, Wong TY, et al. The association of atherosclerosis, vascular risk factors, and retinopathy in adults with diabetes: the atherosclerosis risk in communities study. *Ophthalmology.* 2002;109:1225-34.

39. Asakawa H, Tokunaga K, Kawakami F. Comparison of risk factors of macrovascular complications. Peripheral vascular disease, cerebral vascular disease, and coronary heart disease in Japanese type 2 diabetes mellitus patients. *J Diabetes Complications.* 2000;14:307-13.

40. Beks PJ, Mackaay AJ, de Neeling JN, de Vries H, Bouter LM, Heine RJ. Peripheral arterial disease in relation to glycaemic level in an elderly Caucasian population: the Hoorn study. *Diabetologia.* 1995;38:86-96.

41. Bruno G, Cavallo-Perin P, Bargero G, Borra M, Calvi V, D'Errico N, et al. Prevalence and risk factors for micro- and macroalbuminuria in an Italian population-based cohort of NIDDM subjects. *Diabetes Care.* 1996;19:43-7.

42. Capuano V, Lamaida N, Borrelli MI, Capuano E, Fasolino A, Capuano E, et al. Chronic kidney disease prevalence and trends (1998-2008) in an area of Southern Italy. The data of the VIP project. *G Ital Nefrol.* 2012;29:445-51.

43. Unnikrishnan RI, Rema M, Pradeepa R, Deepa M, Shanthirani CS, Deepa R, et al. Prevalence and risk factors of diabetic nephropathy in an urban South Indian population: the Chennai Urban Rural Epidemiology Study (CURES 45). *Diabetes Care.* 2007;30:2019-24.

44. Premalatha G, Shanthirani S, Deepa R, Markovitz J, Mohan V. Prevalence and risk factors of peripheral vascular disease in a selected South Indian population. The Chennai Urban Population Study. *Diabetes Care.* 2000;23:1295-300.

45. Pradeepa R, Rema M, Vignesh J, Deepa M, Deepa R, Mohan V. Prevalence and risk factors for diabetic neuropathy in an urban south Indian population: the Chennai Urban Rural Epidemiology Study (CURES-55). *Diabet Med.* 2008;25:407-12.

46. Mohan V, Deepa R, Shanthirani CS, Premalatha G. Prevalence of coronary artery disease and its relationship to lipids in a selected population in South India: The Chennai Urban Population Study (CUPS No. 5). *J Am Coll Cardiol.* 2001;38:682-7.

47. Sobngwi E, Ndour-Mbaye M, Boateng KA, Ramaiya KL, Njenga EW, Diop SN, et al. Type 2 diabetes control and complications in specialised diabetes care centres of six sub-Saharan African countries: The Diabcare Africa study. *Diabetes Res Clin Pract.* 2012;95:30-6.

48. Weber MB, Oza-Frank R, Staimez LR, Ali MK, Narayan KM. Type 2 diabetes in Asians: prevalence, risk factors, and effectiveness of behavioral intervention at individual and population levels. *Annu Rev Nutr.* 2012;32:417-39.

49. Harris SB, Gittelsohn J, Hanley AJ, Barnie A, Wolever TM, Gao XJ, et al. The prevalence of NIDDM and associated risk factors in native Canadians. *Diabetes Care.* 1997;20:185-7.

50. Lillioja S, Mott DM, Spraul M, Ferraro R, Foley JE, Ravussin E, et al. Insulin resistance and insulin secretory dysfunction as precursors of non-insulin-dependent diabetes mellitus. Prospective studies of Pima Indians. *N Engl J Med.* 1993;329:1988-92.

51. Haffner SM, Miettinen H, Gaskill SP, Stern MP. Decreased insulin secretion and increased insulin resistance are independently related to the 7-year risk of NIDDM in Mexican-Americans. *Diabetes.* 1995;44:1386-91.

52. Sharp PS, Mohan V, Levy JC, Mather HM, Kohner EM. Insulin resistance in patients of Asian Indian and European origin with non-insulin dependent diabetes. *Horm Metab Res.* 1987;19:84-5.

53. Hamman RF, Marshall JA, Baxter J, Kahn LB, Mayer EJ, Orleans M, et al. Methods and prevalence of non-insulin-dependent diabetes mellitus in a biethnic Colorado population. The San Luis Valley Diabetes Study. *Am J Epidemiol.* 1989;129:295-311.

54. Harris MI. Noninsulin-dependent diabetes mellitus in black and white Americans. *Diabetes Metab Rev.* 1990;6:71-90.

55. West KM. Epidemiology of Diabetes and its Vascular Lesions. New York: Elsevier; 1978. pp. 224-79.

56. Amati F, Dube JJ, Coen PM, Stefanovic-Racic M, Toledo FG, Goodpaster BH. Physical inactivity and obesity underlie the insulin resistance of aging. *Diabetes Care.* 2009;32: 1547-9.

57. Chan JC, Malik V, Jia W, Kadowaki T, Yajnik CS, Yoon KH, et al. Diabetes in Asia: epidemiology, risk factors, and pathophysiology. *JAMA.* 2009;301:2129-40.

58. Mohan V, Deepa M, Deepa R, Shanthirani CS, Farooq S, Ganesan A, et al. Secular trends in the prevalence of diabetes and glucose tolerance in urban South India—the Chennai Urban Rural Epidemiology Study (CURES-17). *Diabetologia.* 2006;49:1175-8.

59. Annis AM, Caulder MS, Cook ML, Duquette D. Family history, diabetes, and other demographic and risk factors among participants of the National Health and Nutrition Examination Survey 1999–2002. *Prev Chronic Dis.* 2005;2:A19.

60. Meigs JB, Cupples LA, Wilson PW. Parental transmission of type 2 diabetes: the Framingham Offspring Study. *Diabetes.* 2000;49:2201-7.

61. Radha V, Mohan V. Genetic predisposition to type 2 diabetes among Asian Indians. *Indian J Med Res.* 2007;125:259-74.

62. Kooner JS, Saleheen D, Sim X, Sehmi J, Zhang W, Frossard P, et al. Genome-wide association study in individuals of South Asian ancestry identifies six new type 2 diabetes susceptibility loci. *Nat Genet.* 2011;43:984-9.

63. Huxley R, Barzi F, Stolk R, Caterson I, Gill T, Lam TH, et al.; Obesity in Asia Collaboration. Ethnic comparisons of obesity in the Asia-Pacific region: protocol for a collaborative overview of cross-sectional studies. *Obes Rev.* 2005;6:193-8.

64. Indulekha K, Anjana RM, Surendar J, Mohan V. Association of visceral and subcutaneous fat with glucose intolerance, insulin resistance, adipocytokines and inflammatory markers in Asian Indians (CURES-113). *Clin Biochem.* 2011;44:281-87.

65. Gao H, Salim A, Lee J, Tai ES, van Dam RM. Can body fat distribution, adiponectin levels and inflammation explain differences in insulin resistance between ethnic Chinese, Malays and Asian Indians? Int J Obes (Lond). 2012;36:1086-93.

66. Boyko EJ, Fujimoto WY, Leonetti DL, Newell-Morris L. Visceral adiposity and risk of type 2 diabetes: a prospective study among Japanese Americans. *Diabetes Care*. 2000;23:465-71.

67. Lee IM, Shiroma EJ, Lobelo F, Puska P, Blair SN, Katzmarzyk PT; Lancet Physical Activity Series Working Group. Effect of physical inactivity on major non-communicable diseases worldwide: an analysis of burden of disease and life expectancy. *Lancet*. 2012;380:219-29.

68. Joubert J, Norman R, Lambert EV, Groenewald P, Schneider M, Bull F, et al.; South African Comparative Risk Assessment Collaborating Group. Estimating the burden of disease attributable to physical inactivity in South Africa in 2000. *S Afr Med J*. 2007;97:725-31.

69. Lee DC, Park I, Jun TW, Nam BH, Cho SI, Blair SN, et al. Physical activity and body mass index and their associations with the development of type 2 diabetes in Korean men. *Am J Epidemiol*. 2012;176:43-51.

70. Schenk S, Horowitz JF. Acute exercise increases triglyceride synthesis in skeletal muscle and prevents fatty acid-induced insulin resistance. *J Clin Invest*. 2007;117:1690-8.

71. Shepherd PR, Kahn BB. Glucose transporters and insulin action—implications for insulin resistance and diabetes mellitus. *N Engl J Med*. 1999;341:248-57.

72. Grøntved A, Rimm EB, Willett WC, Andersen LB, Hu FB. A prospective study of weight training and risk of type 2 diabetes mellitus in men. *Arch Intern Med*. 2012;172:1306-12.

73. Hu FB. Globalization of diabetes: the role of diet, lifestyle, and genes. *Diabetes Care*. 2011;34:1249-57.

74. Mohan V, Radhika G, Sathya RM, Tamil SR, Ganesan A, Sudha V. Dietary carbohydrates, glycaemic load, food groups and newly detected type 2 diabetes among urban Asian Indian population in Chennai, India (Chennai Urban Rural Epidemiology Study 59). *Br J Nutr*. 2009;102:1498-506.

75. Wang Y, Mi J, Shan XY, Wang QJ, Ge KY. Is China facing an obesity epidemic and the consequences? The trends in obesity and chronic disease in China. *Int J Obes (Lond)*. 2007;31:177-88.

76. Shetty PS. Nutrition transition in India. *Public Health Nutr*. 2002;5:175-82.

77. Matsumura Y. Nutrition trends in Japan. *Asia Pac J Clin Nutr*. 2001;10(suppl):S40-7.

78. Kosulwat V. The nutrition and health transition in Thailand. *Public Health Nutr*. 2002; 5:183-9.

79. Haag M, Dippenaar NG. Dietary fats, fatty acids and insulin resistance: short review of a multifaceted connection. *Med Sci Monit*. 2005;11(12):RA359-67.

80. Villegas R, Liu S, Gao YT, Yang G, Li H, Zheng W, et al. Prospective study of dietary carbohydrates, glycemic index, glycemic load, and incidence of type 2 diabetes mellitus in middle-aged Chinese women. *Arch Intern Med*. 2007;167:2310-6.

81. Murakami K, Sasaki S, Takahashi Y, Okubo H, Hosoi Y, Horiguchi H, et al. Dietary glycemic index and load in relation to metabolic risk factors in Japanese female farmers with traditional dietary habits. *Am J Clin Nutr*. 2006;83:1161-9.

82. Radhika G, Van Dam RM, Sudha V, Ganesan A, Mohan V. Refined grain consumption and the metabolic syndrome in urban Asian Indians (Chennai Urban Rural Epidemiology Study 57). *Metabolism*. 2009;58:675-81.

83. Radhika G, Sathya RM, Ganesan A, Saroja R, Vijayalakshmi P, Sudha V, et al. Dietary profile of urban adult population in South India in the context of chronic disease epidemiology (CURES-68). *Public Health Nutr*. 2011;14:591-8.

84. Fajans SS, Conn JW. Prediabetes, subclinical diabetes, and latent clinical diabetes: interpretation, diagnosis and treatment. In: Leibel BS, Wrenshall GA (Eds). On the Nature and Treatment of Diabetes. New York: Excerpta Media; 1965. pp. 641-56.

85. Remein QR, Wilkerson HL. The efficiency of screening tests for diabetes. *J Chronic Dis.* 1961;13:6-21.

86. Classification and diagnosis of diabetes meUitus and other categories of glucose intolerance. National Diabetes Data Group. *Diabetes.* 1979;28:1039-57.

87. World Health Organization. Diabetes mellitus. Report of a WHO study group. *World Health Organ Tech Rep Ser.* 1985;727:1-113.

88. American Diabetes Association Expert Committee. Report of the Expert Committee on the Diagnosis and Classification of Diabetes Mellitus. *Diabetes Care.* 1997;20:1183-97.

89. McCance DR, Hanson RL, Charles MA, Jacobsson LT, Pettitt DJ, Bennett PH, et al. Comparison of tests for glycated haemoglobin and fasting and two hour plasma glucose concentrations as diagnostic methods for diabetes. *BMJ.* 1994;308:1323-8.

90. Engelgau MM, Thompson TJ, Herman WH, Boyle JP, Aubert RE, Kenny SJ, et al. Comparison of fasting and 2-hour glucose and HbA_1c levels for diagnosing diabetes: diagnostic criteria and performance revisited. *Diabetes Care.* 1997;20:785-91.

91. Report of the expert committee on the diagnosis and classification of diabetes mellitus. Expert Committee on the Diagnosis and Classification of Diabetes Mellitus. *Diabetes Care.* 2003;26 Suppl 1:S5-20.

92. Expert Committee. International Expert Committee report on the role of the A1c assay in the diagnosis of diabetes. *Diabetes Care.* 2009;32:1327-34.

93. Executive summary: Standards of medical care in Diabetes—2010: current criteria for the diagnosis of diabetes. *Diabetes Care.* 2010;33(Supp 1):S4-10.

94. World Health Organization. (2011). Use of glycated haemoglobin (HbA1c) in the diagnosis of diabetes mellitus. Abbreviated report of a WHO consultation. [online]. Available from http://www.who.int/diabetes/publications/diagnosis_diabetes2011/en/index.html [Accessed May, 2013].

95. Mostafa SA, Davies MJ, Srinivasan BT, Carey ME, Webb D, Khunti K. Should glycated haemoglobin (HbA1c) be used to detect people with type 2 diabetes mellitus and impaired glucose regulation? *Postgrad Med J.* 2010;86:656-62.

96. Cowie CC, Rust KF, Byrd-Holt DD, Gregg EW, Ford ES, Geiss LS, et al. Prevalence of diabetes and high risk for diabetes using A1c criteria in the U.S. population in 1988–2006. *Diabetes Care.* 2010;33:562-8.

97. Mohan V, Vijayachandrika V, Gokulakrishnan K, Anjana RM, Ganesan A, Weber MB, et al. A1C cut points to define various glucose intolerance groups in Asian Indians. *Diabetes Care.* 2010;33:515-9.

98. Hu Y, Liu W, Chen Y, Zhang M, Wang L, Zhou H, et al. Combined use of fasting plasma glucose and glycated hemoglobin A1c in the screening of diabetes and impaired glucose tolerance. *Acta Diabetol.* 2010;47:231-6.

99. Mostafa S, Khunti K, Kilpatrick E, Webb D, Srinivasan B, Gray L, et al. Diagnostic performance of using one- or two-HbA1c cut-point strategies to detect undiagnosed type 2 diabetes and impaired glucose regulation within a multi-ethnic population. *Diab Vasc Dis Res.* 2013;10:84-92.

100. Joshi SR, Saboo B, Vadivale M, Dani SI, Mithal A, Kaul U, et al.; Site Investigators. Prevalence of diagnosed and undiagnosed diabetes and hypertension in India— results from the Screening India's Twin Epidemic (SITE) study. *Diabetes Technol Ther.* 2012;14:8-15.

101. Griffin SJ, Little PS, Hales CN, Kinmonth AL, Wareham NJ. Diabetes risk score: towards earlier detection of type 2 diabetes in general practice. *Diabetes Metab Res Rev.* 2000;16:164-71.

102. Tabaei BP, Herman WH. A multivariate logistic regression equation to screen for diabetes: development and validation. *Diabetes Care.* 2002;25:1999-2003.

103. Lindstrom J, Tuomilehto J. The diabetes risk score: a practical tool to predict type 2 diabetes risk. *Diabetes Care.* 2003;26:725-31.

104. Glumer C, Carstensen B, Sandbaek A, Lauritzen T, Jorgensen T, Borch-Johnsen K. A Danish diabetes risk score for targeted screening: The Inter99 study. *Diabetes Care.* 2004;27:727-33.

105. Colagiuri S, Hussain Z, Zimmet P, Cameron A, Shaw J. Screening for type 2 diabetes and impaired glucose metabolism: the Australian experience. *Diabetes Care.* 2004;27:367-71.

106. Mohan V, Deepa R, Deepa M, Somannavar S, Datta M. A simplified Indian Diabetes Risk Score for screening for undiagnosed diabetic subjects. *J Assoc Physicians India.* 2005;53:759-63.

107. Ramachandran A, Snehalatha C, Vijay V, Wareham NJ, Colagiuri S. Derivation and validation of diabetes risk score for urban Asian Indians. *Diabetes Res Clin Pract.* 2005;70:63-70.

108. Aekplakorn W, Bunnag P, Woodward M, Sritara P, Cheepudomwit S, Yamwong S, et al. A risk score for predicting incident diabetes in the Thai population. *Diabetes Care.* 2006;29:1872-7.

109. Al-Lawati JA, Tuomilehto J. Diabetes risk score in Oman: a tool to identify prevalent type 2 diabetes among Arabs of the Middle East. *Diabetes Res Clin Pract.* 2007;77:438-44.

110. Bang H, Edwards AM, Bomback AS, Ballantyne CM, Brillon D, Callahan MA, et al. Development and validation of a patient self-assessment score for diabetes risk. *Ann Intern Med.* 2009;151:775-83.

111. Gao WG, Dong YH, Pang ZC, Nan HR, Wang SJ, Ren J, et al. A simple Chinese risk score for undiagnosed diabetes. *Diabet Med.* 2010;27:274-81.

112. Doi Y, Ninomiya T, Hata J, Hirakawa Y, Mukai N, Iwase M, et al. Two risk score models for predicting incident Type 2 diabetes in Japan. *Diabet Med.* 2012;29:107-14.

113. Lee YH, Bang H, Kim HC, Kim HM, Park SW, Kim DJ. A simple screening score for diabetes for the Korean population: development, validation, and comparison with other scores. *Diabetes Care.* 2012;35:1723-30.

114. Girach A, Vignati L. Diabetic microvascular complications—can the presence of one predict the development of another? *J Diabetes Complications.* 2006;20:228-37.

115. Pradeepa R, Anjana RM, Unnikrishnan R, Ganesan A, Mohan V, Rema M. Risk factors for microvascular complications of diabetes among South Indian subjects with type 2 diabetes—the Chennai Urban Rural Epidemiology Study (CURES) Eye Study-5. *Diabetes Technol Ther.* 2010;12:755-61.

116. El-Asrar AM, Al-Rubeaan KA, Al-Amro SA, Moharram OA, Kangave D. Retinopathy as a predictor of other diabetic complications. *Int Ophthalmol.* 2001;24:1-11.

117. Barr EL, Wong TY, Tapp RJ, Harper CA, Zimmet PZ, Atkins R, et al.; AusDiab Steering Committee. Is peripheral neuropathy associated with retinopathy and albuminuria in individuals with impaired glucose metabolism? The 1999-2000 AusDiab. *Diabetes Care.* 2006;29:1114-6.

118. Emerging Risk Factors Collaboration. Diabetes mellitus, fasting blood glucose concentration, and risk of vascular disease: a collaborative meta-analysis of 102 prospective studies. *Lancet.* 2010;375:2215-22.

119. Barr EL, Zimmet PZ, Welborn TA, Jolley D, Magliano DJ, Dunstan DW, et al. Risk of cardiovascular and all-cause mortality in individuals with diabetes mellitus, impaired fasting glucose, and impaired glucose tolerance: the Australian Diabetes, Obesity, and Lifestyle Study (AusDiab). *Circulation.* 2007;116:151-7.

120. Juutilainen A, Lehto S, Ronnemaa T, Pyorala K, Laakso M. Retinopathy predicts cardiovascular mortality in type 2 diabetic men and women. *Diabetes Care.* 2007;30:292-9.

121. Cheung N, Rogers S, Couper DJ, Klein R, Sharrett AR, Wong TY. Is diabetic retinopathy an independent risk factor for ischemic stroke? *Stroke.* 2007;38:398-401.

122. Cheung N, Wang JJ, Rogers SL, Brancati F, Klein R, Sharrett AR, et al.; ARIC (Atherosclerosis Risk In Communities) Study Investigators. Diabetic retinopathy and risk of heart failure. *J Am Coll Cardiol.* 2008;51:1573-8.

123. Patel A, MacMahon S, Chalmers J, Neal B, Billot L, Woodward M, et al.; ADVANCE Collaborative Group. Intensive blood glucose control and vascular outcomes in patients with type 2 diabetes. *N Engl J Med.* 2008;358:2560-72.

124. Zoungas S, Patel A, Chalmers J, de Galan BE, Li Q, Billot L, et al.; ADVANCE Collaborative Group. Severe hypoglycemia and risks of vascular events and death. *N Engl J Med.* 2010;363:1410-8.

125. Ma RC, Tong PC. Epidemiology of type 2 diabetes. In: Holt RG, Cockram CS, Flyvbjerg A, Goldstein BJ (Eds). Textbook of Diabetes, 4th edition. USA: Wiley-Blackwell—A John Wiley & Sons, Ltd. Publication; 2010. p. 45.

126. Cusick M, Meleth AD, Agrón E, Fisher MR, Reed GF, Knatterud GL, et al.; Early Treatment Diabetic Retinopathy Study Research Group. Associations of mortality and diabetes complications in patients with type 1 and type 2 diabetes: early treatment diabetic retinopathy study report no. 27. *Diabetes Care.* 2005;28:617-25.

127. Sasaki A, Uehara M, Horiuchi N, Hasegawa K, Shimizu T. A 15-year follow-up study of patients with non-insulin dependent diabetes mellitus (NIDDM) in Osaka, Japan. Long-term prognosis and causes of death. *Diabetes Res Clin Pract.* 1996;34:47-55.

128. Mohan V, Shanthirani CS, Deepa M, Deepa R, Unnikrishnan RI, Datta M. Mortality rates due to diabetes in a selected urban south Indian population—the Chennai Urban Population Study [CUPS-16]. *J Assoc Physicians India.* 2006;54:113-7.

129. Zargar AH, Wani AI, Masoodi SR, Bashir MI, Laway BA, Gupta VK, et al. Causes of mortality in diabetes mellitus: data from a tertiary teaching hospital in India. *Postgrad Med J.* 2009;85:227-32.

130. Tchobroutsky G. Relation of diabetic control to development of microvascular complications. *Diabetologia.* 1978;15:143-52.

131. Brinchmann-Hansen O, Dahl-Jorgensen K, Hanssen KF, Sandvik L. The response of diabetic retinopathy to 41 months of multiple insulin injections, insulin pumps, and conventional insulin therapy. *Arch Ophthalmol.* 1988;106:1242-6.

132. The DCCT Research Group. The effect of intensive treatment of diabetes on the development and progression of long-term complications in insulin-dependent diabetes mellitus. *N Engl J Med.* 1993;329:977-86.

133. The DCCT Research Group. Effect of intensive diabetes management on macrovascular events and risk factors in the Diabetes Control and Complication Trial. *Am J Cardiol.* 1995;75:894-903.

134. The DCCT Research Group. The relationship of glycemic exposure (HbA1c) to the risk of development and progression of retinopathy in the Diabetes Control and Complications Trial. *Diabetes.* 1995;44:968-83.

135. United Kingdom Prospective Diabetes Study (UKPDS) Group. Intensive blood-glucose control with sulphonylureas or insulin compared with conventional treatment and risk of complications in patients with type 2 diabetes (UKPDS 33). *Lancet*. 1998;352:837-53.

136. Stratton IM, Adler AI, Neil HA, Matthews DR, Manley SE, Cull CA, et al. Association of glycaemia with macrovascular and microvascular complications of type 2 diabetes (UKPDS 35): prospective observational study. *BMJ*. 2000;321:405-12.

137. The Diabetes Control and Complications Trial (DCCT)/Epidemiology of Diabetes Interventions and Complications (EDIC) Research Group. Effect of intensive therapy on the microvascular complications of type 1 diabetes mellitus. *JAMA*. 2002;287:2563-9.

138. Nathan DM, Cleary PA, Backlund JY, Genuth SM, Lachin JM, Orchard TJ, et al.; Diabetes Control and Complications Trial/Epidemiology of Diabetes Interventions and Complications (DCCT/EDIC) Research Group. Intensive diabetes treatment and cardiovascular disease in patients with type 1 diabetes. *N Engl J Med*. 2005;353:2643-53.

139. Hoerger TJ, Segel JE, Gregg EW, Saaddine JB. Is glycemic control improving in U.S. adults? *Diabetes Care*. 2008;31:81-6.

140. Action to Control Cardiovascular Risk in Diabetes Study Group, Gerstein HC, Miller ME, Byington RP, Goff DC Jr, Bigger JT, Buse JB, et al. Effects of intensive glucose lowering in type 2 diabetes. *N Engl J Med*. 2008; 358:2545-59.

141. ADVANCE Collaborative Group, Patel A, MacMahon S, Chalmers J, Neal B, Billot L, Woodward M, et al. Intensive blood glucose control and vascular outcomes in patients with type 2 diabetes. *N Engl J Med*. 2008;358:2560-72.

142. Duckworth W, Abraira C, Moritz T, Reda D, Emannele N, Reaven PD, et al.; VADT Investigators. Glucose control and vascular complications in veterans with type 2 diabetes. *N Engl J Med*. 2009;360:129-39.

143. Skyler JS, Bergenstal R, Bonow RO, Buse J, Deedwania P, Gale EA, et al; American Diabetes Association; American College of Cardiology Foundation; American Heart Association. Intensive glycemic control and the prevention of cardiovascular events: implications of the ACCORD, ADVANCE, and VA Diabetes Trials: a position statement of the American Diabetes Association and a Scientific Statement of the American College of Cardiology Foundation and the American Heart Association. *J Am Coll Cardiol*. 2009;53:298-304.

144. Inzucchi SE, Bergenstal RM, Buse JB, Diamant M, Ferrannini E, Nauck M, et al. Management of hyperglycaemia in type 2 diabetes: a patient-centered approach. Position statement of the American Diabetes Association (ADA) and the European Association for the Study of Diabetes (EASD). *Diabetologia*. 2012;55:1577-96.

145. Herman WH, Teutsch SM, Geiss LS: The Carter Center of Emory University: closing the gap: the problem of diabetes mellitus in the United States. *Diabetes Care*. 1985; 8:391-406.

146. Tuomilehto J, Lindstrom J, Eriksson JG, et al. Finnish Diabetes Prevention Study Group. Prevention of Type 2 diabetes mellitus by changes in lifestyle among subjects with impaired glucose tolerance. *N Engl J Med*. 2001; 344: 1343-50.

147. Li G, Hu Y, Yang W, et al. Effects of insulin resistance and insulin secretion on the efficacy of interventions to retard development of type 2 diabetes mellitus: the DA Qing IGT and Diabetes Study. *Diabetes Res Clin Pract*. 2002; 58:193 - 200.

148. Knowler WC, Barrett-Connor E, Fowler SE, Hamman RF, Lachin JM, Walker EA, et al.; Diabetes Prevention Program Research Group. Reduction in the incidence of type 2 diabetes with lifestyle intervention or metformin. *N Engl J Med*. 2002;346:393-403.

149. Knowler WC, Hamman RF, Edelstein SL, Barrett-Connor E, Ehrmann DA, Walker EA, et al.; Diabetes Prevention Program Research Group. Prevention of type 2 diabetes with troglitazone in the Diabetes Prevention Program. *Diabetes*. 2005;54:1150-6.

150. Chiasson JL, Josse RG, Gomis R, et al. Acarbose for prevention of type 2 diabetes mellitus: the STOP-NIDDM randomized trial. *Lancet.* 2002;359:2072-7.

151. DREAM (Diabetes REduction Assessment with ramipril and rosiglitazone Medication) Trial Investigators, Gerstein HC, Yusuf S, Bosch J, Pogue J, Sheridan P, Dinccag N, et al. Effect of rosiglitazone on the frequency of diabetes in patients with impaired glucose tolerance or impaired fasting glucose: a randomized controlled trial. *Lancet.* 2006;368:1096-105.

152. DeFronzo RA, Tripathy D, Schwenke DC, Banerji M, Bray GA, Buchanan TA, et al; ACT NOW Study. *N Engl J Med.* 2011;364:1104-15.

153. Ramachandran A, Snehalatha C, Mary S, Mukesh B, Bhaskar AD, Vijay V. The Indian Diabetes Prevention Programme shows that lifestyle modification and metformin prevent type 2 diabetes in Asian Indian subjects with impaired glucose tolerance (IDPP-1). *Diabetologia.* 2006;49:289-97.

154. Kosaka K, Noda M, Kuzuya T. Prevention of type 2 diabetes by lifestyle intervention: a Japanese trial in IGT males. Diabetes Res. *Clin Pract.* 2005;67:152-62.

Management of Diabetes in Primary Care

3

Chapter

Kathleen E Kendle, Jayendra H Shah

ABSTRACT

Connections are crucial to humans. We thrive upon them in countless ways. Chronic disease management is certainly no exception. It is well established that an observed process tends to improve chronic disease management. Management of diabetes is such a process. Patients who are observed in some fashion tend to do better than those who do not. The methods by which we observe diabetics, particularly those not requiring insulin engenders some debate. Cost-effective methods for managing diabetes are elusive given the perpetual emergence of new drugs, each more sophisticated than the last, all with a costly price tag in common. How well do they work, for how long, and at what cost? Complicating matters are the aging baby boomer demographic, the obesity epidemic and the impending shortage of primary care providers. In this chapter, authors review the concept of "Medical Home" in the management of diabetes, importance of patient-physician relationship for adherence of diabetic regimen, use of motivational interview in diabetes management, and overall prevention aspect of this chronic disease.

INTRODUCTION

Connections are crucial to humans. We thrive upon them in countless ways. Chronic disease management is certainly no exception. It is well established that a monitored process tends to improve chronic disease management. Management of diabetes is such a process. Patients who are monitored in some fashion tend to do better than those who do not. The methods by which we monitor diabetics, particularly those not requiring insulin engenders some debate. Cost-effective methods for managing diabetes are elusive given the perpetual emergence of new drugs, each more sophisticated than the last, all with a costly price tag in common. How well do they work, for how long and at what cost? As of 2011, there were 25.8 million persons with diabetes in the United States. The costs for managing diabetes exceeded $174 million in 2007.[1] Complicating matters are the aging baby boomer demographic, the obesity epidemic, and the impending shortage of primary care providers.

Many factors are responsible for metabolic control in the patients with diabetes.[2] However, for the purpose of this chapter, we will review the patients' adherence to diabetic regimens and the patient-physician relationship.

COMPLIANCE AND ADHERENCE

In clinical practice, the term compliance is frequently interchanged for adherence. In their reports, Kurtz[3] and Churkoney and Hart[4] described that majority of diabetic patients are not compliant or adherent to their treatment regimen. They reported that compliance or adherence to all aspect of diabetes care was observed only in a small number of diabetic patients. Also, a great deal of variability has been observed to compliance or adherence in different aspect of diabetes treatment. In diabetic patients, 19–30% variance in compliance or adherence was seen in the exercise program[5,6] where as the compliance and adherence in the frequency and accuracy of taking insulin showed a variance of 20–80%.[4,7] Similarly, a variance in compliance or adherence of 57–70% was seen in self-monitoring of blood glucose (SMBG).[4,8]

In their article, Haynes et al.[9] defined compliance as "the extent to which a person's behavior coincides with medical or health advice". In this context, in diabetic patients, "behavior" means making several lifestyle changes, performing SMBG, adhering to prescribed diet, taking insulin injections, and/or oral medications. The word compliance indicates that patients follow their physicians' instructions. In compliance, the physician defines the patient's conformity to medical goals, whereas the word adherence (as defined by Lutfey and Wishner) "characterizes the patients as independent, intelligent, and autonomous people, who take more active and voluntary roles in defining and pursuing goals for their medical treatment".[10] Alternatively, McNabb defined adherence as "the degree to which a patient follows a predetermined set of behaviors or actions (established cooperatively by the patient and provider) to care for diabetes on a daily basis".[11] Therefore, in order to achieve patient's adherence to diabetic treatment regimens, the patients as well as all health care providers play an equally important role.

PATIENT-PHYSICIAN RELATIONSHIP

In the management of type 2 diabetes, the interaction between the patient and physician is important. Poor communication between the patient and physician may lead to poor patient compliance. Lawler and Viviani[12] reported that when a survey of diabetic patients and their primary care physicians was taken, a significant dissociation was observed between what physicians thought they recommended and what patients understood. In this survey, 95% of physicians reported that they referred their patients to ophthalmologist or optometrist yet only 43% of the patients understood that their primary care physicians recommended referral. Similarly, 78% of physicians reported that they ordered HbA1c test, but only 33% of patients thought that their physicians ordered the test (Table 1).[12]

It is also important to understand geographic, cultural, and economic features of the community in which the patient lives before recommending a diabetic regimen. The access barriers like distance, transportation, and society's beliefs play an important role in the treatment compliance of diabetic patients in the rural community.[13]

The important role of the patient-physician relationship in the adherence to diabetes treatment has been proposed by Ciechanowski and associates.[14] The attachment theory of Bowlby[15] was used by these investigators. Bowlby proposed that patients internalize earlier experiences with their primary care providers and determine whether others, i.e., physicians, can be trusted to provide care (view of others) or they themselves are worthy of care (view of self). Bartholomew and Horowitz described four attachment categories in adults: (1) secure, (2) dismissing, (3) preoccupied, and (4) fearful (Table 2).[14,16]

A dismissing attachment in a diabetic patient had significantly worse glucose control than in diabetic patients with other categories.[14] With a dismissing attachment, these diabetic patients developed a positive view of self and become compulsively self-reliant. Since they developed a negative view of others, they became uncomfortable being close to or trusting others. Those diabetic patients with a dismissing attachment style who rated their patient-physician communication as poor had even significantly higher HbA1c than those who rated their communication as good.[14] Therefore, in

TABLE 1: Physicians' Recommendation and Patients' Perception	
Physicians	**Patients**
SMBG: 98%	SMBG: 73%
HbA1c: 78%	HbA1c: 33%
Frequency of HbA1c (3–12 months): 71%	Frequency of HbA1c (3–12 months): 29%
Referred to eye specialist 95%	Referred to eye specialist 43%

SMBG, self-monitoring of blood glucose.
Source: Adapted from Lawler FH, Viviani N. Patient and physician perspectives regarding treatment of diabetes: compliance with practice guidelines. *J Fam Pract.* 1997;44:369-73.

TABLE 2: Categories of Attachment
• Secure—positive view of self and others
• Dismissing—positive view of self, negative view of others
• Preoccupied—negative view of self, positive view of others (clingy)
• Fearful—negative view of self and others

Source: Adapted from Ciechanowski PS, Katon WJ, Russo JE, Walker EA. The patient-provider relationship: attachment theory and adherence to treatment in diabetes. *Am J Psychiatry.* 2001;158:29-35.

the compliance or adherence of diabetes treatment regimen the patient-physician relationship plays an important role.

MEDICAL HOME CONCEPT IN PRIMARY CARE

If we are to improve outcomes in patients with diabetes, we must find a health care delivery model which leverages resources, improves outcomes while holding down costs. Patient-centered medical home is one health care delivery model poised to deliver on the demands of chronic disease management.

There have, to date, been many number of medical homes developed in a variety of settings throughout American health care.[17] The medical home philosophy is based upon the tenets of access, care coordination, practice redesign, patient activation, and team based care. Medical home encourages the use of technology to proactively identify patients who may require intervention even before they seek it out. The health care delivered in "medical home" concept also known in the VA medical centers as Patient Aligned Care Team (PACT) is provided by a team of individuals. Importantly, the patient is seen as a crucial member of the team. Motivational interviewing and health coaching, described in subsequent sections, prepare the patient for their role. The team is composed of a provider (either a physician or nurse practitioner or physician assistant), nursing staff, a pharmacist, nutritionist, social worker, and a clerical individual. Kathleen Wyne's article entitled "information technology for the treatment of diabetes: improving and controlling costs" reminds us that patients studied in the Diabetes Control and Complications Trial (DCCT) are best treated in a collaborative fashion by a team of health care providers with frequent contacts.[18] All members of the team are trained and willing to maximize their skills to achieve excellent patient care. Internal medicine and family practice trainings will soon incorporate medical home features into their residency programs.

In addition to clinical skills, providers must be proficient in communication and their teams and patients must find them approachable. Providers must be willing to lead or support that team member who emerges as the leader. Providers of medical home primary care will also embrace nontraditional methods of appointments, such as phone visits, group visits, and email. Payer systems must morph to support these changes. Importantly, providers will delegate some task to other team members. Among these tasks are the day-to-day connections made with patients who have diabetes. The nursing elements of the medical home center their activities on coordinating health care for patients, patient education, and problem solving. Medical home practices within the Veterans Health Administration (VHA) have found it useful to develop protocols and scopes of practice that allow nursing staff a variety of abilities. Useful among them is the ability to make alterations to insulin doses based upon fasting and postprandial blood glucose data. Additionally, nursing staff provide comprehensive patient education for insulin starts, basic nutrition, sick day protocol, hyper/hypoglycemia, and basic pathophysiology of diabetes. At one site, nursing staff complete a basic course consisting of 14 hours of didactic material and are paired with a mentor physician. This process allows them to execute the diabetic scope of practice. This allows nursing staff to participate in all-important process of connecting with diabetic patients for providing comprehensive care. While certified diabetes educator (CDE) training is desirable, it is not necessary to assist the diabetic patient in a meaningful way and to promote high quality outcomes in a primary care clinic setting.

The core members of the medical home unit, the teamlet, include a provider, nurse and clerk. They are assisted by other health care members, specifically the clinical pharmacist, dietician, and social worker. The role of the clinical pharmacist, with a scope of practice is to maximally leverage the provider's resources. The management of hypertension, hypercholesterolemia, and diabetes can be taken on by a clinical pharmacist. Data indicate excellent cost-effective outcomes with a disease based pharmacy management.[19] With the assistance of the pharmacist, who is able to manage routine aspects of chronic disease, the provider is freed to manage acute exacerbations of chronic disease or new complaints and processes. This division of primary care means both provider and pharmacist work in collaboration to the top of their efficiencies. This is a common theme among medical homes.

Traditionally, diabetic patients have been seen face to face on a 3-month schedule. This convention likely originated in part because of the physiology of the glycosylated hemoglobin. Components of medical home now allow clinicians to intervene more frequently if needed. Innovations in technology allow practitioners to monitor patients and be proactive about making interventions. Email or secure messaging with patients allows members of the health care team to communicate frequently with patients, inquire about adherence to diet, exercise, and medication regimens. Patients can ask questions and a sense of connectedness is cultivated. Home telehealth and televideo technologies also allow for frequent communication and intervention. Generally, these technologies depend on a device, which requires phone access in some fashion. Patients are queried with a series of questions regarding their health status at a particular interval. Care coordinators then can access this information, look for concerning patterns, and alert a clinician to changes in the patient status. This technology has been shown by Polisena and colleagues to decrease hospitalization rates.[20]

Electronic consult (e-consult) offers another adjunct to the care of diabetic patients. This modality actually can leverage the expertise of the diabetic expert. Practices with integrated electronic medical records such as the VHA can use this technology to improve efficiency for patients and providers. If the consulting primary care provider believes a face-to-face encounter is not required to answer the clinical question, the diabetic consultant can review the chart and make recommendations. The e-consultant may act as a resource to the PACT nurse care coordinators who directly interface with the patients. In this way, PACT nurse care coordinators do not have to be CDE to be effective.

Effective advancements in the care of diabetes can be achieved with the use of computerized diabetes registries (see Chapter: Diabetes Registries). Bu and colleagues published a computer simulation suggesting that over a 10-year period, diabetic registries could save $14.5 billion.[21] In this simulation, registries increased retinopathy screening from a baseline of 14.2 to 61.5%. In addition, glycosylated hemoglobin, total cholesterol and systolic blood pressure all were lowered. Adverse microvascular and macrovascular outcomes decreased. There are a number of registry examples around the country; it is in their systematic regular use that the care of diabetes could be revolutionized. It has also been suggested that adherence to drug and lifestyle regimens will probably have a dramatic impact on diabetes outcomes. As the connection between the medical team and patient improves, a diabetic registry for a medical home team could make a major influence on adherence to diabetes management.

MOTIVATIONAL INTERVIEW

The model of medical home relies, in part, upon an activated patient, to take a lead role in managing their own health care. In this way, the resources of the clinical team are maximally leveraged. Motivational interviewing plays a key role in guiding patients toward positive behavior change. Unlike traditional medical models of delivering medical advice, motivational interviewing seeks to uncover and capitalize on the patient's own priorities and confidence. Motivational interviewing is not an appropriate method for delivering all types of medical advice, particularly that centered around catastrophic results; however, in the context of healthy decisions, it is very helpful. Learning and applying motivational interviewing takes practice and initially may seem like a lengthy endeavor in the setting of a busy primary care practice, however, its results are well worth any initial investment of time.

Motivational interviewing was first described by Miller and Rollnick in 1995 and was described in the context of substance and alcohol abuse counseling.[22] In this model, the primary care provider helps to facilitate positive behavior change. Basic principles of motivational interviewing include respecting the patient's autonomy and lifestyle. The clinician seeks the patient's permission to discuss positive healthy behavior changes regarding the care of their diabetes. Once the patient has given permission, the discussion can begin. The provider is more of a coach and helps the patient discover their own motivation for change and connect with the internal motivation to make such a change. Much of the interaction focuses on keeping the patient talking about behavior change. The conversational exchange should resemble more of a dance than a wrestling match. Providers should avoid mounting resistance to negative comments made by the patient and instead look for ways to keep the conversation going and listen for change talk. In this way, the small seeds of behavior change are cultivated and nurtured to grow by the patient. "It is the patient who should be voicing the arguments for change." All members of the health care team can use concepts of motivational interviewing. Training by a counselor experienced in motivational interviewing is useful as these approaches are counterintuitive to the traditional model of patient education.

NUTRITIONAL SUPPORT

No discussion of primary care management of diabetes would be complete without focusing on the importance of nutritional support. The provider can provide some rudimentary information; however, the team dietician and nurse care coordinator have greater opportunities to delve into the topic in greater depth (see Chapter: Nutritional Care). The need for routine meals at regular intervals consisting of fewer simple carbohydrates and fat will also serve to frame the discussion regarding weight loss and exercise. The intricacies of dietary recommendations will not be discussed here, however, access to clinicians that can provide this expertise is of great importance to the medical team. Similarly, the role of weight loss and exercise in the control and prevention of diabetes is a cornerstone of therapy and the wise activated patient will eventually embrace them. The Finnish Diabetes Prevention Study demonstrated a significant reduction in the incidence of progression to diabetes in patients near 10-pound weight loss which persisted over the 7 years of follow-up.[23]

DEPRESSION AND DIABETES

The identification and treatment of depression will have a substantial impact on diabetic outcomes. A meta-analysis of 27 studies looked at the correlation between depression and diabetic complications. The results showed a significant and consistent association between depression and diabetic complications.[24] The prevalence of depression in adults with diabetes ranges from 8.5% to 27.3%. Patients suffering from diabetes may often lack the confidence and motivation to care for themselves or make positive health behavior changes. Depression has been associated with less adherence to medications and lifestyle recommendations.[24] If depression is unidentified, the provider may find themselves frustrated by the apathy displayed by the depressed patient. For some, the diagnosis and treatment of diabetes will be overwhelming. All primary care patients should be screened with a Patient Health Questionnaire-2 (PHQ-2) or similar instrument at some regular interval.[25] Those who screen positive should be followed with a PHQ-9 administered by a clinician. Those patients who have a positive follow-up screen may benefit from an integrated care approach, which may include medication. Within VHA, much has been done to integrate the treatment of depression into primary care. The primary care provider can begin medication and consult with embedded mental health staff to follow the patient. They in turn will connect with the patient to discuss the importance of medication adherence if applicable, develop a self-care plan and readminister the PHQ-9 at various intervals. If worrisome signs or symptoms develop, the integrated mental health clinician identifies those and works with the primary care provider and mental health expert to devise a plan to address the patient's needs. Once treated, the depressed diabetic patient is ready to take on the responsibility of caring for themselves and their disease.

CONCLUSION

Prevention is a key aspect of the medical home model's approach to diabetes; if not in the prevention of the disease itself, in the prevention of the complications which come as a result of the chronic disease. The clinical team that put forth a concerted coordinated effort to manage hyperlipidemia, hypertension, and other comorbidities will have a significant impact on outcomes for their patients. Approximately 60% of adults with diabetes have high blood pressure. Although reductions in blood pressure can lead to reductions in risk of coronary artery disease and death, we know from the Action to Control Cardiovascular Risk in Diabetes (ACCORD) study that reductions in systolic blood pressure less than 120 mmHg did not reduce outcomes as compared with systolic blood pressures less than 140 mmHg.[26] Control of hyperlipidemia and low-density lipoprotein level of less than 100 is desirable in diabetic patients.[27] Pharmacists and nurses can participate in a meaningful fashion using scopes of practice to manage disease. The pharmacists, using a skills based scope, could use a diabetic registry to identify patients with uncontrolled parameters and plan interventions. Similarly, nursing staff can use the registry in concert with the provider to ensure that all patients are offered standard preventive interventions such as an annual flu and pneumococcal vaccinations, colonoscopy, Pap smear, and mammogram.

REFERENCES

1. Centers for Disease Control and Prevention. (2011). National diabetes fact sheet: national estimates and general information on diabetes and prediabetes in the United States. Atlanta, Georgia.
2. Shah JH, Murata GH, Duckworth WC, Hoffman RM, Wendel CS. Factors affecting compliance in type 2 diabetic patients: experience from diabetes outcomes in veterans study (DOVES). *Int J Diabetes Dev Ctries*. 2003;23:75-82.
3. Kurtz MS. Adherence to diabetic regimens: empirical status and clinical applications. *Diabetes Educ*. 1990;16:50-9.
4. Churkoney KA, Hart LK. The relationship between health belief model and compliance of persons with diabetes mellitus. *Diabetes Care*. 1980;3:594-8.
5. Kravitz RL, Hays RD, Sherbourne CD, DiMatteo MR, Rogers WH, Ordway L, et al. Recall of recommendations and adherence to advice among patients with chronic medical conditions. *Arch Intern Med*. 1993;153:1869-78.
6. Kamiya A, Ohsawa I, Fujii T, Nagai M, Yamanouchi K, Oshida Y, et al. A clinical survey of exercise therapy for diabetic outpatients. *Diabetes Res Clin Pract*. 1995;27:141-5.
7. Watkins JD, Roberts DE, Williams TF, Martin DA, Coyle V. Observation of medication errors made by diabetic patients in the home. *Diabetes*. 1967;16:882-5.
8. Gonder-Frederick LA, Julian DM, Cox DJ, Clarke WL, Carter WR. Self-measurement of blood glucose. Accuracy of self-reported data and adherence to recommended regimen. *Diabetes Care*. 1988;11:579-85.

9. Haynes RB, Taylor WR, Sackett DL. Compliance in Health Care, 1st edition. Baltimore, MD: The Johns Hopkins University Press; 1979.

10. Lutfey KE, Wishner WJ. Beyond "compliance" is adherence. Improving the prospect of diabetes care. *Diabetes Care.* 1999;22:635-9.

11. McNabb WL. Adherence in diabetes: can we define it and can we measure it? *Diabetes Care.* 1997;20:215-8.

12. Lawler FH, Viviani N. Patient and physician perspectives regarding treatment of diabetes: compliance with practice guidelines. *J Fam Pract.* 1997;44:369-73.

13. Srinivas G, Suresh E, Jagadeesan M, Amalraj E, Datta M. Treatment-seeking behavior and compliance of diabetic patients in a rural area of south India. *Ann N Y Acad Sci.* 2002;958:420-4.

14. Ciechanowski PS, Katon WJ, Russo JE, Walker EA. The patient-provider relationship: attachment theory and adherence to treatment in diabetes. *Am J Psychiatry.* 2001;158: 29-35.

15. Bowlby J. Attachment and loss, Vol II: Separation: Anxiety and Anger. New York: Basic Books; 1973.

16. Bartholomew K, Horowitz LM. Attachment styles among young adults: a test of a four-category model. *J Pers Soc Psychol.* 1991;61:226-44.

17. Meyer H. Group Health's move to the medical home: for doctors, it's often a hard journey. Health Aff (Millwood). 2010;29:844-51.

18. Wyne K. Information Technology for the Treatment of Diabetes: Improving Outcomes and Controlling Costs. *J Manag Care Pharm.* 2008;14:S12-7.

19. Johnson KA. The impact of clinical pharmacy services integrated into medical homes on diabetes-related clinical outcomes. *Ann Pharmacother.* 2010;44:1877-86.

20. Polisena J, Tran K, Cimon K, Hutton B, McGill S, Palmer K. Home telehealth for diabetes managment: a systematic review and meta-analysis. *Diabetes Obes Metab.* 2009;11: 913-30.

21. Bu D, Pan E, Walker J, Adler-Milstein J, Kendrick D, Hook JM, et al. Benefits of information technology-enabled diabetes management. *Diabetes Care.* 2007;30:1137-42.

22. Rollnick S, Miller WR. What is motivational interviewing? Behavioural and Cognitive Psychotherapy. 1995;23:325-34.

23. Lindström J, Louheranta A, Mannelin M, Rastas M, Salminen V, Eriksson J, et al. The Finnish Diabetes Prevention Study (DPS): lifestyle intervention and 3-year results on diet and physical activity. *Diabetes Care.* 2003;26:3230-6.

24. Egede LE. Effect of depression on self-management behaviors and health outcomes in adults with type 2 diabetes. *Curr Diabetes Rev.* 2005;1:235-43.

25. O'Connor EA, Whitlock EP, Beil TL, Gaynes BN. Screening for depression in adult patients in a primary care settings: a systematic evidence review. *Ann Intern Med.* 2009;151: 793-803.

26. ACCORD Study Group, Cushman WC, Evans GW, Byington RP, Goff DC, Grimm RH. Effects of intensive blood-pressure control in type 2 diabetes mellitus. *N Engl J Med.* 2010;362:1575-85.

27. National Institutes of Health (NIH), National Heart, Lung, and Blood Institute. (2002). Detection, Evaluation, and Treatment of High Blood Cholesterol in Adults (Adult Treatment Panel III). NIH Publication.

Use of HbA1c in Clinical Practice

Hemraj B Chandalia

ABSTRACT

HbA1c is that fraction of hemoglobin to which glucose has been attached at the amino acid valine of the beta chain. Glucose also gets attached to other amino acids of the hemoglobin, the estimation of which gives total glycated hemoglobin or glycosylated hemoglobin (GHb), but the major site is the amino acid valine. The total GHb is 1.5–2% above HbA1c. HbA1c has been extensively studied and standardized. Hence, for all clinical purposes, currently we confine to HbA1c. The process of glycation of hemoglobin molecule is a post-translational, substrate concentration dependent, irreversible phenomenon. A single sample averages the blood glucose values witnessed by the mixed population of erythrocytes over their life span, thus faithfully reflecting the glycemic status for the past 2–3 months. This chapter describes the methods of HbA1c determination, its relationship to plasma glucose, and its use in the clinical practice.

WHAT IS HBA1C?

HbA1c is that fraction of hemoglobin to which glucose has been attached at the amino acid valine of the beta chain. Glucose also gets attached to other amino acids of the hemoglobin, the estimation of which gives total glycated hemoglobin or glycosylated hemoglobin (GHb), but the major site is the amino acid valine. The total GHb is 1.5-2% above HbA1c. HbA1c has been extensively studied and standardized. Hence, for all clinical purposes, currently we confine to HbA1c. The process of glycation of hemoglobin molecule is a post-translational, substrate concentration dependent, irreversible phenomenon. A single sample averages the blood glucose values witnessed by the mixed population of erythrocytes over their life span, thus faithfully reflecting the glycemic status for the past 2-3 months.[1]

METHODS TO ESTIMATE HBA1C

HbA1c moves faster in the electrophoretic systems than HbA_0 (non-glycated adult hemoglobin), hence it can be estimated by its electrophoretic mobility. HbA1c also has a different ionic change, which makes its separation possible on cationic resins. The boronic acid affinity method employs the structural characteristics to measure HbA1c. HbA1c has stronger affinity to boronic acid; hence it elutes later than HbA_0. Lastly, immunological methods can be employed to estimate HbA1c. These assays use monoclonal antibodies to HbA1c and an agglutinator, measuring the inhibition of HbA1c antibody agglutination by the HbA1c present in the sample.

All these methods have been made traceable to the National Glycohemoglobin Standardization Program (NGSP). The same methods were used in large studies, like the Diabetes Control and Complications Trial (DCCT) and the UK Prospective Diabetes Study (UKPDS). More recently, the International Federation of Clinical Chemistry (IFCC) has isolated HbA1c in its pure form. This is achieved by an enzymatic cleavage of the β-N-terminal hexapeptides of HbA1c and HbA and their separation and quantitation.[2]

The initial process of glycation results in an unstable compound called Schiff base or preglycohemoglobin which can either dissociate or by Amadori rearrangement convert into a stable ketamine. Preglycohemoglobin, a transitory product reflects recent glycemic events and has similar electrophoretic mobility as GHb and thus cannot be separated from the glycohemoglobin in electrophoretic systems. A process of saline incubation removes preglycohemoglobin. IFCC demonstrated that actual HbA1c is 1.5–2% lower than that obtained from NGSP methods. Most equipments currently in use to estimate HbA1c are now standardized to IFCC standard, but report NGSP values. To avoid confusion, presently NGSP values should be used for clinical purposes. As the IFCC values are lower, their use has resulted in complacency in patients and subsequent deterioration of metabolic control.[3] As the relationship of ambient blood glucose to HbA1c is more firmly established by recent studies, it may be possible to transform all data to mean blood glucose (MBG). As most patients and clinicians are tuned to NGSP values, it is recommended that these continue to be used in the near future. Interconversion of these parameters is possible (Table 1).[4] HbA1c is often expressed in HbA1c reports as MBG. IFCC has further proposed that HbA1c values be expressed in mmol of GHb per mol of unglycated component (Table 2).[5]

TABLE 1: Interconversion of MBG and HbA1c	
1	MBG (mmol/L) = 1.84 × IFCC.HbA1c
	MBG (mmol/L) = 1.98 × DCCT (NGSP).HbA1c - 4.29
2	NGSP.HbA1c = 0.915 (IFCC.HbA1c) + 2.15%
3	IFCC.HbA1c (mmol/mol) = [DCCT.HbA1c (%) - 2.15] × 10.929

MBG, mean blood glucose; IFCC, the International Federation of Clinical Chemistry; NGSP, the National Glycohemoglobin Standardization Program; DCCT, the Diabetes Control and Complications Trial.

TABLE 2: Relationship of HbA1c with Mean Plasma Glucose		
	Mean plasma glucose	
A1c (%)	mg/dL	mmol/L
6	126	7.0
7	154	8.6
8	183	10.2
9	212	11.8
10	240	13.4
11	269	14.9
12	298	16.5

Source: American Diabetes Association. *Diabetes Care.* 2011;34(suppl):S18.

CLINICAL USE OF HBA1C

HbA1c is now considered a gold standard for determining the long-term glycemic control. It is essential to employ this parameter in long-term clinical follow-up and research studies.

There are numerous advantages of employing this parameter. It can be estimated during anytime of day, regardless of the meal timings. It is not influenced by any recent events, like the meal just prior to reporting for the test or previous 2–3 days. Discrepancies between GHb and blood glucose values reported by patients are expected, as self-monitoring of blood glucose (SMBG) may not be an accurate procedure and falsification of data is possible by patients. GHb and blood glucose values were measured in 4,203 patients and interpreted in a study as indicative of good, fair and poor control.[1] The interpretation by these 2 parameters was in agreement in 51.3%, one-step different (e.g., good by one method, showing fair by other method) in 43% and 2-step different (e.g., good by one method, showing poor by other method) in 5.7% of patients. In 63% of patients showing discrepant values, GHb showed poorer control than postprandial blood glucose values, thus indicating that a large number of patients diet a little better on the day of testing to produce better blood glucose values. This brings out the importance of GHb as a non-manipulable and reliable parameter in assessing metabolic control as compared to SMBG or one-point blood glucose estimation.

Initially, it was thought that a single HbA1c value reflects the glycemic control of the past 3 months. However, further studies have shown that the glycemia in the past 1 month contributes 50%, past 2 months 90%, and past 3 months 100% toward the HbA1c value. Thus, it primarily reflects the metabolic control over the past 2 months.[6] Dissipation rate of an elevated HbA1c value has been calculated.[7] In a group of type 2 diabetics, the blood glucose levels were lowered steadily. In these patients, it was found that GHb declined at 2, 4, 6, 8, and 10 weeks by 1%, 0.7%, 0.5%, 0.5%, and 0.1%, respectively. If hyperglycemia is controlled predictably and consistently, the drop in HbA1c is quite significant even in a month's time. Hence, in many such clinical situations, a 1-month follow-up HbA1c estimation is justified.

It has been clearly demonstrated that HbA1c reflects the MBG. It has been questioned whether fasting or prandial blood glucose finds predominant expression in the HbA1c value. Whenever there is global hyperglycemia, the HbA1c values are very high, for example, in the range of 10–12%. When glycemic control is achieved and fasting blood glucose is controlled, the HbA1c drops to about 8%. At that point, the postprandial blood glucose continues to be high. Currently, most clinics are making a serious effort to move the average HbA1c of the clinic population from about 8–8.5% down to 6.5–7%. This process entails addressing the issue of prandial hyperglycemia.[8]

Although HbA1c faithfully reflects the MBG, it does not give any insight into glycemic excursions.[9] Thus, 2 very dissimilar blood glucose profiles obtained by continuous glucose monitoring system (CGMS) may produce same HbA1c values. It is important clinically to identify these glycemic excursions, because endothelial damage and oxidative processes may be accelerated by these short-term prandial peaks. These facts bring out the complementarities of HbA1c estimation, SMBG, and CGMS.

HBA1C TARGETS

The long-term vascular complications correlate closely with the HbA1c values. In the DCCT study, the HbA1c was about 2% lower in the intensively treated group versus the conventionally treated group. In the UKPDS, the difference between the HbA1c values of the standard and intensively treated group was 1%. In these studies, the incidence of renal, retinal, and peripheral nerve disease was lowered significantly. This was more evident for microvascular disease than macrovascular disease. It is estimated from the DCCT data that 1% lowering of HbA1c translates into 30% reduction of microvascular complications and neuropathy.[10]

In the UKPDS,[11] 1% lowering of HbA1c in the intensive policy group as compared to the conventional policy group resulted in 35% reduction in microvascular complications and 16% reduction in the incidence of myocardial infarction.

Most investigators suggest an HbA1c target of less than 7% to be achieved in most diabetics. However, there is a need for individualizing the targets. Overall, targets can be lower in type 2 diabetes mellitus (DM), especially in the first 2–5 years of the disease. At that stage, it is easier to achieve these targets without producing hypoglycemia. Strategically, it is more important to achieve stricter metabolic control during the early years of diabetes as compared to the later years. It has been shown in the follow-up studies of both UKPDS and DCCT that the metabolic memory of early good control reflects favorably in the long-term outcomes.[12,13] In a long-standing type 2 diabetic with vascular complications, however, the targets should be somewhat relaxed. Speedy control of their diabetes and pushing them toward lower targets of less

TABLE 3: HbA1c Targets		
Type 2 DM	Initial 2–5 years of disease	<6.5%
	5–10 years of disease	<7%
	> 10 years of disease with cardiovascular, renal, retinal, neurological complications	<7.5%
Type 1 DM	With standard insulin therapy	<7.5%
	With intensified insulin therapy or insulin pump therapy	<7%
Pregnancy	Gestational DM	<6%
	Pregestational type 2 DM	<6.5%
	Type 1 DM	<7%

than 6% HbA1c can worsen the outcomes. This was amply demonstrated in several studies.[14-16] However, carefully addressing the comorbid conditions and controlling glycemia slowly produce improved outcomes.[17] The key message is to control as strictly as possible, without producing significant hypoglycemia (Table 3). Currently, only 30–35% of diabetics achieve HbA1c goals in most centers round the world.

In type 1 DM, the achievable targets of HbA1c even with multiple doses basal-bolus insulin regimens are about 7–7.5%. With the use of insulin pump therapy, it may be possible to achieve targets below 7% in type 1 DM.

The targets are stricter in pregnancy with diabetes. It is advisable to set targets about 1.5% lower than those recommended in the non-pregnant state. The ambient blood glucose is low in non-diabetic pregnant women. Hence, lower targets are advised. There are several other factors modifying the HbA1c value in pregnancy, e.g., iron deficiency and altered erythrokinetics. Not withstanding these facts, a value of HbA1c less than 6% is achievable in gestational diabetes, less than 6.5% in type 2 DM with pregnancy and less than 7% in type 1 DM with pregnancy. In the last instance, the target may only be achieved by the use of an insulin pump. It is advisable to estimate HbA1c every month in pregnant diabetic because the glycemic control is closely related to macrosomia and fetal outcomes and as discussed above upto 50% of HbA1c value is determined by the previous 1 month of glycemia.

HBA1C IN RENAL DISEASE

The HbA1c value seen in chronic renal failure is a resultant of several opposing factors; altered erythrocyte survival, concomitant iron and erythropoietin deficiency, and the presence of carbamylated hemoglobin which electrophoretically demonstrates similar properties as HbA1c. However, most modern HbA1c methods, mainly the high-performance liquid chromatography (HPLC) and boronic acid affinity methods, are not vitiated by the presence of carbamylated hemoglobin.

HBA1C IN HEMOGLOBINOPATHIES

Hemoglobinopathies are highly rampant in most populations. A few important and frequent ones are thalassemia and sickle-cell disease. The prevalence and type of hemoglobinopathies in one population is different from that in other. Hemoglobinopathies alter the HbA1c by several mechanisms: altered erythrokinetics and altered electrophoretic mobility. For this reason, reference A1c values in any population need to be established. In hemolytic anemia, without diabetes, an estimation of HbA1c may be used to estimate the severity of the hemolytic process.[7]

GENETIC FACTORS DETERMINING HBA1C VALUES

It has been postulated that the rate of glycation may exhibit genetic polymorphism.[18] Although this has been described, its rarity makes it an unimportant issue. More important factor may be genetic variability in erythrokinetics. This may alter the reference range in a given population and hence, requires to be studied further.

USE OF HBA1C IN DIAGNOSIS OF DIABETES

Use of HbA1c in the diagnosis of diabetes was examined long ago,[19] with the conclusion that the sensitivity is fair and specificity is good. More recently, this issue has been examined afresh, with similar conclusions. A value of less than 6.1% is considered normal; 6.1–6.5% indicative of impaired glucose tolerance and greater than 6.5% diagnostic of diabetes.[20]

It has been argued that use of HbA1c in the diagnosis of diabetes has certain advantages over the use of fasting blood glucose (FBG) or oral glucose tolerance test (OGTT) (Table 4). The coefficient of variation (CV) of HbA1c assay has narrowed down considerably over the years, partly due to the efforts of NGSP and more recently, participation of IFCC. In many countries, the CV of HbA1c assay is less than or equal to 2%. This test does not require preparation of the patient. The sample is stable, thus minimizing pre-analytical errors. Hence, it appears highly suited for epidemiological purposes in field practice. On the other hand, the blood glucose estimation methods have come under close scrutiny. A large pre-analytical error is possible because of rapid glycolysis at room temperature even in a sample collected

TABLE 4: Use of HbA1c in the Diagnosis of Diabetes	
Advantages	• Patient preparation not required
	• Stable sample; minimum preanalytical error
	• Coefficient of variation (CV) ≤2%
	• Specificity 90%
Disadvantages	• Expensive
	• Sensitivity (60%); less than oral glucose tolerance test (OGTT)

in the fluoride tube. The CV of estimation is also described to be 5–10%. The postglucose blood glucose requires additional time to conduct the test. For these reasons, the HbA1c has received great attention in diagnosing diabetes. However, the cost of HbA1c estimation is higher than that of blood glucose estimation. The points of care method have not demonstrated enough accuracy to be adopted for diagnosis. In the ultimate analysis, the use of HbA1c for diagnostic purposes needs to be further examined.

REFERENCES

1. Chandalia HB. Monitoring glycemic control: long-term parameters. In: Tripathy BB, Chandalia HB, Das AK, Rao PV, Madhu SV, Mohan V, (Eds). RSSDI Textbook of Diabetes Mellitus, 2nd edition. New Delhi: Jaypee Brothers Medical Publishers (P) Ltd; 2012. pp. 587-93.
2. Kobold U, Jeppsson JO, Dülffer T, Finke A, Hoelzel W, Miedema K. Candidate reference methods for hemoglobin A1c based on peptide mapping. *Clin Chem.* 1997;43:1944-51.
3. Hoelzel W, Weykamp C, Jeppsson JO, Miedema K, Barr JR, Goodall I, et al. IFCC reference system for measurement of hemoglobin A1c in human blood and the national standardization schemes in the United states, Japan, and Sweden: a method-comparison study. *Clin Chem.* 2004;50:166-74.
4. Chandalia HB. Standardization of hemoglobin A1c. *Int J Diab Dev Ctries.* 2010;30:109-10.
5. Goldstein DE, Little RR, Lorenz RA, Malone JI, Nathan D, Peterson CM, et al. Tests of glycemia in diabetes. *Diabetes Care.* 2004;27:1761-73.
6. Tahara Y, Shima K. Kinetics of HbA1c, glycated albumin, and fructosamine and analysis of their weight functions against preceding plasma glucose level. *Diabetes Care.* 1995;18: 440-7.
7. Chandalia HB, krishnaswamy PR. Glycated hemoglobin. *Curr Sci.* 2002;83:1522-32.
8. Monnier L, Lapinski H, Colette C. Contributions of fasting and postprandial plasma glucose increments to the overall diurnal hyperglycemia of type 2 diabetic patients: variations with increasing levels of HbA(1c). *Diabetes Care.* 2003;26:881-5.
9. Derr R, Garrett E, Stacy GA, Saudek CD. Is HbA(1c) affected by glycemic instability? *Diabetes Care.* 2003;26:2728-33.
10. The Diabetes Control and Complications Trails Research Group. The effect of intensive treatment of diabetes on the development and progression of long-term complications in insulin-dependent diabetes mellitus. *N Engl J Med.* 1993;329:977-1036.
11. UK Prospective Diabetes Study (UKPDS) Group. Intensive blood-glucose contol with sulphonylureas or insulin compared with conventional treatment and risk of complications in patients with type 2 Diabetes (UKPDS 33). *Lancet.* 1998;352:837-53.
12. Epidemiology of Diabetes Intervention and Complications (EDIC). Design, implementation, and preliminary results of a long-term follow-up of the Diabetes Control and Complications Trial cohort. *Diabetes Care.* 1999;22:99-111.
13. Holman RR, Paul SK, Bethel MA, Matthews DR, Neil HA. 10-year follow-up of intensive glucose control in type 2 diabetes. *N Engl J Med.* 2008;359:1577-89.
14. ADVANCE Collaborative Group, Patel A, MacMahon S, Chalmers J, Neal B, Billot L, et al. Intensive blood glucose control and vascular outcomes in patients with type 2 diabetes. *N Engl J Med.* 2008;358:2560-72.

15. The ACCORD Study Group, Cushman WC, Evans GW, Byington RP, Goff DC, Grimm RH, et al. Effects of intensive blood-pressure control in type2 diabetes mellitus. *N Engl J Med*. 2010;362:1575-85.

16. Duckworth W, Abraira C, Moritz T, Reda D, Emanuele N, Reaven PD, et al. Glucose control and vascular complications in veterans with type 2 diabetes. *N Engl J Med*. 2009;360: 129-39.

17. Gaede P, Lund-Andersen H, Parving HH, Pedersen O. Effect of a multifactorial intervention on mortality in type 2 diabetes. *N Engl J Med*. 2008;358:580-91.

18. Gloria-Bottini F, Antonacci E, Cozzoli E, De Acetis C, Bottini E. The effect of genetic variability on the correlation between blood glucose and glycated hemoglobin levels. *Metabolism*. 2011;60:250-5.

19. Chandalia HB, Khera S, Bhargav A. Use of glycosylated hemoglobin in diagnosis of diabetes. *Diabetes Research and Clinical Practice*. 1982;Suppl 1:S93.

20. Rohlfing CL, Little RR, Wiedmeyer HM, England JD, Madsen R, Harris MI, et al. Use of GHb (HbA1c) in screening for undiagnosed diabetes in the US population. *Diabetes Care*. 2000;23:187-91.

Self-monitoring of Blood Glucose

5

Chapter

Jayendra H Shah

ABSTRACT

This chapter discusses how self-monitoring of blood glucose (SMBG) is a hallmark in the glycemic management of type 1, insulin requiring type 2, and pregnant diabetic patients. It describes that although controversies exists concerning benefits of SMBG in the management of non-insulin requiring diabetic patients, recent studies have shown clear improvement in the glycemic control and argued for preventing long-term complication of diabetes and ultimately improved quality of life. The author reasons that once patients and providers agree on the benefits of SMBG then the monitoring will help in overall glycemic management and health care outcome of diabetes. Evidence suggests that structured SMBG, and incorporating its finding into day-to-day management of diabetes, improves glycemic control. The chapter further outlines how parsimonious approach in the use of strips for SMBG will decrease undue patient suffering and financial burden for the patients, health care institutions, and insurance providers. The author strongly makes a case that "cookbook" approaches to any diabetes management regimen often are unworkable as each patient's ethnicity, his/her glycemic state, comorbidities, and other circumstances are unique. A generalized guideline is described in the chapter so appropriate modification can be made to tailor unique management regimen for a specific patient.

INTRODUCTION

Glycemic control of diabetes is important in preventing complication of diabetes. It is generally agreed that microvascular complications (retinopathy, nephropathy, and neuropathy) can be prevented or delayed if blood glucose levels are kept near normal levels.[1-3] Although a controversy exists whether "tight" glycemic control can prevent or delay macrovascular complications, several organizations have recommended optimum glycemic control, a glycohemoglobin (HbA1c) level below 7.0% [American

Diabetes Association (ADA), American Association of Clinical Endocrinologists (AACE), and Normoglycemia in Intensive Care Evaluation (NICE)].[4-6] Self-monitoring of blood glucose (SMBG) is essential in achieving the optimum glycemic control. Therefore, SMBG has become routine in day-to-day management of patients with type 1 diabetes, insulin-requiring type 2 diabetes and diabetes during pregnancy. The SMBG in noninsulin-treated diabetic patient remains controversial. The benefits of SMBG in patients treated with oral hypoglycemic agents (OHAs) have been debated and are not clearly established.[7-10] However, majority of cross-sectional studies are inadequately powered and failed to control for severity of disease, did not provide treatment options or overtly against SMBG. In contrast, best designed studies show a strong positive correlation between intensity of SMBG and glycemic control.[11,12] These studies showed that if the analysis of data failed to adjust for the risk factors for poor glycemic control then benefits of SMBG would be missed. It is evident that some of the risk factors for poor glycemic control can be controlled with pharmacologic treatment and SMBG, the other factors such as patient's attitude, unhealthy behaviors and comorbid conditions are difficult to control.

The ADA in their guideline has recommended that all insulin-treated diabetic patients should perform SMBG and in patients treated with OHA it is desirable to perform SMBG. The guideline has not been specific about optimal frequency of SMBG but it was recommended that it should be sufficient to reach the desired glycemic goals.[4] Despite benefits of SMBG in insulin-treated diabetic patients, there remains reluctance by providers for rationally prescribing SMBG and by patients in performing SMBG. In a survey by Harris et al., only less than 10% of the diabetic patients were performing SMBG two or more times and 39% of the patients performed SMBG once a day.[13] There is also controversy whether SMBG is effective. Some studies show minimal beneficial effect of SMBG whereas others have shown clear evidence of the effectiveness of SMBG.[8,14-20] On patients perspective, SMBG appears to be one of the most demanding aspect of self-care as it creates pain, anxiety and frustration. It also causes disruption of daily routine and significant out-of-pocket expense. Furthermore, SMBG readings are often ignored by busy physicians. Internationally, the cost of strips used for SMBG out numbers the cost of OHA and insulin treatment. However, if one assumes that SMBG helps better glycemic control and prevents such complications as blindness, end-stage renal disease, and amputation, then front-end monitoring cost may be justified.

FUNCTIONS OF MONITORING

Once both physician and patient see benefit of SMBG, then the monitoring creates a positive influence in health management. It involves patients in refocusing on their health care, empowering them and shifting the locus of control on self. SMBG alerts the patients of hypo- and hyperglycemia and the need for medical assistance. It also provides them the immediate feedback for change in lifestyle. SMBG also provides patients with reassurance and reinforcement when the SMBG values are acceptable. For physicians, SMBG can be used for the diagnosis of hyper- or hypoglycemia and only way to tract the acute changes in clinical status. The physician can diagnose and correlate patient's symptoms and measure patient's adherence to the treatment plan. Using SMBG readings, physicians can evaluate effects of diet and exercise recommendations as well as titrate doses of insulin and OHA. Although SMBG was developed for screening, diagnosing, and tracking the status of diabetes, it is only evaluated for its therapeutic effect. This is akin to examining an ability of hematocrit measurement to treat anemia!

SMBG AND PREDICTING HYPERGLYCEMIA, HYPOGLYCEMIA, AND GLYCEMIC CONTROL

One can question whether SMBG is beneficial in type 2 diabetic patient and whether it can accurately assess glycemic control that leads to improved health care outcomes.[21] We feel that SMBG is effective when it targets a specific pathophysiologic process in diabetes and is linked to structured intervention. The SMBG is the only way of acutely identifying when patient is hyperglycemic, confirming that patient's hypoglycemic symptoms are indeed due to low blood glucose levels and to forecast the risk of hypoglycemia.

We evaluated usefulness of SMBG in several Diabetes Outcomes in Veterans Studies (DOVES).[22-26] One of these observational studies evaluated the usefulness of SMBG in predicting hyperglycemia, hypoglycemia, and glycemic control in type 2 diabetic patients treated with insulin.[22,23] The patients were selected randomly from 3 different hospitals. The patients were required to participate in a monitoring period of 8 weeks where they performed 4 times a day SMBG; before breakfast, lunch and dinner and at bedtime. We measured HbA1c at baseline and 4, 8, 26, 39, and 52 weeks interval. The glucose meters, provided by the study, were downloaded for glucose data at 4- and 8-week interval.

We defined the compliance for SMBG as number of SMBG performed divided by number of SMBG determination requested. Overall compliance was high in the study of patients for first 6 weeks and started to decline during 7–8 weeks. The compliance was inversely correlated to week 8 HbA1c.[22]

There was a good linear correlation was observed between week 8 HbA1c and mean SMBG blood glucose during 8 weeks. Several studies[27-30] have also observed similar excellent correlation between glucose monitoring and HbA1c (Table 1). Severe hyperglycemia, as defined as monitored blood glucose greater than 400 mg/dL (>22.2 mmol/L) was observed in 1% of all SMBG samples and occurred at least in 43% of patients during 8 weeks of observation period. Moderate hyperglycemia, defined as monitored blood glucose value greater than 200 mg/dL (>11.1 mmol/L) but less than 400 mg/dL (22.2 mmol/L) was observed in 30% SMBG samples and occurred at least once in the 99% of the patients during the 8 weeks of observation period.

TABLE 1: Correlation Between Average Daily Blood Glucose During SMBG and HbA1c				
Author (Reference)	Year	Method	Number of samples	Coefficient
Paisey[27]	1980	Capillary	7–8	0.93
Svendsen[28]	1982	Capillary	7	0.98
Rohlfing[29]	2002	Capillary	7	0.82
Bonora[30]	2002	SMBG	6	0.69
Shah[22]	2003	SMBG	4	0.79

SMBG, self-monitoring of blood glucose; HbA1c, glycosylated hemoglobin.

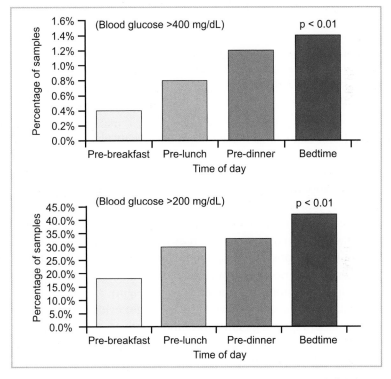

FIGURE 1 Risk of hyperglycemic events. Hyperglycemic events as defined as moderate hyperglycemia, blood glucose levels between 200 mg/dL (11.1 mmol/L) and 400 mg/dL (22.2 mmol/L) and severe hyperglycemia, blood glucose level more than 400 mg/dL (22.2 mmol/L) in type 2 insulin-treated diabetic patients who performed SMBG four times a day. The hyperglycemic events were more common during bedtime and predinner SMBG.

Hyperglycemia at both levels (>200 mg/dL and >400 mg/dL; 11.1 mmol/L and 22.2 mmol/L) were most common at bedtime (Figure 1). Hypoglycemia defined as monitored blood glucose less than 60 mg/dL (3.3 mmol/L) was observed in 1.7% of all SMBG samples and occurred at least once in 53% of patients during 8 weeks of

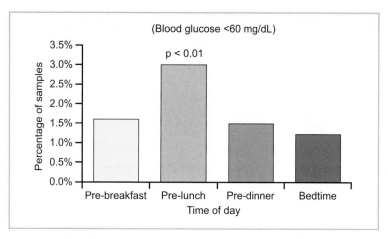

(Blood glucose <60 mg/dL)

FIGURE 2 Risk of hypoglycemic events. Hypoglycemic events as defined as blood glucose levels less than 60 mg/dL (3.3 mmol/L) in type 2 insulin-treated diabetic patients who performed SMBG four times a day. The hypoglycemic events were more common during prelunch SMBG.

observation period. Frequently the patients were unaware of hypoglycemia. Although hypoglycemia was observed during all four determination of SMBG, it was most common before lunch SMBG determination (Figure 2).

The study patients were treated with insulin for an average of 8 years, received insulin twice a day and were stable on insulin regimen for at least 2 months prior to enrolling in the study. During the observation period no changes in the insulin doses were made nor was a change in diet or exercise advised. Also, all patients maintained same weight during the observation period. Despite no changes in these variables HbA1c levels significantly declined from baseline value at 4 and 8 weeks and remained at significantly low level from baseline at 52 week (Figure 3). The exact explanation for this interesting benefit of intensive SMBG was not evident. We speculated that immediate feedback of intensive SMBG prompted patients to alter the carbohydrate content of their diet, thus improving their glycemic control. Such beneficial effect of intensive SMBG has been also observed by other investigators.[31]

From this study, we concluded that in insulin-treated type 2 diabetic patients: (1) higher the compliance in performing intensive SMBG, lower the HbA1c, i.e. better glycemic control; (2) a beneficial effect on glycemic control was observed during intensive SMBG period. This beneficial effect lasted for a longer time after discontinuation of the intensive SMBG; (3) hyperglycemia is most commonly observed at bedtime in patients taking insulin twice a day, whereas occurrence of hypoglycemia was most common before lunch. These SMBG observations may lead clinicians to alter the insulin treatment in such a way to decrease occurrence of hyperglycemia and hypoglycemia to improve glycemic control. Similar to our observation, an observation study performed in 31,000 patients at the Kaiser Permanente Group in

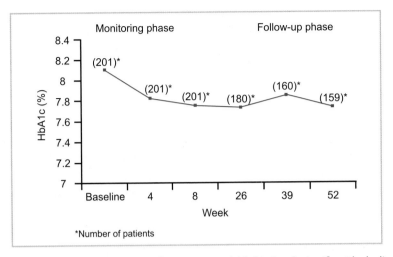

FIGURE 3 Effect of intensive SMBG on glycemic control. HbA1c levels significantly declined from baseline value at 4 and 8 weeks (monitoring phase) and remained at significantly low level from baseline at the 52 week (end of observation phase). The number of patients followed at the time period is depicted in the parentheses.

Northern California also demonstrated the benefits of SMBG.[12] This study observed that regardless of treatment with OHAs or insulin, SMBG improved glycemic control in dose response manner when multivariate adjusted analysis was used. In our another observational study of 2,572 patients with type 2 diabetes, who received glucose meter monitoring strips, on OHAs and/or insulin were followed for 2 years to determine the benefits of SMBG.[11] The study found that in stable patients as well as those required treatment intensification, SMBG was inversely associate with glycemic control (more use of SMBG, lower the HbA1c). The SMBG effect was more pronounced on the patient with poor glycemic control. The study estimated that effect of SMBG on glycemic control (HbA1c) was comparable to that observed with either OHAs or insulin therapy.

RANDOMIZED TRIALS TO ESTABLISH BENEFITS OF SMBG

The observational studies have some limitations as they have been performed in certain groups of patients, for example, patients of significantly older age and with multitude of comorbidities. It is also possible that patients who monitor their blood glucose more frequently have healthy behaviors. Therefore, it is difficult to definitely prove with the observational studies that SMBG improves glycemic control or determine specific mechanism by which SMBG exerts its effect. Nevertheless, the observational studies showing beneficial effect of SMBG[11,12,19,22-26] and meta-analysis of some randomized trials[9,10] lead to the need for a well-designed prospective multicenter randomized trial to establish the cause effect relationship between the SMBG and glycemic control, if risk factors are reasonably controlled.

We recently conducted a randomized controlled study to evaluate the effect of structured SMBG on glycemic control.[32] In this study, we focused on the health care providers instead of patients to drive the glycemic control using targeted SMBG (instead of random SMBG used in previous studies). The intervention was done by specific treatment algorithms using oral agents or insulin preparations. The study was open label randomized trial carried out at three medical centers. Intervention and control patients were stable with their HbA1c above 7.5%. The providers were randomized as either interventional group or control group. The control provider's patients performed SMBG ad libitum and they were provided routine care as before. Intervention provider's patients performed SMBG seven times daily (before and 2 hours after breakfast, lunch, dinner, and at bedtime) for 3 days prior to visit with their providers. Interventional providers were free to choose their treatment and also educated for various algorithms for treatment. Targeted fasting and postprandial glucose excursions were used to arrive at specific algorithms of long acting and fast acting insulin, or intermediate acting insulin plus regular insulin or combination of OHAs. The structured SMBG was used to guide the treatment as well as minimize the hypoglycemic events. Initial data in 36 interventional and 30 control patients showed no differences in mean age, baseline HbA1c, sex, ethnicity, number of OHAs used, and total units of insulin used. At 3 months, standard group showed slight (0.2%) and insignificant (p = 0.21) decline in the HbA1c. In contrast, the interventional group showed a 1.0%, a significant (p < 0.0001) decline in HbA1c from baseline. Seven hypoglycemic events in the standard group were significantly (p = 0.02) higher than two hypoglycemic events observed in the intervention group. Thus, structured SMBG with standard treatment orders were associated with rapid improvement in the glycemic control in insulin-treated type 2 diabetic patients. The intensive treatment with structured SMBG decreased the risk of hypoglycemia during first 3 months of intervention.

McIntosh et al. did a systematic review and meta-analysis of benefits of SMBG performed by diabetic patients managed without insulin treatment.[33] They observed small but significant improvement in glycemic control in these patients. However, this improvement was not associated with any lifestyle changes or with improvement in quality of life. Recently, in poorly controlled, noninsulin-treated type 2 diabetic patients, a structured SMBG significantly reduced HbA1c levels.[31] In this prospective cluster-randomized multicenter study, the structured testing group performed seven-point SMBG over three consecutive days, with an end point to assess HbA1c at the end of 12 months. They concluded that the structured use of SMBG significantly improved glycemic control and general well-being in noninsulin-treated type 2 diabetic patients. Those patients who became nonadherent in performing SMBG at the end of the study, the significant improvement in the HbA1c was lost.

BURDEN OF SMBG

Certainly, inconvenience, pain, and suffering of performing SMBG are significant burden for diabetic patients. But the out-of-pocket cost for the glucose strips needed for SMBG surpasses all burdens of this task to the patients with diabetes. At times, the cost for SMBG may become more than the cost for pharmacologic treatment of diabetes. The SMBG can also create significant financial drain on the health care institutions that are required to provide glucose meter strips to their patients and the insurance payers alike. The studies have found that SMBG in noninsulin-treated type 2 diabetic patients is associated with no significant differences in outcomes, higher cost of treatment and lower quality of life.[34] Such studies have found SMBG to be not cost effective in the management of non-insulin-treated diabetic patient. However, such a contention is challenged by others stating improved glycemic control in these patients ultimately leads to decreased complications thus decreasing the health care cost and in fact improved quality of life.[31,35-37]

CONCLUSION AND RECOMMENDATIONS

SMBG is hallmark in the glycemic management of type 1, insulin-requiring type 2 and pregnant diabetic patients. Although controversies exist concerning benefits of SMBG in the management of noninsulin-requiring diabetic patients, recent studies have shown clear improvement in the glycemic control and argued for preventing long-term complication of diabetes and ultimately improved quality of life. Once patients and providers agree on the benefits of SMBG then the monitoring will help in overall glycemic management and health care outcome of diabetes. Evidence suggests that structured SMBG, and incorporating its finding into day-to-day management of diabetes, improves glycemic control. A parsimonious approach in the use of strips for SMBG will decrease undue patient suffering and financial burden for the patients, health care institutions and insurance providers.

We strongly feel that a "cookbook" approach to any diabetes management regimen often is unworkable as each patient's ethnicity, his/her glycemic state, comorbidities, and other circumstances are unique. A generalized guideline is described so appropriate modification can be made to tailor unique management regimen for a specific patient. We recommend that during uncontrolled glycemic state of diabetes (HbA1c above 7.0%) staggering pre- and 2-hour postmeal SMBG for 1–2 weeks prior to patient's visit to physician can provide assessment of patient's glycemic state at various time of the day to logically choose and/or alter nutritional and pharmacologic treatment to achieve targeted glycemic control. For example, during uncontrolled glycemic state a patient may be asked to do SMBG before and 2 hours after breakfast on Monday and Thursday, before and 2 hours after lunch on Tuesday and Friday, before and 2 hours after dinner on Wednesday and Saturday and fasting and at bedtime SMBG on Sunday. Since this parsimonious regimen requires SMBG only twice a day, we have observed good adherence by the patients in performing SMBG. In type 1 and insulin-requiring type 2 diabetic patients fasting and preprandial targeted blood glucose be 110 mg/dL (6.1 mmol/L) or less and 2-hour postprandial blood glucose be 140 mg/dL (7.8 mmol/L) or less. It is important to target blood glucose excursion occurring between pre- and 2-hour postprandial period. Once a reasonable glycemic control (HbA1c less than 7.0%) is achieved then an appropriate SMBG frequency according to patient's glycemic variability and agreeable adherence plan between the patients and their physicians should be established to maintain proper glycemic control. In pregnant diabetic patient, an aggressive approach for SMBG is needed to achieve proper glycemic control rapidly. Daily SMBG for pre- and 2-hour post- major meals may be required to establish proper glycemic control. We recommend that fasting and preprandial blood glucose to be maintained at 95 mg/dL (5.3 mmol/L) or less and 2-hour postprandial blood glucose be maintained at 120 mg/dL (6.7 mmol/L) or less. Detailed SMBG guideline for pregnant diabetic patients is outlined in the Chapter "Care of Pregnant Diabetic Patient".

REFERENCES

1. The Diabetes Control and Complications Trial Research Group. The effect of intensive treatment of diabetes on the development and progression of long-term complications in insulin-dependent diabetes mellitus. *N Engl J Med*. 1993;329(14):977-86.
2. UK Prospective Diabetes Study (UKPDS) Group. Intensive blood-glucose control with sulphonylureas or insulin compared with conventional treatment and risk of complications in patients with type 2 diabetes (UKPDS 33). *Lancet*. 1998;352:837-53.
3. Ohkubo Y, Kishikawa H, Araki E, Miyata T, Isami S, Motoyoshi S, et al. Intensive insulin therapy prevents the progression of diabetic microvascular complications in Japanese patients with non-insulin-dependent diabetes mellitus: a randomized prospective 6-year study. *Diabetes Res Clin Pract*. 1995;28(2):103-17.
4. Expert Committee on the Diagnosis and Classification of Diabetes Mellitus. American Diabetes Association: clinical practice recommendations 2002. *Diabetes Care*. 2002;25 Suppl 1:S1-147.
5. Rodbard HW, Jellinger PS, Davidson JA, Einhorn D, Garber AJ, Grunberger G, et al. Statement by an American Association of Clinical Endocrinologists/American College of Endocrinology consensus panel on type 2 diabetes mellitus: an algorithm for glycemic control in type 2 diabetes. *Endocr Pract*. 2009;15:540-59.
6. NICE. National Collaborating Centre for Chronic Conditions. Type 2 diabetes: National clinical guideline for management in primary and secondary care (update). London: Royal College of Physicians; 2008. pp. 47-51.
7. Faas A, Schellevis FG, Van Eijk JT. The efficacy of self-monitoring of blood glucose in NIDDM subjects. A criteria-based literature review. *Diabetes Care*. 1997;20:1482-6.
8. Coster S, Gulliford MC, Seed PT, Powrie JK, Swaminathan R, et al. Self-monitoring in type 2 diabetes mellitus: a meta-analysis. *Diabet Med*. 2000;17:755-61.
9. Welschen LM, Bloemendal E, Nijpels G, Dekker JM, Heine RJ, Stalman WA, et al. Self-monitoring of blood glucose in patients with type 2 diabetes who are not using insulin: a systematic review. *Diabetes Care*. 2005;28:1510-7.

10. Sarol JN, Nicodemus NA, Tan KM, Grava MB. Self-monitoring of blood glucose as part of a multi-component therapy among non-insulin requiring type 2 diabetes patients: a meta-analysis (1966-2004). *Curr Med Res Opin*. 2005;21:173-84.

11. Murata GH, Duckworth WC, Shah JH, Wendel CS, Mohler MJ, Hoffman RM. Blood glucose monitoring is associated with better glycemic control in type 2 diabetes: a database study. *J Gen Intern Med*. 2009;24(1):48-52.

12. Karter AJ, Parker MM, Moffet HH, Spence MM, Chan J, Ettner SL, et al. Longitudinal study of new and prevalent use of self-monitoring of blood glucose. *Diabetes Care*. 2006;29:1757-63.

13. Harris MI. Health care and health status and outcomes for patients with type 2 diabetes. *Diabetes Care*. 2000;23:754-8.

14. Oki JC, Flora DL, Isley WL. Frequency and impact of SMBG on glycemic control in patients with NIDDM in an urban teaching hospital clinic. *Diabetes Educ*. 1997;23:419-24.

15. Harris MI. Frequency of blood glucose monitoring in relation to glycemic control in patients with type 2 diabetes. *Diabetes Care*. 2001;24:979-82.

16. Evans JM, Newton RW, Ruta DA, MacDonald TM, Stevenson RJ, Morris AD. Frequency of blood glucose monitoring in relation to glycaemic control: observational study with diabetes database. *BMJ*. 1999;319:83-6.

17. Rindone JP, Austin M, Luchesi J. Effect of home blood glucose monitoring on the management of patients with non-insulin dependent diabetes mellitus in the primary care setting. *Am J Manag Care*. 1997;3:1335-8.

18. Polonsky W, Fisher L, Schikman C, Hinnen D, Parkin C, Jelsovsky Z, et al. The value of episodic, intensive blood glucose monitoring in non-insulin treated persons with type 2 diabetes: design of the Structured Testing Program (STeP) study, a cluster-randomized, clinical trial. *BMC Fam Pract*. 2010;11:37.

19. Karter AJ, Ackerson LM, Darbinian JA, D'Agostino RB, Ferrara A, Liu J, et al. Self-monitoring of blood glucose levels and glycemic control: the Northern California Kaiser Permanente Diabetes registry. *Am J Med*. 2001;111:1-9.

20. Schiel R, Müller UA, Rauchfub J, Sprott H, Müller R. Blood-glucose self-monitoring in insulin treated type 2 diabetes mellitus: a cross-sectional study with an intervention group. *Diabetes Metab*. 1999;25:334-40.

21. Kennedy L. Self-monitoring of blood glucose in type 2 diabetes: time for evidence of efficacy. *Diabetes Care*. 2001;24:977-8.

22. Shah JH, Murata GH, Duckworth WC, Hoffman RM, Wendel CS. Factors affecting compliance in type 2 diabetes: experience from the Diabetes Outcomes in Veterans Study (DOVES). *Int J Diabetes Dev Ctries*. 2003;23:75-82.

23. Hoffman RM, Shah JH, Wendel CS, Duckworth WC, Adam KD, Bokhari SU, et al. Evaluating once- and twice-daily self-monitored blood glucose testing strategies for stable insulin-treated patients with type 2 diabetes: the Diabetes Outcomes in Veterans Study. *Diabetes Care*. 2002;25:1744-8.

24. Murata GH, Shah JH, Wendel CS, Hoffman RM, Adam KD, Bokhari SU, et al. Risk factor management in stable, insulin-treated patients with type 2 diabetes: the Diabetes Outcomes in Veterans Study. *J Diabetes Complications*. 2003;17(4):186-91.

25. Murata GH, Shah JH, Hoffman RM, Wendel CS, Adam KD, Solvas PA, et al. Intensified blood glucose self-monitoring improves glycemic control in stable, insulin-treated veterans with type 2 diabetes: the Diabetes Outcomes in Veterans Study (DOVES). *Diabetes Care*. 2003;26:1759-63.

26. Murata GH, Hoffman RM, Shah JH, Wendel CS, Duckworth WC. A probabilistic model for predicting hypoglycemia in type 2 diabetes mellitus: the Diabetes Outcomes in Veterans Study (DOVES). *Arch Intern Med.* 2004;164:1445-50.

27. Paisey RB, Macfarlane DG, Sherriff RJ, Hartog M, Slade RR, White DA. The relationship between blood glycosylated haemoglobin and home capillary blood glucose levels in diabetics. *Diabetologia.* 1980;19:31-4.

28. Svendsen PA, Lauritzen T, Søegaard U, Nerup J. Glycosylated haemoglobin and steady-state mean blood glucose concentration in type 1 (insulin-dependent) diabetes. *Diabetologia.* 1982;23:403-5.

29. Rohlfing CL, Wiedmeyer HM, Little RR, England JD, Tennill A, Goldstein DE. Defining the relationship between plasma glucose and HbA(1c): analysis of glucose profiles and HbA(1c) in the Diabetes Control and Complications Trial. *Diabetes Care.* 2002;25:275-8.

30. Bonora E. Postprandial peaks as a risk factor for cardiovascular disease: epidemiological perspectives. *Int J Clin Pract Suppl.* 2002;(129):5-11.

31. Polonsky WH, Fisher L, Schikman CH, Hinnen DA, Parkin CG, Jelsovsky Z, et al. Structured self-monitoring of blood glucose significantly reduces A1c levels in poorly controlled, noninsulin-treated type 2 diabetes: results from the Structured Testing Program study. *Diabetes Care.* 2011;34:262-7.

32. Shah JH, Wendel CS, Fotieo GG, Plummer EV, Murata GH. Structured SMBG with standard treatment improves glycemic control in insulin-treated type 2 diabetics. Presented at and in the program of the International Diabetes Federation meeting, World Diabetes Congress, Dubai, UAE December 6, 2011.

33. McIntosh B, Yu C, Lal A, Chelak K, Cameron C, Singh SR, et al. Efficacy of self-monitoring of blood glucose in patients with type 2 diabetes mellitus managed without insulin: a systematic review and meta-analysis. *Open Med.* 2010;4(2):e102-13.

34. Simon J, Gray A, Clarke P, Wade A, Neil A, Farmer A. Cost effectiveness of self-monitoring of blood glucose in patients with non-insulin treated type 2 diabetes: economic evaluation of data from the DiGEM trial. *BMJ.* 2008;336:1177-80.

35. Tunis SL, Minshall ME. Self-monitoring of blood glucose in type 2 diabetes: cost-effectiveness in the United States. *Am J Manag Care.* 2008;14:131-40.

36. Palmer AJ, Dinneen S, Gavin JR, Gray A, Herman WH, Karter AJ. Cost-utility analysis in a UK setting of self-monitoring of blood glucose in patients with type 2 diabetes. *Curr Med Res Opin.* 2006; 22: 861-872.

37. Gray A, Raikou M, McGuire A, Fenn P, Stevens R, Cull C, et al. Cost effectiveness of an intensive blood glucose control policy in patients with type 2 diabetes: economic analysis alongside randomized controlled trial (UKPDS 41). United Kingdom Prospective Diabetes Study Group. *BMJ.* 2000;320:1373-8.

Nutritional and Exercise Management of Diabetes

6
Chapter

Jayendra H Shah

"Foods which promote longevity, intelligence, vigor, health, happiness, and cheerfulness and which are appealing, substantial, and naturally agreeable are dear to spiritual people."

(Bhagavad Gita: Chapter 17, Verse 8)

"Take thou also unto thee wheat, and barley, and beans, and lentils, and millet, and fitches, and put them in one vessel, and make thee bread thereof, according to the number of the days that thou shalt lie upon thy side, three hundred and ninety days shalt thou eat thereof."

(King James Bible: Ezekiel 4:9)

ABSTRACT

In the management of diabetes, the patients understanding of the disease (knowledge) and nutritional and exercise considerations are as important as pharmacologic treatment. Yet, the nutritional and exercise aspect of management are poorly understood by the patients and their health care providers. Overall adherence to nutritional recommendation is poor in both type 1 and type 2 diabetic patients. The findings of poor nutritional and exercise compliance has been confirmed by studies from other countries indicating universal difficulties in adhering to lifestyle changes recommendations in the treatment of diabetes. Therefore, it is important to understand the factors which influence the lifestyle changes in diabetic patients. If diabetic patients can be educated that how their nutritional habits contribute to the glycemic control and eventually to micro- and macrovascular complications, then their adherence to recommended diet could improve. If the food intake in diabetic patient can be regularly and reliably measured then nutritional counseling could be more effective. Unfortunately, conflicting information from various reports have created confusion on effectiveness of particular nutritional method for both patients and clinicians. It is important to establish specific nutritional and exercise goal for each patient to make recommendation effective. Also, healthy behavior and lifestyle changes frequently depend on establishing goals which are personally relevant and attainable by the patient. In this chapter, the author discusses various methods to establish goals and evidence based recommendations for nutrition and exercise therapy for diabetic patients.

INTRODUCTION

Over 5,000 years ago, holy scripts *Bhagavad Gita* and Vedas in India have observed profound effect of diet on mind and body of human being by describing "purity of mind follows purity of diet". Ayurvedic medicine in ancient India, 600 BC has also recognized the effect of diet on mind and body and overall well-being. King James Bible also reveals importance of good diet for humans. In recent years, importance of diet in the prevention and management of diabetes, obesity, colon cancer and cardiovascular disease has been recognized.

In the management of diabetes, the patients understanding of the disease (knowledge) and nutritional and exercise considerations are as important as pharmacologic treatment. Yet, the nutritional and exercise aspect of management are poorly understood by the patients and their health care providers. Overall adherence to nutritional recommendation is poor in both type 1 and type 2 diabetic patients. In our prospective observational study,[1] the Diabetes Outcome in Veterans Study (DOVES), noncompliance to the American Diabetes Association (ADA) recommended nutritional guideline[2] was common among insulin-treated type 2 diabetic patients. In this study, ADA recommended limits for cholesterol and saturated fatty acids (SFAs) consumption was met by only 2.1% of patients with metabolic syndrome. Of all the patients, the ADA standard for carbohydrate and monosaturated fatty acid was met by 25.2%, standard for SFA met by 9.5%, standard for cholesterol met by 25.2%, and standard for daily sodium consumption was met by 30.6% of patients. It was interesting to note that 99.2% of the patients met the ADA guideline for alcohol consumption! Similar to our observation, other studies have found high rate of noncompliance to prescribed diet and exercise.[3-5] The findings of poor nutritional and exercise compliance in these studies have been confirmed by studies from other countries indicating universal difficulties in adhering to lifestyle changes recommendations in the treatment of diabetes.[6,7] Therefore, it is important to understand the factors which influence the lifestyle changes in diabetic patients. If diabetic patients can be educated that how their nutritional habits contribute to the glycemic control and eventually to micro- and macrovascular complications, then their adherence to recommended diet could improve. If the food intake in diabetic patient can be regularly and reliably measured then nutritional counseling could be more effective. Unfortunately, conflicting information from various reports has created confusion on effectiveness of particular nutritional method for both patients and clinicians. In recent years,

ADA and other investigators have critically reviewed and published guidelines on evidence-based medical nutrition therapy for diabetic patients.[8,9] It is clear that "one recommendation fit all" kind of nutrition and exercise recommendation does not work as the need and personal circumstances for each diabetic patient are different. It is important to establish specific nutritional and exercise goal for each patient to make recommendation effective. Also, healthy behavior and lifestyle changes frequently depend on establishing goals which are personally relevant and attainable by the patient.[10-12] In general, the goals for nutritional and exercise therapy for diabetic patients are:

- To achieve and maintain appropriate body weight. As we know that majority of type 2 diabetic patients are overweight or obese, the nutritional and exercise recommendations work hand in hand for weight reduction and maintenance
- To maintain near normal glycemic control, avoiding hyper- or hypoglycemia, in harmony with personal and cultural preferences as well as pharmacological (oral agents and insulin) treatment
- To prevent micro- and macrovascular complications of diabetes by maintaining recommended blood pressure and normal lipid levels.

For the purpose of this chapter, we will discuss various methods and evidence-based recommendations of nutrition and exercise treatment for diabetic patients.

FOOD FREQUENCY QUESTIONNAIRE

As stated above, if the food intake is regularly and reliably measured in diabetic patients then medical nutritional therapy may be more effective. By using food frequency questionnaire (FFQ), we can easily measure daily food intake by diabetic patient. It is a valid method for evaluating diet habit of the patient and does not require detail interview by clinician.[1,13-15] However, in diabetic patients it is difficult to validate a FFQ because several metabolic parameters cannot be correlated with one macronutrient as these metabolic parameters are affected by other behaviors (depression, cognitive dysfunctions, inadequate diabetes knowledge, complication of diabetes) and by the disease itself and pharmacologic treatment.[16,17] We validated Fred Hutchinson Cancer Research Center FFQ[18] in insulin-treated type 2 diabetic patients by quantitative assessment of nutrient intake, rating the patient's diet quality by acceptable standards, correlating adherence to these standards and metabolic parameters, and excluding non-nutritional causes of poor diabetic control.[1] We used following ADA clinical practice recommendations[2] to compare nutritional consumption reported on the FFQ by diabetic patients:

- Carbohydrate and monounsaturated fatty acid (MUFA) calories contribution 60–70% of total calories
- Saturated fatty acids calories contribution less than 7% of total calories
- Protein 15–20% of total caloric intake in diabetic patient without chronic kidney disease

- Salt consumption should be less than 2,400 mg per day
- Cholesterol consumption should be less than 300 mg per day if serum low-density lipoprotein (LDL) cholesterol was less than or equal to 2.59 mmol/L or less than 200 mg per day if serum LDL cholesterol was greater than 2.59 mmol/L
- Alcohol intake should be limited to two drinks per day for men and one drink per day for women.

From FFQ, we estimated adherence to ADA nutritional recommendation in type 2 insulin-treated diabetic patients. The differences in the macronutrient consumption correlated with various metabolic parameters such as body mass index (BMI), HbA1c, serum total and LDL cholesterol, and serum triglycerides. In all cases, the least adherent patient with ADA nutritional recommendation was found to have poorest metabolic control of diabetes. These observations could not be attributed to the differences in the duration of diabetes, intensity of pharmacotherapy or levels of physical activity. In addition, patients adherent to ADA nutritional recommendation were more likely achieve metabolic targets of HbA1c, BMI, total, and LDL cholesterol than those patients who were nonadherent. These findings suggest that the patients' nutritional habits contributed to obesity and poor diabetic control were identified by FFQ analysis. In this study, we also evaluated psychological determinants of dietary adherence. We observed that those patients with positive attitude about diabetes, fewer social obligations and firm belief that nutritional management improves diabetes were adherent to dietary standards recommended by ADA. The patients who were less adherent to dietary recommendations were depressed, which have been attributed to adverse self-care behaviors.[19-21] These nonadherent patients were younger with high BMI who have been reported to have poor prognosis.[20] We also found that in obese patients, with or without metabolic syndrome, only small number of patients were adherent to ADA nutritional recommendation, specifically to total calorie, fat and SFA consumption. This finding has implications for providing better nutritional education to prevent macrovascular complication of diabetes.

The adherence to nutritional recommendation is a complex issue and requires concerted efforts between a dietician, psychologist and social worker. The dietician can emphasize healthy ADA recommended diet and its effect on better metabolic control and identify methods to achieve the nutritional goals. A social worker may help to involve family-oriented nutritional training, correct social barriers in achieving nutritional goal and explore alternative aspects to achieve the nutritional goals for working patients. A psychologist can provide motivational interview and help in the treatment of depression.

We recommend that diabetic patients should be encouraged to use ADA recommended diet of macronutrients. The FFQ should be used to identify dietary habits of diabetic patients and their nonadherence to prescribed diet. The FFQ can help dietician to work with patients to achieve nutritional goals according to patient's personal preferences, social and family environment. This also requires periodic reassessment and dietary modification by dietician to solicit better adherence by the patient.

PHYSICAL ACTIVITY, WEIGHT REDUCTION, AND MAINTENANCE

Majority of type 2 diabetic patients are overweight or obese. These patients frequently have insulin resistance, hyperlipidemia and hypertension. Initial weight loss of 5–10% in these patients can improve glycemic control, hyperlipidemia, and hypertension.[22,23] It was reported in a meta-analysis of 103 studies involving 10,455 subjects that the metabolic control was improved with exercise intervention.[24] The studies have also demonstrated an inverse association between exercise capacity and all-cause mortality in diabetic patients. This effect was independent of BMI.[25,26] Aerobic or resistance exercise can improve glycemic control, but the maximum effect was observed when aerobic and resistance exercise were combined.[27] However, since duration of exercise was also increased; it was not clear whether the combination of the type of exercise or duration of exercise was responsible for the increased benefit. Another meta-analysis showed that aerobic exercise significantly lowered LDL cholesterol by 5%.[28] Lowering of other lipids did not reach significant level. Several studies have shown that significant improvement in the dyslipidemia and hypertension by inducing weight reduction by nutritional therapy with or without medications used for weight loss.[29-34] Regular physical activities have shown to improve glycemic control, hypertension, reduction in cardiovascular risk, and overall well-being independent of weight reduction. Also, in type 1 diabetic patients, increased physical activity was shown to improve dyslipidemia and glycemic control.[35] However, in patients with type 1 diabetic (and some type 2 diabetic patients treated with insulin), moderate exercise is associated with the risk of hypoglycemia during and 31 hours after exercise.[36] In these patients, 30–50% down adjustment of premeal insulin during planned moderate exercise is recommended. In case, the insulin dose was not reduced or exercise activity was unplanned then increase in 15–30 g of carbohydrate meal should be consumed before and after 60 minutes of moderate exercise.[37] Since hypoglycemia can occur up to 31 hours after exercise, blood glucose should be monitored before bedtime on the day the moderate exercise activity was done in the early afternoon or evening. Appropriate dietary supplementation should be given for bedtime blood glucose level of less than 130 mg/dL (7.21 mmol/L). Also, if before exercise blood glucose level is less than 100 mg/dL (5.55 mmol/L) then appropriate amount of carbohydrate (e.g., 15–30 g) should be consumed before commencing the exercise.

In patients with type 2 diabetes, 90–150 minutes of accumulated moderate intensity aerobic exercise/activity per week and resistance exercise 3 times a week is recommended to improve glycemic control, dyslipidemia and hypertension. This improvement may occur with or without weight loss. This level of physical activity also leads to improved well-being feeling, decreases cardiovascular risks and morbidity and mortality from all-causes. The patients with diabetes can accomplish the recommended activity/exercise by walking for 3–4 hours per week. Tenasescu et al. have reported that walking at least half an hour a day was associated with 18% lower risk of new diagnosis of coronary artery disease.[38] Generally, walking is a safe exercise activity compared to other forms of exercise. In one survey, 1.5% of persons reported injuries during walking.[39] It is, therefore, important for patients with diabetes to wear good fitting shoes, provide good feet care, proper safe place to walk, and appropriate environment protection to minimize injuries. Choosing a companion for regular walking improves the pleasure and personal well-feeling. In patients, receiving insulin, especially in type 1 diabetic patients, blood glucose monitoring before and after exercise, down adjustment of insulin dose and if needed, addition of carbohydrate meal as outlined above is recommended.

It should be emphasized that both increase in physical activity and decreased total caloric intake are most effective in achieving weight loss. A sustained weight loss of 5–10% of initial body weight in overweight and obese diabetic patients is a reasonable goal. Such reduction in body weight has been associated with tangible benefit in improving blood glucose levels, lowering of blood pressure, increasing high-density lipoprotein (HDL) cholesterol levels and decreasing LDL cholesterol and triglyceride levels.[22,23,40,41] In patients with diabetes, significant weight reduction has been associated with 28% reduction in cardiovascular morbidity and 25% all-cause mortality.[42] Once initial goal of 5–10% weight reduction is achieved further goal for weight reduction depends on its impact on reduction in fasting blood glucose, individual's motivation for weight reduction and lifestyle changes and family support. Some of the simple methods to increase activities and burn more calories are outlined in table 1. We briefly discussed the activity and exercise strategy for weight reduction. Discussion and recommendations in following sections will outline other strategies that impact on weight reduction.

CONSUMPTION OF CALORIES

The daily caloric requirement in an individual varies greatly with the gender, age, level of daily activity, BMI, and state of sickness or well-being. In general, the hepatic output of glucose determines fasting blood glucose. Caloric restriction in overweight or obese diabetic patients has initial effect on fasting blood glucose even before any significant weight loss.[43,44] But weight loss has the ultimate effect on the long-term reduction on the fasting blood glucose level.[45] The caloric restriction with increased activities/exercise, thus have beneficial effect on the glycemic control in diabetic patients.

To estimate caloric intake, one can use different formulas available. The simple way to estimate caloric need is to assume that the patient needs 10 calories per pound of ideal body weight to maintain daily metabolism. We can add 3–5 calories per pound of body weight for mild for moderately active lifestyle and 7–10 calories per pound of very active lifestyle. We can also further adjust the calories according to patient's need, type of diabetes, pharmacologic treatment and weight loss goals. In our experience, other recommended complex formulas[46,47] to estimate caloric need, essentially yield the same effect on weight reduction. When calculated, the rough caloric need according to ideal body weight, most overweight or obese individual

TABLE 1: How Body May Burn More Calories

Build muscle
- For every extra pound of muscle, body uses around 50 extra calories a day

Aerobic exercise
- For several hours after aerobic exercise more calories are burned

Move more
- Tap feet
- Swing legs
- Drum fingers
- Stand up and stretch
- Move head from side to side
- Change position
- Wriggle and fidget
- Pace up and down
- Use stairs frequently
- Park in the furthest corner of the car park
- Stand up when talking on the phone
- Clench and release muscle

Eat spicy food
- Spicy food, especially chili, can raise metabolic rate up to 50% up to 3 hours after meal

Eat little and often
- Eating small, regular meals will keep metabolism going faster than larger, less frequent meals

lose weight. The ideal body weight for man and woman can be estimated according to the determinations made by the Metropolitan Life insurance tables or as outlined by Close and associates[4] as follows:

- Ideal body weight for men 60 inches (152 cm) tall is estimated to be 106 pounds (48 kg). For each additional inch (2.5 cm) in height add 6 pounds (2.7 kg) for ideal body weight
- Ideal body weight for women 60 inches (152 cm) tall is estimated to be 100 pounds (45 kg). For each inch (2.5 cm) in the height difference (higher or lower) add or subtract 5 pounds (2.3 kg) ideal body weight.

It is important to emphasize that the ADA recommended macronutrient should be used for calorie distribution.[2] Also, we have observed that prescribing less than 1,000 or even 1,200 calorie consumption per day is not practical and frequently not followed by patients in out-patient clinics. The strategies of educating patients on counting calories and fat content of the diet as well as keeping diaries help in increasing adherence to the prescribed calorie diet.[48,49] Also, in patients whose diabetes is controlled by diet and/or oral agents, frequent small meals may help to increase metabolism and burn more calories (Table 1).

CONCEPT OF MEAL REPLACEMENT

The Action for Health in Diabetes (Look AHEAD)[48] and the Diabetes Prevention Program[49] have used the concept of meal replacement in the form of portion-control servings of conventional food, liquid shakes or food bars. Metz and associates have shown that in patients with type 2 diabetes, prepackaged meal replacement resulted in the desired weight loss to a greater degree, lower HbA1c levels, increased compliance with diet and overall improved feeling of well-being.[30] Similarly, in a group of patients with type 2 diabetes, 12 weeks meal replacement diet with liquid meals caused greater weight loss and better glycemic control than same calorie conventional diet.[50] Several investigators have shown that the concept of meal replacement works in reducing and maintaining weight, improving glycemic control and reducing cardiovascular risk factors for prolong period.[51-53] This concept is very effective in highly motivated patients who are able afford the cost of meal replacement. Therefore, the meal replacement nutritional therapy may be useful in certain group of patients with type 2 diabetes. In certain ethnic groups and countries meal replacement nutritional therapy may not be acceptable or affordable.

FOOD EXCHANGE SYSTEM

The food exchange system originally consisted of six groups: (1) starch/bread, (2) meat and meat substitutes, (3) vegetables, (4) fruits, (5) milk, and (6) fat, was jointly developed by ADA, and US Public Health Service.[54] The portion of food listed in each group contained similar calories and same amount of carbohydrates, fat, and protein and, therefore, exchangeable. In order to create consistency with carbohydrate content, these groups are further simplified into 3 groups: (1) carbohydrates, (2) meat and meat substitutes, and (3) fat. These groups also list foods that have high sodium and fiber content. The food exchange is excellent concept to keep consistency of macronutrients. However, many patients (and sometimes their primary care providers!) find it is difficult to understand this concept and follow it in their day-to-day life. In our experience, we have observed poor adherence in following food exchange system by diabetic patients.

MACRONUTRIENT CONTENT OF DIET

The optimal content of carbohydrate, fat, and protein in a diet is controversial. High-carbohydrate diet compared with diet high in MUFA diet has shown to be associated with modest increase in blood pressure.[55] However, high-fat and high-protein diet may have deleterious effect on cardiovascular system promoting risk for atherosclerosis[56] and kidney, promoting risk for diabetic nephropathy. In the comparison of low-fat and high-carbohydrate (72%) vegan diet with ADA recommended carbohydrate (48%) diet, Barnard and associates observed that glycemic and lipid control was better in high-carbohydrate, low-fat vegan diet.[57,58] No differences in glycemic control, lipid levels, HbA1c levels, and body weight were observed in a study where patients with type 2 diabetes were followed for 1 year with higher carbohydrate (47% and 52%) versus low-carbohydrate (39%) diet.[59] In another study, patients with type 2 diabetic patients were followed for 1 year with high-carbohydrate (60%) and low-fat (25%) diet or moderate-carbohydrate (45%) and high-fat (40%) diet. In both groups, the improvement in blood pressure, fasting blood glucose, HDL cholesterol, HbA1c, waist circumference, and weight loss were similar.[60] In American Indian patients with type 2 diabetes, higher intake of total fat, saturated and polyunsaturated fatty acids, and low-carbohydrate diet was associated with worsening of glycemic control.[61] The Diabetes Control and Complications Trial (DCCT) in type 1 diabetes showed that diet low in carbohydrate and high in total and saturated fats was associated with poorer glycemic control, independent of BMI and exercise.[62] In a 4-year Mediterranean diet study, newly diagnosed patients with type 2 diabetes were randomly assigned to a diet with 50% complex carbohydrate, 30% mono- and polyunsaturated fat (Mediterranean-style diet) or assigned to a low-fat diet. The patients assigned to Mediterranean diet less likely to required oral diabetic medication to control hyperglycemia.[63] Also, this study showed that HDL cholesterol levels were consistently higher and triglyceride levels were lower in the patients consuming Mediterranean diet. The studies comparing high-protein (28–30%) versus low-protein (15–16%) diets in diabetic patients with normal renal function showed no differences in the glycemic control and showed similar degree of weight loss.[64-66] It has been reported that glomerular filtration rate (GFR) and albumin excretion rate (AER) were improved in diabetic patients with macroalbuminuria when placed on daily 0.8 g per kg protein diet. This improved effect was not seen in patients with normo- or microalbuminuria.[67] However, in type 1 and 2 diabetic patients with overt and insipient nephropathy low-protein diet failed to show improvement in GFR and AER.[68]

The research does not support any particular percentage of macronutrients distribution in the diet for patients with diabetes. Therefore, consumption of macronutrients based on dietary reference intake for healthy eating is recommended for diabetic patients.[9] In patients with diabetes who are treated with diet alone, treated with oral agents or fixed insulin doses should consume carbohydrate with consistent distribution during the day. In patients with type 1 and type 2 diabetes who are using insulin pump therapy or who adjust their mealtime insulin dose should consume carbohydrates in proportion to the insulin dose. Also, glycemic control is improved if insulin dose is adjusted to planned carbohydrate intake in balance with fat and protein intake. Diets too low in carbohydrates are not recommended as they are unpalatable and frequently eliminate foods with minerals, vitamins and fiber. Dietary carbohydrates from whole grains, legumes, low-fat milk, fruits and vegetables with low glycemic index are recommended (Table 2). To prevent and treat cardiovascular diseases in diabetic patients, a decreased consumption of total fat and saturated and hydrogenated fat is recommended. Mono- and polyunsaturated fats, especially

TABLE 2: Glycemic Index of Common Food Items		
Food item	Glycemic index	Rating
Grains and cereals		
White rice (steamed)	High	98
Basmati rice	Medium	58
Barley (cracked)	Low	50
Cornflakes	High	83
Bran	Low	42
Shredded wheat	Medium	69
Cheerios	High	74
Rice Krispies	High	82
Pasta		
Spaghetti (white)	Medium	55
Spaghetti (whole wheat)	Low	37
Macaroni	Low	47
Breads		
White bread	High	71
Whole grain bread	Low	50
Multigrain bread	Low	47
Rye bread	Medium	65
Wheat tortilla	Low	30
Pita bread	Medium	57
Hamburger bun (white)	Medium	61
Pastries		
Doughnut	High	78
Bagel	High	72
Croissant	Medium	67
Shortbread biscuit	Medium	64
Beans and legumes		
Kidney beans (cooked from dried)	Low	29
Lentils (cooked from dried)	Low	29
Kidney beans (canned)	Low	52
Chickpeas (canned)	Low	42
Red lentils	Low	26
Vegetables		
Carrots	Low	49
Green beans	Low	15

Contd...

Contd...

TABLE 2: Glycemic Index of Common Food Items		
Food item	**Glycemic index**	**Rating**
Eggplant	Low	15
Green peas	Low	50
Potato (baked)	High	85
Broccoli	Low	15
Spinach	Low	15
Tomatoes	Low	15
Pumpkin	High	75
Zucchini	Low	15
Sweet potato (baked)	Low	45
Corn	Low	55
Fruits		
Bananas	Low	52
Oranges	Low	44
Apples	Low	38
Pineapple	Medium	66
Pears	Low	38
Strawberries	Low	40
Cherries	Low	22
Watermelon	High	72
Cantaloupe melon	Medium	67
Green grapes	Low	46
Peaches	Low	42
Kiwifruit	Low	52
Grapefruit	Low	25
Dates	High	102

- Low glycemic index foods (rating 55 or less)
- Medium glycemic index foods (rating between 56 and 69)
- High glycemic index foods (rating 70 or more)

omega-3 fatty acids have protective effect on cardiovascular disease. The consumption of saturated fat should be less than 7% of total daily calorie intake. Total daily cholesterol intake should be less than 200 mg. In type 1 and type 2 diabetic patients with normal renal function, protein intake of 15–20% of daily calorie consumption is recommended. In patients with diabetic nephropathy, optimum daily intake of protein should not exceed 0.8 g per kg of body weight.

GLYCEMIC INDEX AND GLYCEMIC LOAD

Many foods may contain same amount of carbohydrates but their glycemic effect may be very different. Thus, in the nutritional treatment of diabetes, understanding the concept of glycemic index (glycemic quality) and glycemic load (glycemic quantity) is important. Glycemic index is calculated by the impact of a particular food containing 50 g of carbohydrate on blood glucose in comparison with the elevation in blood glucose caused by 50 g of a reference carbohydrate, e.g. glucose or white bread.[69,70] Certain grains, such as barley or converted rice, nuts, non-starchy vegetable, and legumes have low glycemic index. In contrast, white bread, potato and candies have high glycemic index (Table 2). The blood glucose response to carbohydrate containing food is also dependent on quantity (glycemic load) of the food. The glycemic load of a particular food containing carbohydrate can be calculated as the product of glycemic index value and total amount of carbohydrate content of the food.[71,72] In general, food containing high fibers have low glycemic index and load values. Buyken and associates showed positive correlation between low glycemic index diet and improved glycemic control in 2,810 patients with type 1 diabetes from 31 European clinics.[73] In randomized trials performed in patients with type 1 and 2 diabetes, the low glycemic diets were effective in reducing HbA1c when compared with ADA recommended diet but with high glycemic foods.[74] However, another trial has failed to show differences between low and high glycemic foods on glycemic control.[75] Variability of glycemic index for same carbohydrate in same individual at different times as well as between the subjects has been reported.[76] In recent years, studies have implicated additional role of glycemic index and glycemic load in the development of coronary artery disease, cancers and type 2 diabetes.[77,78]

For patients and clinicians, the glycemic index and glycemic load are difficult to understand and remember. Also, labels on food packages do not contain information on glycemic load and combining different foods in a meal may complicate the issue further. Difficulties arise when food containing high glycemic food is combined with food with low glycemic index and/or with fat and ingested in a meal. For example, rice with high glycemic index when ingested in a meal combined with low glycemic index legumes with addition of butter or ghee (refined butter) would have different glycemic effect than if the rice is consumed alone as a meal. Understanding glycemic index values of different foods may help the patient in smart selection of meal containing low glycemic value food or combining meals with low, medium and high glycemic index foods. For example, choosing sweet potato (low glycemic index value) versus a regular white potato (high glycemic index value) in a meal is a smart food choice for diabetic patients. High glycemic index foods are not necessarily bad. For example, watermelon has high glycemic index value but glycemic load in one cup of watermelon would not be much as watermelon volume comprise mainly of water.

DIETARY FIBER

Dietary fibers are heterogeneous plant materials which enzymes in the human gastrointestinal tract are unable to digest. The plant dietary fibers can be soluble or insoluble in water. The structural fibers of the plant are insoluble in water. Cellulose in coarse bran, hemicellulose in bran cereal, and whole grain bread and lignin in many fruits are examples of structural insoluble fibers. Water soluble fibers, such as pectins are found in fruits and vegetables such as banana, carrots, apples, and oranges. Water soluble fibers as gums are found in oat meal and as mucilage as psyllium hydrophilic mucilloid. The water insoluble fibers accelerate gastric emptying time and intestinal transit time as well as absorb water to increase fecal bulk. This mechanical effect causes frequency of bowel movements. In contrast, water soluble fibers may increase the bulk but also increase viscosity and stickiness by their gel forming properties to cause delay in gastric emptying and intestinal transit time. An interruption in the enterohepatic circulation of bile salts by soluble fibers cause increased excretion of bile salts and hence cholesterol in the feces. It has been postulated that soluble and insoluble fibers can inhibit dietary cholesterol absorption by trapping it and excreting in feces.[79-81] High fiber content of some common foods is outlined in table 3.[80,82]

In patients with diabetes, several reports have shown beneficial effects of fiber on glycemic control. In a study, patients compliant with daily 50 g consumption of

TABLE 3: Food Items with High Fiber Content		
Food	Serving	Fiber amount (g)
Kidney beans	½ cup	9.7
Pinto beans	½ cup	8.9
All bran cereals	1/3 cup	8.4
Lima beans	½ cup	8.3
Peas (cooked)	½ cup	6.7
Pear	Medium	4.0
Apple	Large	4.0
Broccoli	½ cup	3.5
Orange	Small	3.2
Strawberries	1 cup	3.1
Banana	Medium	3.0
Cornflakes	¾ cup	2.6
Eggplant (raw)	½ cup	2.5
Peach	Medium	2.3
Sweet potato (raw)	½ medium	2.1
Cabbage (raw)	½ cup	2.1

fiber show 2% reduction in HbA1c.[83] Other studies have shown improved 24-hour glycemic profiles with high fiber consumption compared to low fiber consumption[84,85] and even lowering of postprandial glucose levels with meal containing high fiber meals.[86] Several studies compared the effect of low fiber (5–20 g) versus high fiber (30–53 g) content with different amount of macronutrients percentages in the diet. Improvement in glycemic control with high fiber diet[87,88] as well as no difference in glycemic control with high fiber diet[89,90] was observed in these studies. In addition to improving the glycemic control, high fiber diets are effective in reducing cholesterol levels in diabetic patients.[84,88,90] We recommend that patients with diabetes should consume more than 25 g of fiber per day. Ten to fifteen gram of this fiber source should be as soluble fiber.

SUGAR SUBSTITUTES (NON-NUTRITIVE SWEETENERS)

Several non-nutritive sweeteners are available as sugar substitutes for use in the diet for diabetic patients. Saccharin, aspartame, sucralose and stevia are most commonly used sugar substitutes and are approved by US Food and Drug Administration (FDA). The FDA has set guidelines for these sugar substitutes, the acceptable average daily intake (ADI) a subject can safely consume over the lifetime.[91] In general, limited human studies have shown that these non-nutritive sweeteners when added to diet of the diabetic patient exerted no effect on glycemic control in patients with diabetes.[92,93] It is important to realize that aspartame is made of two amino acids, phenylalanine and aspartic acid chemically bonded by methanol. Both amino acids dissociate when aspartame is heated or kept for longer period of time in solution (i.e., diet drinks containing aspartame). If needed, in the preparation of hot meal, aspartame should be added after the meal is cooked. Permissible ADI for saccharin for children is 500 mg per day and for adult 1,000 mg per day; for aspartame 50 mg per kg of body weight per day; and for sucralose 5 mg per kg of body weight. For stevia ADI has not been determined. The patients with diabetes may use the FDA approved sugar substitutes of their choice and consume in moderation the recommended amount of acceptable daily intake. The patients should be educated when buying prepared food items that the label on the food item stating "sugar-free" may not be necessarily "calorie-free".

CONCLUSION AND RECOMMENDATIONS

Nutritional counseling is an important aspect of management of diabetes. A good assessment of patient's food habits by FFQ or a simple food diary is essential in planning for nutritional therapy. Dietician assumes an important role in outlining the nutritional goal and educating the patient in achieving the goal. The patient's primary care provider should be aware of these nutritional goals, understands difficulties and barriers the patient may encounter and willing to facilitate in patient overcoming these difficulties and barriers. Appropriate help from social worker is important to help patient overcome personal, family, and work barriers. A motivational interview from patient's primary care provider and help from a psychologist can also be useful in achieving nutritional goals. Ultimately, it is the patient who should be comfortable with the dietary goals and his or her determination on adhering to the acceptable dietary goals.

It is important to customize the diet for a diabetic patient keeping in mind patient's dietary preferences, working situation, social environment and ethnicity. Ideally, a balanced diet with adequate carbohydrate, protein and fat distribution of total calorie consumption is recommended. As a guideline, 60–70% calories be comprised of carbohydrate and MUFA. The patient should be encouraged to consume carbohydrate in the form of whole grains, legumes, fruits, and low-fat milk and milk products. Fiber intake should be more than 25 g/day. In diabetic patients without chronic kidney disease, 15–20% of calories to be consumed as proteins in the diet. In patient with chronic kidney disease, the protein intake should be reduced to 0.8 g per kg of body weight. Saturated fat should not be consumed more that 7% of total calories. Salt intake should be limited to no more than 2,400 mg/day and cholesterol intake should be less than 200 mg per day. FDA approved sugar substitutes may be taken in moderation according to acceptable daily intake level. It is important to understand that buying prepared food items with label "sugar-free" may not be "calorie-free".

The total calorie consumption should be tailored with daily activity and exercise level for weight reduction and maintenance goals. Knowledge of glycemic index and glycemic load will help in appropriate meal planning with insulin therapy. Prepared meal concept may help patient in the weight reduction plan. Although complicated, understanding of food exchange may help diabetic patient further in achieving nutritional goals.

REFERENCES

1. Murata GH, Shah JH, Duckworth WC, Wendel CS, Mohler MJ, Hoffman RM. Food frequency questionnaire results correlate with metabolic control in insulin-treated veterans with type 2 diabetes: the Diabetes Outcomes in Veterans Study. *J Am Diet Assoc.* 2004;104:1816-26.
2. Franz MJ, Bantle JP, Beebe CA, Brunzell JD, Chiasson JL, Garg A, et al. Evidence-based nutrition principles and recommendations for the treatment and prevention of diabetes and related complications. *Diabetes Care.* 2003;26(Suppl 1):S51-61.
3. Hernández-Ronquillo L, Téllez-Zenteno JF, Garduño-Espinosa J, González-Acevez E. Factors associated with therapy noncompliance in type-2 diabetes patients. *Salud Publica Mex.* 2003;45:191-7.
4. Close EJ, Wiles PG, Lockton JA, Walmsley D, Oldham J, Wales JK. The degree of day-to-day variation in food intake in diabetic patients. *Diabet Med.* 1993;10:514-20.
5. Neuhouser ML, Miller DL, Kristal AR, Barnett MJ, Cheskin LJ. Diet and exercise habits of patients with diabetes, dyslipidemia, cardiovascular disease or hypertension. *J Am Coll Nutr.* 2002;21:394-401.

6. Toeller M, Klischan A, Heitkamp G, Schumacher W, Milne R, Buyken A, et al. Nutritional intake of 2868 IDDM patients from 30 centers in Europe. EURODIAB IDDM Complications Study Group. *Diabetologia*. 1996;39:929-39.

7. Eeley EA, Stratton IM, Hadden DR, Turner RC, Holman RR. UKPDS 18: estimated dietary intake in type 2 diabetic patients randomly allocated to diet, sulphonylurea or insulin therapy. UK Prospective Diabetes Study Group. *Diabet Med*. 1996;13:656-62.

8. American Diabetes Association, Bantle JP, Wylie-Rosett J, Albright AL, Apovian CM, Clark NG, et al. Nutritional recommendations and interventions for diabetes: a position statement of the American Diabetes Association. *Diabetes Care*. 2008;31(Suppl 1):S61-78.

9. Franz MJ, Powers MA, Leontos C, Holzmeister LA, Kulkarni K, Monk A, et al. The evidence for medical nutrition therapy for type 1 and type 2 diabetes in adults. *J Am Diet Assoc*. 2010;110:1852-89.

10. Bandura A. Social Foundations of Thought and Action. Englewood Cliffs: Prentice-Hall; 1986.

11. Hampson SE, Glasgow RE, Foster LS. Personal models of diabetes among older adults: relationship to self-management and other variables. *Diabetes Educ*. 1995;21:300-7.

12. Glasgow RE, Hampson SE, Strycker LA, Ruggiero L. Personal-model beliefs and social-environmental barriers related to diabetes self-management. *Diabetes Care*. 1997;20:556-61.

13. Hu FB, Rimm E, Smith-Warner SA, Feskanich D, Stampfer MJ, Ascherio A, et al. Reproducibility and validity of dietary patterns assessed with a food-frequency questionnaire. *Am J Clin Nutr*. 1999;69:243-9.

14. Riley MD, Blizzard L. Comparative validity of a food frequency questionnaire for adults with IDDM. *Diabetes Care*. 1995;18:1249-54.

15. Feskanich D, Rimm EB, Giovannucci EL, Colditz GA, Stampfer MJ, Litin LB, et al. Reproducibility and validity of food intake measurements from a semiquantitative food frequency questionnaire. *J Am Diet Assoc*. 1993;93:790-6.

16. Murata GH, Shah JH, Wendel CS, Hoffman RM, Adam KD, Bokhari SU, et al. Risk factor management in stable, insulin-treated patients with type 2 diabetes: the Diabetes Outcomes in Veterans Study. *J Diabetes Complications*. 2003;17:186-91.

17. Murata GH, Shah JH, Adam KD, Wendel CS, Bokhari SU, Solvas PA, et al. Factors affecting diabetes knowledge in type 2 diabetic veterans. *Diabetologia*. 2003;46:1170-8.

18. Kristal AR, Abrams BF, Thornquist MD, Disogra L, Croyle RT, Shattuck AL, et al. Development and validation of a food use checklist for evaluation of community nutrition interventions. *Am J Public Health*. 1990;80:1318-22.

19. Marcus MD, Wing RR, Guare J, Blair EH, Jawad A. Lifetime prevalence of major depression and its effect on treatment outcome in obese type II diabetic patients. *Diabetes Care*. 1992;15:253-5.

20. Wing RR, Marcus MD, Blair EH, Epstein LH, Burton LR. Depressive symptomatology in obese adults with type II diabetes. *Diabetes Care*. 1990;13:170-2.

21. Turner RC, Cull CA, Frighi V, Holman RR. Glycemic control with diet, sulfonylurea, metformin, or insulin in patients with type 2 diabetes mellitus: progressive requirement for multiple therapies (UKPDS 49). UK Prospective Diabetes Study (UKPDS) Group. *JAMA*. 1999;281:2005-12.

22. Pasanisi F, Contaldo F, de Simone G, Mancini M. Benefits of sustained moderate weight loss in obesity. *Nutr Metab Cardiovasc Dis*. 2001;11:401-6.

23. Albright A, Franz M, Hornsby G, Kriska A, Marrero D, Ullrich I, et al. American College of Sports Medicine position stand. Exercise and type 2 diabetes. *Med Sci Sports Exerc.* 2000;32:1345-60.

24. Conn VS, Hafdahl AR, Mehr DR, LeMaster JW, Brown SA, Nielsen PJ. Metabolic effects of interventions to increase exercise in adults with type 2 diabetes. *Diabetologia.* 2007; 50:913-21.

25. McAuley PA, Myers JN, Abella JP, Tan SY, Froelicher VF. Exercise capacity and body mass as predictors of mortality among male veterans with type 2 diabetes. *Diabetes Care.* 2007;30:1539-43.

26. Church TS, Cheng YJ, Earnest CP, Barlow CE, Gibbons LW, Priest EL, et al. Exercise capacity and body composition as predictors of mortality among men with diabetes. *Diabetes Care.* 2004;27:83-8.

27. Sigal RJ, Kenny GP, Boulé NG, Wells GA, Prud'homme D, Fortier M, et al. Effects of aerobic training, resistance training, or both on glycemic control in type 2 diabetes: a randomized trial. *Ann Intern Med.* 2007;147:357-69.

28. Kelley GA, Kelley KS. Effects of aerobic exercise on lipids and lipoproteins in adults with type 2 diabetes: a meta-analysis of randomized-controlled trials. *Public Health.* 2007;121(9): 643-55.

29. Dhindsa P, Scott AR, Donnelly R. Metabolic and cardiovascular effects of very-low-calorie diet therapy in obese patients with type 2 diabetes in secondary failure: outcomes after 1 year. *Diabet Med.* 2003;20:319-24.

30. Mertz JA, Stern JS, Kris-Etherton P, Reusser ME, Morris CD, Hatton DC, et al. A randomized trial of improved weight loss with a prepared meal plan in overweight and obese patients: impact on cardiovascular risk reduction. *Arch Intern Med.* 2000;160:2150-8.

31. Miles JM, Leiter L, Hollander P, Wadden T, Anderson JW, Doyle M, et al. Effect of orlistat in overweight and obese patients with type 2 diabetes treated with metformin. *Diabetes Care.* 2002;25:1123-8.

32. Redmon JB, Raatz SK, Reck KP, Swanson JE, Kwong CA, Fan Q, et al. One-year outcome of a combination of weight loss therapies for subjects with type 2 diabetes: a randomized trial. *Diabetes Care.* 2003;26:2505-11.

33. Derosa G, Cicero AF, Murdolo G, Ciccarelli L, Fogari R. Comparison of metabolic effects of orlistat and sibutramine treatment in type 2 diabetic obese patients. *Diabetes Nutr Metab.* 2004;17:222-9.

34. Wolf AM, Conaway MR, Crowther JQ, Hazen KY, L Nadler J, Oneida B, et al. Translating lifestyle intervention to practice in obese patients with type 2 diabetes: Improving Control with Activity And Nutrition (ICAN) study. *Diabetes Care.* 2004;27: 1570-6.

35. Herbst A, Kordonouri O, Schwab KO, Schmidt F, Holl RW; DPV Initiative of the German Working Group for Pediatric Diabetology Germany. Impact of physical activity on cardiovascular risk factors in children with type 1 diabetes: a multicenter study of 23,251 patients. *Diabetes Care.* 2007;30:2098-100.

36. Guelfi KJ, Jones TW, Fournier PA. New insights in managing the risk of hypoglycaemia associated with intermittent high-intensity exercise in individuals with type 1 diabetes mellitus: implications for existing guidelines. *Sports Med.* 2007;37:937-46.

37. Rachmiel M, Buccino J, Daneman D. Exercise and type 1 diabetes mellitus in youth: review and recommendations. *Pediatr Endocrinol Rev.* 2007;5:656-65.

38. Tanasescu M, Leitzmann MF, Rimm EB, Hu FB. Physical activity in relation to cardiovascular disease and total mortality among men with type 2 diabetes. *Circulation.* 2003;107:2435-9.

39. Powell KE, Heath GW, Kresnow MJ, Sacks JJ, Branche CM. Injury rates from walking, gardening, weightlifting, outdoor bicycling, and aerobics. *Med Sci Sports Exerc.* 1998; 30:1246-9.

40. Look AHEAD Research Group, Pi-Sunyer X, Blackburn G, Brancati FL, Bray GA, Bright R, et al. Reduction in weight and cardiovascular disease risk factors in individuals with type 2 diabetes: one-year results of the look AHEAD trial. *Diabetes Care.* 2007;30:1374-83.

41. Wing RR, Jeffery RW. Effect of modest weight loss on changes in cardiovascular risk factors: are there differences between men and women or between weight loss and maintenance? *Int J Obes Relat Metab Disord.* 1995;19:67-73.

42. Williamson DF, Thompson TJ, Thun M, Flanders D, Pamuk E, Byers T. Intentional weight loss and mortality among overweight individuals with diabetes. *Diabetes Care.* 2000;23:1499-504.

43. Henry RR, Scheaffer L, Olefsky JM. Glycemic effects of intensive caloric restriction and isocaloric refeeding in noninsulin-dependent diabetes mellitus. *J Clin Endocrinol Metab.* 1985;61:917-25.

44. Wing RR, Blair EH, Bononi P, Marcus MD, Watanabe R, Bergman RN. Caloric restriction per se is a significant factor in improvements in glycemic control and insulin sensitivity during weight loss in obese NIDDM patients. *Diabetes Care.* 1994;17:30-6.

45. UK Prospective Diabetes Study 7: response of fasting plasma glucose to diet therapy in newly presenting type II diabetic patients, UKPDS Group. *Metabolism.* 1990;39:905-12.

46. Escott-Stump S. Nutrition and Diagnosis-Related Care, 5th edition. Hagerstown, MD: Lippincott Williams & Wilkins; 2002.

47. Institutes of Medicine, Food and Nutrition Board. Dietary reference intakes for energy, carbohydrate, fiber, fat, fatty acids, cholesterol, protein, and amino acids. Washington, DC: National Academies Press; 2002.

48. Ryan DH, Espeland MA, Foster GD, Haffner SM, Hubbard VS, Johnson KC, et al. Look AHEAD (Action for Health in Diabetes): design and methods for a clinical trial of weight loss for the prevention of cardiovascular disease in type 2 diabetes. *Control Clin Trials.* 2003;24:610-28.

49. Diabetes Prevention Program (DPP) Research Group. The Diabetes Prevention Program (DPP): description of lifestyle intervention. *Diabetes Care.* 2002;25:2165-71.

50. Yip I, Go VL, DeShields S, Saltsman P, Bellman M, Thames G, et al. Liquid meal replacements and glycemic control in obese type 2 diabetes patients. *Obes Res.* 2001;9(Suppl 4):341S-47S.

51. Flechtner-Mors M, Ditschuneit HH, Johnson TD, Suchard MA, Adler G. Metabolic and weight loss effects of long-term dietary intervention in obese patients: four-year results. *Obes Res.* 2000;8:399-402.

52. Quinn Rothacker D. Five-year self-management of weight using meal replacements: comparison with matched controls in rural Wisconsin. *Nutrition.* 2000;16:344-8.

53. Pi-Sunyer FX, Maggio CA, McCarron DA, Reusser ME, Stern JS, Haynes RB, et al. Multicenter randomized trial of a comprehensive prepared meal program in type 2 diabetes. *Diabetes Care.* 1999;22:191-7.

54. Pastors JG, Waslaski J, Gunderson H. Diabetes meal-planning strategies. In: Ross TA, Boucher JL, O'Connell BS (Eds). American Dietetic Association Guide to Diabetes Medical Nutrition Therapy and Education. Chicago, IL: American Dietetic Association; 2005. p. 201.

55. Shah M, Adams-Huet B, Bantle JP, Henry RR, Griver KA, Raatz SK, et al. Effect of a high-carbohydrate versus a high—cis-monounsaturated fat diet on blood pressure in patients with type 2 diabetes. *Diabetes Care.* 2005;28:2607-12.

56. Nordmann AJ, Nordmann A, Briel M, Keller U, Yancy WS, Brehm BJ, et al. Effects of low-carbohydrate vs low-fat diets on weight loss and cardiovascular risk factors: a meta-analysis of randomized controlled trials. *Arch Intern Med.* 2006;166:285-93.

57. Barnard ND, Gloede L, Cohen J, Jenkins DJ, Turner-McGrievy G, Green AA, et al. A low-fat vegan diet elicits greater macronutrient changes, but is comparable in adherence and acceptability, compared with a more conventional diabetes diet among individuals with type 2 diabetes. *J Am Diet Assoc.* 2009;109:263-72.

58. Turner-McGrievy GM, Barnard ND, Cohen J, Jenkins DJ, Gloede L, Green AA. Changes in nutrient intake and dietary quality among participants with type 2 diabetes following a low-fat vegan diet of a conventional diabetes diet for 22 weeks. *J Am Diet Assoc.* 2008; 108:1636-45.

59. Wolever TM, Gibbs AL, Mehling C, Chiasson JL, Connelly PW, Josse RG, et al. The Canadian Trial of Carbohydrates in Diabetes (CCD), a 1-year controlled trial of low-glycemic-index dietary carbohydrate in type 2 diabetes: no effect on glycated hemoglobin but reduction in C-reactive protein. *Am J Clin Nutr.* 2008;87:114-25.

60. Brehm BJ, Lattin BL, Summer SS, Boback JA, Gilchrist GM, Jandacek RJ, et al. One year comparison of high-monounsaturated fat diet with a high-carbohydrate diet in type 2 diabetes. *Diabetes Care.* 2009;32:215-20.

61. Xu J, Eilat-Adar S, Loria CM, Howard BV, Fabsitz RR, Begum M, et al. Macronutrient intake and glycemic control in a population-based sample of American Indians with diabetes: the Strong Heart Study. *Am J Clin Nutr.* 2007;86:480-7.

62. Delahanty LM, Nathan DM, Lachin JM, Hu FB, Cleary PA, Ziegler GK, et al. Association of diet with glycated hemoglobin during intensive treatment of type 1 diabetes in the Diabetes Control and Complications Trial. *Am J Clin Nutr.* 2009;89:518-24.

63. Esposito K, Maiorino MI, Ciotola M, Di Palo C, Scognamiglio P, Gicchino M, et al. Effects of a Mediterranean-style diet on the need for antihyperglycemic drug therapy in patients with newly diagnosed type 2 diabetes: a randomized trial. *Ann Intern Med.* 2009;151:306-14.

64. Parker B, Noakes M, Luscombe N, Clifton P. Effect of a high-protein diet, high-mono-unsaturated fat weight loss diet on glycemic control and lipid levels in type 2 diabetes. *Diabetes Care.* 2002;25:425-30.

65. Brinkworth GD, Noakes M, Parker B, Foster P, Clifton PM. Long-term effect of advise to consume high-protein, low-fat diet, rather than a conventional weight-loss diet, in obese adults with type 2 diabetes: one-year follow-up of a randomised trial. *Diabetologia.* 2004;47:1677-86.

66. Nuttall FQ, Gannon MC, Saeed A, Jordan K, Hoover H. The metabolic response of subjects with type 2 diabetes to a high-protein, weight-maintenance diet. *J Clin Edocrinol Metab.* 2003;88:3577-83.

67. Velázquez López L, Sil Acosta MJ, Goycochea Robles MV, Torres Tamayo M, Castañeda Limones R. Effect of protein restriction diet on renal function and metabolic control in patients with type 2 diabetes: a randomized clinical trial. *Nutr Hosp.* 2008;23:141-7.

68. Dussol B, Lovanna C, Raccah D, Darmon P, Morange S, Vague P, et al. A randomized trial of low-protein diet in type 1 and in type 2 diabetes mellitus patients with incipient and overt nephropathy. *J Ren Nutr.* 2005;15:398-406.

69. Wolever TM, Nguyen PM, Chiasson JL, Hunt JA, Josse RG, Palmason C, et al. Determinants of diet glycemic index calculated retrospectively from diet records of 342 individuals with non-insulin-dependent diabetes mellitus. *Am J Clin Nutr.* 1994;59:1265-9.

70. Jenkins DJ, Wolever TM, Taylor RH, Barker H, Fielden H, Baldwin JM, et al. Glycemic index of foods: a physiological basis for carbohydrate exchange. *Am J Clin Nutr.* 1981;34:362-6.

71. Liu S, Willett WC, Stampfer MJ, Hu FB, Franz M, Sampson L, et al. A prospective study of dietary glycemic load, carbohydrate intake, and risk of coronary heart disease in US women. *Am J Clin Nutr.* 2000;71:1455-61.

72. Liu S. Insulin resistance, hyperglycemia and risk of major chronic diseases: a dietary perspective. Proceedings of the Nutrition Society of Australia. 1998;22:140-50.

73. Buyken AE, Toeller M, Heitkamp G, Karamanos B, Rottiers R, Muggeo M, et al. Glycemic index in the diet of European outpatients with type 1 diabetes: relations to glycated hemoglobin and serum lipids. *Am J Clin Nutr.* 2001;73:574-81.

74. Brand-Miller J, Hayne S, Petocz P, Colagiuri S. Low-glycemic index diets in the management of diabetes: a meta-analysis of randomized controlled trials. *Diabetes Care.* 2003; 26:2261-7.

75. Ma Y, Olendzki BC, Merriam PA, Chiriboga DE, Culver AL, Li W, et al. A randomized clinical trial comparing low-glycemic index versus ADA dietary education among individuals with type 2 diabetes. *Nutrition.* 2008;24:45-56.

76. Vega-López S, Ausman LM, Griffith JL, Lichtenstein AH. interindividual variability and intraindividual reproducibility of glycemic index values for commercial white bread. *Diabetes Care.* 2007;30:1412-7.

77. Dumesnil JG, Turgeon J, Tremblay A, Poirier P, Gilbert M, Gagnon L, et al. Effect of a low-glycemic index—low-fat—high protein diet on the atherogenic metabolic risk profile of abdominally obese men. *Br J Nutr.* 2001;86:557-68.

78. Franz MJ, Bantle JP, Beebe CA, Brunzell JD, Chiasson JL, Garg A, et al. Evidence-based nutrition principles and recommendations for the treatment and prevention of diabetes and related complications. *Diabetes Care.* 2002;25:148-98.

79. Anderson JW. Fiber and health: an overview. *Am J Gastroenterol.* 1986;81:892-7.

80. Shah JH. The use of fiber in dietary management of diabetes and hyperlipidemia. In: Chandalia HB, Shah JH, (editors). Endocrinology, Diabetes and Metabolism. The Research Society, J.J. Group of Hospitals and Grant Medical College, Mumbai, India. 1996. pp. 208-17.

81. Jenkins DJ. Dietary fibre, diabetes, and hyperlipidaemia. Progress and prospects. *Lancet.* 1979;2:1287-90.

82. Anderson JW, Bridges SR. Dietary fiber content of selected foods. *Am J Clin Nutr.* 1988; 47:440-7.

83. Giacco R, Parillo M, Rivellese AA, Lasorella G, Giacco A, D'Episcopo L, et al. Long-term dietary treatment with increased amounts of fiber-rich low-glycemic index natural foods improves blood glucose control and reduces the number of hypoglycemic events in type 1 diabetic patients. *Diabetes Care.* 2000;23:1461-6.

84. Chandalia M, Garg A, Lutjohann D, von Bergmann K, Grundy SM, Brinkley LJ. Beneficial effects of high dietary fiber intake in patients with type 2 diabetes mellitus. *N Engl J Med.* 2000;342:1392-8.

85. Kinmonth AL, Angus RM, Jenkins PA, Smith MA, Baum JD. Whole foods and increased dietary fiber improve blood glucose control in diabetic children. *Arch Dis Child.* 1982;57: 187-94.

86. Del Toma E, Lintas C, Clementi A, Marcelli M. Soluble and insoluble dietary fibre in diabetic diets. *Eur J Clin Nutr.* 1988;42:313-9.

87. McCulloch DK, Mitchell RD, Ambler J, Tattersall RB. A prospective comparison of "conventional" and high carbohydrate/high fibre/low fat diets in adults with established type 1 (insulin-dependent) diabetes. *Diabetologia.* 1985;28:208-12.

88. Stevens J, Burgess MB, Kaiser DL, Sheppa CM. Outpatient management of diabetes mellitus with patient education to increase dietary carbohydrate and fiber. *Diabetes Care.* 1985;8:359-66.

89. Milne RM, Mann JI, Chisholm AW, Williams SM. Long-term comparison of three dietary prescriptions in the treatment of NIDDM. *Diabetes Care.* 1994;17:74-80.

90. Anderson JW, Zeigler JA, Deakins DA, Floore TL, Dillon DW, Wood CL, et al. Metabolic effects of high-carbohydrate, high-fiber diets for insulin-dependent diabetic individuals. *Am J Clin Nutr.* 1991;54:936-43.

91. American Dietetic Association. Position of the American Dietetic Association: use of nutritive and nonnutritive sweeteners. *J Am Diet Assoc.* 2004;104:255-75.

92. Grotz VL, Henry RR, McGill JB, Prince MJ, Shamoon H, Trout JR, et al. Lack of effect of sucralose on glucose homeostasis in subjects with type 2 diabetes. *J Am Diet Assoc.* 2003;103:1607-12.

93. Maki KC, Curry LL, Reeves MS, Toth PD, McKenney JM, Farmer MV, et al. Chronic consumption of rebaudioside A, a steviol glycoside, in men and women with type 2 diabetes mellitus. *Food Chem Toxicol.* 2008;46(Suppl 7):S47-53.

Oral Agents in the Treatment of Diabetic Patients

7
Chapter

Stephen P Thomson

ABSTRACT

Oral diabetes medications (ODM) have a prominent role in the treatment of adults with diabetes mellitus (DM) type 2. Several billion dollars are used each year to treat tens of millions of patients around the globe. Oral hypoglycemic agents are often started at the time of diagnosis of diabetes because so few people are successful with the far superior treatment of weight loss and adequate exercise. This chapter emphasizes the practical and cost-effective use of oral diabetes medications. The following section presents an algorithm for the use of ODM within the overall sequence for the evaluation and treatment of DM. The sections that follow discuss the individual medications, their use for the prevention of DM, during hospitalization, during pregnancy, and conclude with how ODM are just one of several necessary components in the overall approach to control DM.

INTRODUCTION

Oral agents have a prominent role in the treatment of adults with diabetes mellitus (DM) type 2. Several billion dollars are spent each year to treat tens of millions of patients around the globe. The presentation and progression of DM often follows a very typical pattern. People with inadequate exercise and excessive caloric consumption slowly develop visceral adiposity, glucose intolerance, and insulin resistance. When this has progressed enough to cause fasting blood glucose of greater than or equal to 7 mmol/L (126 mg/dL) or glycosylated hemoglobin (A1c) greater than or equal to 6.5%, they are given the diagnosis of DM.[1] Oral hypoglycemic agents (OHAs) are often started at the time of diagnosis because few people are successful with the far superior treatment of weight loss and adequate exercise. Monotherapy with metformin is by far the most common initial medication.[1-4] The oral medications have only moderate potency. Often monotherapy can only be used for a few years because DM progresses due to aging and the failure of patients to lose weight and increase exercise. After metformin fails to meet glucose goals, a second oral agent or basal insulin is added to control glucose. Finally, in many patients, DM progresses enough that often all oral agents can be stopped and intensive, relatively high-dose insulin is required to control glucose.

The lack of high quality long-term clinical outcome data for any of the oral DM medications limits the ability to determine the actual overall net benefit of any oral agent.[2,5] Furthermore, there are no high quality long-term studies that provide the "head to head" direct comparisons needed to truly establish the relative effectiveness of the oral DM medications. Thus, oral agents are selected for algorithms and by practitioners for clinical use, based on each agent's limited effect on clinical outcomes, initial and sustained glucose-lowering abilities, side effects, ease of use, and expense.

Many studies done to establish the current oral DM medications and get approval from regulatory authorities used surrogate subclinical end-points, typically glucose-lowering ability, in small studies with short-term durations of 6–12 months. This is a practical approach but it has led to approval of agents with unanticipated but very significant off-target effects. These effects have included liver failure, weight gain, heart failure, bone fractures, and cardiac events that have led to restrictions or removal of oral diabetes medications from the market. These concerns have recently led the Food and Drug Administration (FDA) to require demonstration of glucose-lowering effects and ascertainment of cardiovascular safety prior to approval of new agents.[6] These requirements have the potential to increase the expense of DM drug development but aim to limit the approval and use of medications with significant adverse clinical effects. Practitioners using the newer, more expensive agents should be aware of that the lack of long-term clinical outcome data combined with modest, nonsuperior glucose-lowering effects means these agents may have modest, if any, long-term net clinical benefit. Individuals and societies concerned with cost effectiveness may be asking, "why should we spend many billions of dollars more for nonsuperior newer, expensive medications without clear demonstration of long-term clinical benefit and safety"?[5]

Expense should not be the first consideration. However, when newer and more expensive medications are nonsuperior to well-validated, less expensive medications, as is the case for metformin and the sulfonylurea class compared to the others, it makes little sense to spend money on expensive agents. Diabetes mellitus is no longer just prevalent in developed countries with the most resources to devote to DM treatments.[7] Indeed developing countries have some of the largest numbers of people with DM and have been unable to extend enough resources to fully treat these populations. These facts show how important it is to avoid paying extra for nonsuperior oral diabetes medications. The savings from using more cost-effective metformin and sulfonylurea agents could be used to fund other aspects of DM prevention, control, and treatment programs. Newer, less well-validated and very expensive oral medications should be reserved for those intolerant of metformin or sulfonylurea agents or in limited special situations as described below.

This chapter emphasizes the practical and cost-effective use of oral diabetes medications. There is widespread acceptance of metformin monotherapy as the preferred initial medication. It is as potent as all other oral agents, is associated with less weight gain, seldom causes significant hypoglycemia, has mild and often transient side effects when used correctly, and is much less expensive than second-tier medications. Although there are limited studies showing a positive effect of metformin on long-term clinical outcomes, both metformin and sulfonylurea agents have much more safety and long-term outcome data than the newer, second-tier and much more expensive oral diabetes medications. The following section presents an algorithm for the use of oral diabetes medications within the overall sequence for the evaluation and treatment of DM. Then sections will discuss the individual medications, their use for the prevention of DM, during hospitalization, during pregnancy and conclude with how oral diabetes medications are just one of several necessary components in the overall approach to control DM.

INITIATION AND CHRONIC USE OF ORAL DIABETES MEDICATIONS

Prior to starting oral diabetes medications, the diagnosis of DM should be confirmed and an initial evaluation done to assess possible exclusions for outpatient treatment with oral medications. Patients with DM have a fasting glucose of greater than or equal to 7 mmol/L (126 mg/dL) or A1c greater than or equal to 6.5%. Patients with diabetic ketoacidosis, who are markedly hyperosmolar or are unable to maintain oral hydration are poor candidates for outpatient initiation of oral diabetes agents and should be considered for hospitalization. These patients and those with fasting blood glucose greater than or equal to 13.9 mmol/L (250 mg/dL), random glucose over 16.7 mmol/L (300 mg/dL), A1c greater than 10% or symptoms of polyuria, polydipsia, and weight loss should be considered for insulin treatment rather than oral diabetes medications. A practical and cost-effective algorithm for the treatment of adults with DM is presented in figure 1. It is modeled after the one developed by the American Diabetes Association (ADA) and the European Association for the Study of Diabetes.[8]

Algorithm Step 1

The first steps are lifestyle interventions, elimination of excess caloric intake, and increase in exercise. These interventions are often guided by the provider and associated professionals, often registered dieticians, with experience in behavioral modification therapies. There is increasing realization that success in this and all therapies for DM requires full participation of the patients themselves. Recognizing this central role of the patient, DM care teams should provide patients with self-management education

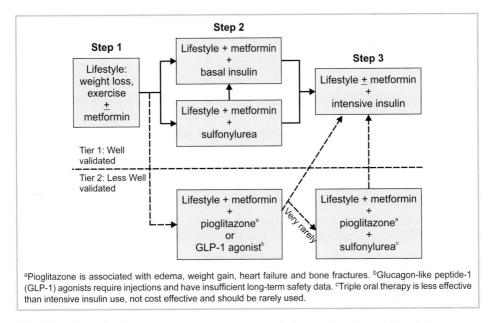

FIGURE 1 Algorithm for the management of glucose in type 2 diabetes. Lifestyle interventions to eliminate excess calories and adequate exercise are needed throughout treatment of diabetes mellitus (DM). Check A1c every 3 months initially and advance to the next step if it is not at goal A1c greater than or equal to 7%. Less well-validated therapies are shown in tier 2.

so that they can develop skills to manage their DM in partnership with their care teams. When the lifestyle interventions are successful, not only does glucose improve, but lipids and blood pressure improve as well. Removal of excess caloric intake and maintenance of adequate exercise should remain a fundamental part of treatment throughout the entire course of the disease as shown in algorithm steps 1, 2, and 3 (Figure 1). Unfortunately, the majority of patients are not completely successful with lifestyle interventions. So it is recommended that metformin should be started concurrently with lifestyle interventions at the time of diagnosis.[8]

Metformin is typically started at lower doses and taken with meals to minimize gastrointestinal adverse effects and then advanced as tolerated. Contraindications for metformin use include renal dysfunction and conditions that may predispose an individual to lactic acidosis such as heart failure, liver disease, or poor tissue perfusion. For those patients with intolerance or contraindications, using low-dose basal insulin as the initial treatment can be considered. Oral diabetes medications other than metformin can also be considered as the first medication when metformin is contraindicated. However, with the exception of the sulfonylurea agents, they do not have long-term safety and clinical outcome data required to become well-validated therapies.

Algorithm Step 2

Patients should move to step 2 interventions after 3 months if they do not obtain or sustain glucose goals with metformin and lifestyle interventions. If patients successfully eliminate excess caloric intake and maintain adequate exercise then they often can delay significant progression of DM and maintain glucose goals using monotherapy for many years. However, most patients exceed their glucose goals within a few years due to a combination of the failure to achieve lifestyle goals, increasing insulin resistance and a decline in endogenous insulin production capacity. These patients will need to add either basal insulin or a sulfonylurea. Either therapy can lower A1c by about 1%. If the A1c is over 8.5%, consider basal insulin because with proper dose adjustment, it can lower A1c more than 1%. The available limited long-term clinical outcome data comparing these therapies do not show a clear advantage of one over the other.[2] Many patients prefer to delay insulin for as long as possible, mainly to avoid the injections and inconvenience, and prefer to add an oral sulfonylurea as the second step. A sulfonylurea or basal insulin may also be needed sooner if there is significant intolerance or contraindication to metformin. Use of metformin and night-time basal neutral protamine Hagedorn (NPH) insulin is associated with slightly less short-term weight gain than the combination of metformin and a sulfonylurea.[9] It is not known if this slight difference in weight leads to significant differences in clinical outcomes. If the combination of a sulfonylurea and metformin do not achieve or sustain glucose goals then the sulfonylurea should be stopped when basal or intensive insulin is added because it is not considered synergistic with insulin use. A sub-study that treated obese patients with DM in the UK Prospective Diabetes Study (UKPDS) found that early addition of metformin to a sulfonylurea therapy might increase the fatality rates.[10] These observations have not been confirmed and the mortality rate is very low; therefore, this potential risk of combination therapy has not been clearly established.

Second-tier therapies are less well validated, mainly because they lack the long-term clinical outcome data that would clearly establish their usefulness. It is clear that the addition of these agents can typically decrease A1c by another 1%. This is similar to the initial 1% decrease seen with metformin and the further 1% decrease seen with more well-validated first-tier agents basal insulin and the oral sulfonylurea class. This additive effect of glucose lowering has made some second-tier therapies quite popular, including the use of tablets combining them with metformin, despite the lack of clinical efficacy data. The most commonly used second-tier oral agents are pioglitazone from the thiazolidinedione (TZD) class and the dipeptidyl peptidase-4 inhibitors (DPP-4)—sitagliptin, vildagliptin in Europe, saxagliptin, and recently linagliptin. The incretin mimetics—exenatide and laraglutide require injection, are expensive and are less commonly used second-tier agents. The precise role of the TZD class is not clear because their use has not shown a net benefit on long-term clinical outcomes. The first agent in this class, troglitazone, was withdrawn from the market due to an association with liver failure, including fatal liver failure. Rosiglitazone was on the market for a decade prior to learning of an association with cardiac events. This association led to it being severely restricted in the US market and removed from European markets. The TZD agents are also associated with bone fractures in women.[1,2]

The oral DPP-4 inhibitors inhibit the enzyme that degrades the main intestinal-derived endogenous human insulinotropic peptide hormones, glucagon-like peptide-1 (GLP-1) and glucose-dependent insulinotropic peptide (GIP). This inhibition of degradation prolongs the action of GLP-1 and GIP, and promotes the release of insulin associated with food ingestion, inhibits glucagon secretion, and decreases gastric motility. These actions decrease serum glucose. The oral DPP-4 inhibitors are weight neutral, unlike the injectable GLP-1 agonist that are associated with moderate weight loss. The DPP-4 inhibitors also inhibit peptides active in the immune system, and side-effects include an increase in nasopharyngitis, headaches, skin reactions, and pancreatitis. Similar to the TZD class, the precise role of oral DPP-4 inhibitors in the management of DM is not clear because of lack of studies on their effect on long-term clinical outcomes.

The other second-tier agents, the injectable GLP-1 agonists, exenatide (approved in the US 2005) and liraglutide (approved in Europe 2009, US 2010), are less commonly used second-tier agents. They increase the release of insulin associated with food ingestion, inhibit glucagon secretion, decrease gastric motility, and reduce appetite and liver fat content. These actions decrease serum glucose and are associated with moderate weight loss. Their gastrointestinal side effects, high cost and need for injection has limited patient acceptance.

Other second-tier, less well-validated oral agents, not shown in the algorithm, can be used in patients unable to tolerate the more widely used agents. These agents include the glinides—repaglinide and nateglinide; the alpha-glucosidase inhibitors—acarbose and miglitol; and colesevelam, a nonabsorbed polymer and bile-acid binder. They all have been shown to decrease glucose in short-term trials. They are used much less often than the other oral medications due to a combination of the lack of long-term clinical outcome data, side-effects and potency only similar to or less than that seen with metformin and expense.

Algorithm Step 3

If glycemic goals are not met or sustained with step 2 therapies—lifestyle, metformin and basal insulin, or sulfonylurea, then patients should start intensive insulin. Most patients lack enthusiasm for move to intensive insulin because of the increase in work required to get good results. They must take multiple injections, use more frequent self-monitoring of blood glucose (SMBG) and take a more consistent approach to meal timing and amounts than when they were taking oral agents or basal insulin. Note that the algorithm suggests ± metformin when advancing to intensive insulin therapy. Some practitioners prefer to continue metformin with intensive insulin, as it may be associated with less weight gain at least in the short term.[9] Other practitioners prefer to use intensive insulin without metformin, citing the lack of long-term data for metformin and intensive insulin on weight loss or improvement in clinical outcomes. There are also concerns that it increases the complexity of treatment in patients that already take many medications. The use of intensive insulin requires multiple daily injections, more intense attention to meal timing and amounts, frequent SMBG, and very careful dose adjustment with an emphasis on avoiding potentially lethal hypoglycemia.

The use of second-tier three oral agents in combination for step 3 is a less well-validated therapy. It is not a preferred treatment because there are no long-term clinical outcome studies that demonstrate a net advantage over alternatives. It is not more effective than insulin in lowering glucose and is more expensive. Some practitioners use it in special circumstances, including for patients performing potentially hazardous duties with an increased need to avoid hypoglycemia. Great care must still be used, however, because the use of 3 oral agents certainly can cause significant hypoglycemia, and has not been shown to offer enhanced protection from hypoglycemia.

GUIDANCE FOR USE OF SPECIFIC ORAL MEDICATIONS

This section will review the general features and use of specific medications. Since there are no high quality long-term studies that provide "head-to-head" direct comparisons of the oral medications, it is not possible to precisely establish their relative effectiveness. Metformin and sulfonylurea agents are first-tier medications based on their limited but positive effect on long-term clinical outcomes, initial and sustained glucose-lowering abilities, side effects, ease of use and expense. The other oral DM medications lack long-term clinical outcome data. Their general features, the data for glucose-lowering ability, side effects, ease of use, and expense will be presented. Most of the oral medications decrease A1c by approximately 1%.[2] Table 1 is a summary of OHA medication dosing, advantages and disadvantages.

Biquanides/Metformin

The main action of metformin is to lower hepatic glucose production and facilitate glucose uptake in peripheral tissues. It does not directly decrease insulin resistance and thus is not a true "insulin sensitizer". The main advantages include: the best long-term outcome data showing both cardiovascular and mortality benefit and safety,[8,10] association with the least amount of weight gain than all of the oral medications, potency as good as any of the other oral agents, very rare association with hypoglycemia, mild gastrointestinal side effects that often decrease over time, easy to use twice-a-day dosing, and very inexpensive. The main disadvantages include: contraindicated with renal insufficiency, and persistent gastrointestinal side effects in

TABLE 1: Main Features of Oral Hypoglycemic Agents (OHAs) and Injectable GLP-1 Agonists

OHA class/agent	Dosing		Advantages	Disadvantages
Biguanide/ Metformin	500 mg once or twice daily increase as needed, tolerated to 2,000–2,550 mg/day in divided doses		Lowers A1c 1%, as potent as any other OHA, safe, low cost	GI side-effects, do not use with renal insufficiency
Sulfonylurea/	*Starting*	*Maximum*	Works rapidly, low cost	Hypoglycemia, especially glibenclamide (glyburide) or chlorpropamide, weight gain, use caution when dosing with renal insufficiency
Glipizide	5 mg daily	20 mg daily		
Glimepiride	1–2 mg	8 mg daily		
Glicazide	80 mg BID	320 mg daily		
Glibencalmide	1.25–5 mg	20 mg daily		
Thiozolidines/	*Starting*	*Maximum*	Additive effect with other OHAs	Fluid retention, CHF, weight gain, fractures, very high cost, potential increase MI (rosiglitazone), bladder cancer, avoid with hepatic impairment
Pioglitazone	15–30 mg daily	45 mg daily		
Rosiglitazone	4 mg daily	8 mg daily		
DPP-4 inhibitor/			Weight neutral	Long-term efficacy and safety not known expensive, use caution and lower dose with significant renal insufficiency
Sitagliptin	100 mg daily			
Vildagliptin	50 mg BID			
Saxaglipitin	2.5–5 mg daily			
Linagliptin	5 mg daily			
Glucosidase inhibitors	*Starting*	*Maximum*	Weight neutral	Long-term efficacy and safety not known TID dosing, GI side-effects, expensive, avoid with significant renal impairment
Acabose	25 mg TID	150 mg daily		
Miglitol	25 mg TID	150 mg daily		
Glinides/	*Starting*	*Maximum*	Fast acting	Long-term efficacy and safety not known weight gain, TID dosing, expensive
Repaglinide	0.5–1 mg	16 mg daily		
Nateglinide	60–120 mg TID	360 mg daily		
GLP-1 agonists/	*Starting*	*Maximum*	Weight loss	Long-term efficacy and safety not known injectable, GI side-effects, very expensive
Exenatide	5 µg BID	10 µg BID		
Liraglutide	0.6 mg	1.2–1.8 mg daily		

some patients particularly when using maximal doses. Metformin can interfere with absorption of vitamin B_{12} but very rarely enough to be associated with anemia. Renal insufficiency, heart failure and conditions associated with poor tissue perfusion may increase the risk of lactic acidosis. Significant lactic acidosis is very rarely associated with metformin use in less than one case per 100,000 patients. Its use with excessive alcohol intake should be avoided as it can increase the effect of metformin on lactic acid metabolism. Metformin should be stopped prior to use of iodinated contrast materials for imaging studies and can be restarted 48 hours later. Taking it with food can decrease gastrointestinal upset. For pregnancy, adverse events have not been seen in animal studies and it is classified as pregnancy category B—no evidence of risk in humans.

Metformin is often started at lower doses, 500 mg once or twice a day, usually one with breakfast and one with the evening meal. If no significant gastrointestinal side effects occur, then in 2 weeks, increase to 1,000 mg twice a day. Clinically-significant responses typically require the use of greater than or equal to 1,000 mg/day. If there is intolerance of the higher doses, then decrease to tolerated dose for several weeks before another trial of the higher doses. The maximum effective dose is often 1,000 mg twice a day; some patients get slightly more effects at the maximum dose of 2,500 mg/day. Most favor use of the cost-effective generic forms. The longer acting forms do not confer additional clinical benefit and are typically less cost effective.

Sulfonylurea—Glipizide, Glimepiride, Gliclazide, Glibenclamide (Glyburide in US and Canada)

These agents are known as "insulin secretagogues" because their main action is to increase insulin release by inhibiting the potassium ATP channel of pancreatic beta cells. These medications were the first widely used oral diabetes medications, and are also known as OHAs. The above agents are the widely used second-generation agents. The first-generation agents—tolbutamide, acetohexamide, tolazamide, and chlorpropamide are less effective, have more side effects, and their use has been largely replaced by the second-generation agents. The main advantages of sulfonylurea agents include: modestly favorable effects on long-term clinical outcomes and safety, initial potency as good as any of the other oral agents, rapid onset of glucose-lowering effects, easy to use once- or twice-a-day dosing, and very inexpensive. The main disadvantages include: rare but potentially serious and prolonged hypoglycemia, more weight gain than metformin, and less maintenance of glucose-lowering effects than metformin.

The sulfonylurea agents are given with meals, once a day for the lower doses and twice a day for the higher doses. At half their maximal doses, they have very nearly maximal glucose-lowering effects. Therefore, maximal doses can generally be avoided. Prolonged, severe and potentially fatal hypoglycemia can rarely occur with any of the sulfonylurea agents but there is a higher association with glibenclamide (called glyburide in the US and Canada) and chlorpropamide. The risk of hypoglycemia increases when sulfonylurea agents are used in the elderly, or those with decreased caloric intake, drugs like ciprofloxicin, ethanol use or those with impaired renal, hepatic, adrenal, or pituitary function. To minimize the risk of severe hypoglycemia, providers should avoid using inpatients with increased risk and especially in the elderly with A1c much below 7%. Sulfonylurea agents for pregnancy are FDA category C—risk cannot be ruled out. Sulfonylurea agents can be used as monotherapy in patients intolerant of metformin. In addition, some providers have successfully used maximal-dose sulfonylurea agents in DM type 2 patients who present with very symptomatic hyperglycemia without ketoacidosis (Davidson 1992).[11]

Thiazolidinedione—Pioglitazone and Rosiglitazone

The TZD class of agents is peroxisome proliferator-activated receptor gamma modulators and act as "insulin sensitizers" to increase the sensitivity of muscle, fat, and liver to insulin. The main advantages of TZDs include: potency and maintenance of glucose-lowering effects similar to metformin,[2] easy to use once-a-day dosing, use in renal insufficiency and FDA approval for use in combination with metformin, sulfonylurea agents, glinides and insulin. The main disadvantages include: lack of studies on their effect on long-term clinical outcomes and safety, fluid retention, weight gain, twofold increase in heart failure, bone fractures, potential increase in myocardial infarction for rosiglitazone and extreme expense. Other potential disadvantages include: increase in risk of bladder cancer, macular edema, and an increase in the chance of pregnancy in premenopausal women who do not have regular monthly periods. The TZD agents have had failures and successes but they remain very controversial. They remain controversial because although they clearly provide glucose lowering by a unique mechanism, they cost billions of dollars each year without showing that they have a positive net long-term beneficial outcome.[5,12]

The first approved agent, troglitazone, was removed from the market after the discovery that is was associated with hepatitis and liver failure, including fatal liver failure. Rosiglitazone was removed from the European market by the European Medicine Agency in September 2010 and severely restricted in the US market by the FDA 10 years after its introduction due to discovery of an association with cardiovascular disease. Pioglitazone does not seem to share these adverse events, and in one prospective study it did not decrease the overall cardiovascular primary end-point but did decrease a secondary cardiovascular disease end-point.[13] However, in June of 2011, the FDA issued a special alert on an ongoing study on the potential increased risk of bladder cancer with pioglitazone.[14] The FDA recommends not using pioglitazone in patients who have active bladder cancer and to use caution in patients with a prior history of bladder cancer since the risk of recurrence induced by pioglitazone is unknown. The TZD class needs further study, particularly on its effect on clinical outcomes rather than the surrogate subclinical outcome of glucose lowering, before many will be convinced they provide enough positive clinical outcomes to justify their expense. The ADA and European Association for the Study of Diabetes consensus statement and algorithm placed pioglitazone as a second-tier agent because of concerns over adverse reactions and lack of long-term clinical outcome data.[8]

Although there have been endorsements for use of pioglitazone as a first-tier agent,[15] it should be used as a second-tier agent only in carefully selected patients (Figure 1). In the US, it must be dispensed with an FDA-approved patient medicine guide, which is available with the product information at http://www.accessdata.fda.gov/drugsatfda_docs/label/2009/021073s037lbl.pdf. Pioglitazone should not be used in patients with heart failure, significant hepatic impairment (transaminases ≥2.3 upper limit of normal), macular edema, and active bladder cancer; during pregnancy; in breastfeeding women, children, or in premenopausal women who do not have regular monthly periods. Thiazolidinediones for pregnancy are FDA category C—risk cannot be ruled out, and should not be used. In Canadian labeling, use with insulin is contraindicated, and the use of triple therapy (pioglitazone in combination with metformin and a sulfonylurea) is not indicated due to increased risk of congestive heart failure. Pioglitazone should be used with caution in patients with high cardiovascular risk, prior history of bladder cancer and those at risk for bone fractures. The FDA recommends monitoring of liver enzymes periodically during treatment and routine ophthalmic examinations.

DDP-4 Inhibitors—Sitagliptin, Vildagliptin, Saxagliptin, and Linagliptin

The main action of the DDP-4 inhibitors is to inhibit the enzyme dipeptidyl peptidase type 4, which inactivates the main intestinal-derived endogenous human insulino-tropic peptide hormones, GLP-1, and glucose-dependent insulinotropic peptide (GIP), the "incretin hormones". This inhibition of degradation prolongs the action of GLP-1 and GIP and promotes the release of insulin associated with food ingestion, inhibits glucagon secretion, and decreases gastric motility. These actions decrease serum glucose elevations after eating. The main advantages of DDP-4 inhibitors include: weight neutrality, easy to use once-a-day dosing, generally well tolerated, no hypoglycemia when used as monotherapy, and approved for use with metformin. The main disadvantages include: lack of studies on long-term clinical outcomes and safety, somewhat less potency than metformin, possible interference with the immune system, an increase in nasopharyngitis, long-term safety not established, and very expensive. Adverse effects have not been seen in animal reproduction studies and DDP-4 inhibitors are in pregnancy risk category B—no evidence of risk in humans. The DDP-4 inhibitors need further study, particularly on their long-term effects on clinical outcomes rather than the surrogate subclinical outcome of glucose lowering in short-term studies, before many will be convinced they provide enough positive clinical outcomes to justify their expense. The ADA and European Association for the Study of Diabetes consensus statement and algorithm did not place the DDP-4 inhibitors in the top tier of oral agents because of concerns over adverse reactions and lack of long-term clinical outcome data.[1,8]

The DDP-4 inhibitors should not be used as a first-tier agent (Figure 1) and do not have enough long-term efficacy or safety data to support widespread use. Some guidelines have placed DDP-4 inhibitors in the first tier.[15] Some practitioners prescribe a combination tablet with DDP-4 inhibitors with metformin. The combination tablets are not associated with an increase in clinical effectiveness over separate tablets and the extra cost is not justified. Some practitioners use DDP-4 inhibitors in patients that do not tolerate, fail, or have contraindications to metformin, sulfonylurea agents, or pioglitazone.

Alpha-Glucosidase Inhibitors—Acarbose and Miglitol

The main actions of the alpha-glucosidase inhibitors are to decrease the digestion of polysaccharides in the proximal small intestine and decrease the postprandial glucose levels. The carbohydrates are absorbed later in the distal intestine. The main advantages of the alpha-glucosidase inhibitors include: weight neutrality and lack of hypoglycemia when used as monotherapy. A potential advantage is a decrease in cardiovascular events. One trial to prevent DM in high-risk individuals showed a decrease in cardiovascular events.[16] Whether this also occurs during use in those with DM is not known. Further studies are needed before they are used for this effect. A Cochrane systematic review found no evidence on morbidity or mortality and no needs for dosages above 50 mg three times a day.[17] The main disadvantages include: lack of studies on long-term clinical outcomes and safety, less potent than metformin, poorly tolerated due to common gastrointestinal side effects, poor ease of use due to three times a day dosing, and expense. Adverse effects have not been seen in animal reproduction studies and the alpha-glucosidase inhibitors are in pregnancy risk category B—no evidence of risk in humans. Only a small amount of the alpha-glucosidase inhibitors are absorbed systemically, which limits exposure to the fetus. These agents have mainly been studied in Europe and Japan and have much more use there than in other parts of the world. Miglitol has been studied less than acarbose but appears to have very similar effects. Their effect on lipids have been reported as decreasing low-density lipoprotein (LDL) and increasing high-density lipoprotein (HDL) but a meta-analysis found no overall beneficial effect on lipid concentrations.[17]

The alpha-glucosidase inhibitors are typically started at a low dose and with the first bite of the meal. For acarbose, 25 mg can be started with one or three main meals per day, then uptitrated to 50–100 mg three times a day as needed for effect on glucose and as allowed by gastrointestinal side effects. The gastrointestinal side effects: diarrhea, abdominal pain, abdominal bloating, and increase in flatulence occur frequently and are the main factors limiting patient acceptance of these medications. The gastrointestinal side effects are dose related and tend to decrease with time. Thus, slow uptitration of the dose can help minimize them. They are not recommended for use in patients with significant renal insufficiency. Some practitioners use them in patients that do not tolerate, fail, or have contraindications to metformin, sulfonylurea agents, or pioglitazone.

The alpha-glucosidase inhibitors need further study, particularly on their long-term effects on clinical outcomes rather than the surrogate subclinical outcome of glucose lowering in short-term studies, before many will be convinced that they provide enough positive clinical outcomes to justify their use and expense. The ADA and European Association for the Study of Diabetes consensus statement and algorithm did not place the alpha-glucosidase inhibitors in the top tier of oral agents because of their moderate potency, poor ease of use and lack of long-term clinical outcome data.[8,17]

Glinides—Repaglinide and Nateglinide

The main actions of the glinides are to increase insulin secretion by binding to a different site on the beta-cell potassium-ATP receptor than where the sulfonylurea agents bind. They are sometimes referred to as "non-sulfonylurea secretagogues" to reflect their similarities to the oral sulfonylurea agents. Their main advantages are modest: rapid onset of action, potency almost as good as the sulfonylurea agents (especially repaglinide) and the ability to use in patients with an intolerance of sulfonylurea. The main disadvantages include: lack of studies on long-term clinical outcomes and safety, somewhat less potency than metformin in maintenance of glucose-lowering effects, weight gain, hypoglycemia that is slightly less than sulfonylurea agents, poor ease of use due to 2–4 times a day dosing, and very expensive. In addition, adverse effects have been seen in animal reproduction studies; therefore, the glinides are in pregnancy risk category C—risk cannot be ruled out. They should be used cautiously in those with significant renal or hepatic insufficiency, especially nateglinide because it has more renal clearance. Repaglinide is mainly metabolized in the liver and as such, some practitioners prescribe it to those with renal insufficiency and intolerance to sulfonylurea agents.

The glinides are given about 15 minutes prior to each main meal. For example, repaglinide can be started at 0.5 mg with each meal, from 2 to 4 meals per day and increase up to 4 mg as tolerated and required for desired effect on glucose. Glinides should not be taken without a meal to decrease the risk for significant hypoglycemia. Some practitioners use them in patients that do not tolerate, fail, or have contraindications to metformin, sulfonylurea agents, or pioglitazone.

The glinides need further study, particularly on their long-term effects on clinical outcomes rather than the surrogate subclinical outcome of glucose lowering in short-term studies, before many will be convinced that they provide enough positive clinical outcomes to justify their use and expense. The ADA and European Association for the

Study of Diabetes consensus statement and algorithm did not place the glinides in the top tier of oral agents because of their moderate potency, poor ease of use, and lack of long-term clinical outcome data.

Bile Acid Binder—Colesevelam

The main mechanism of the bile acid sequestrant to improve glucose is unknown. In trials up to 6-month duration, it slightly reduced A1c by 0.3–0.4%, less than half of that seen with metformin and most other oral diabetes agents. Although it lowers LDL cholesterol, it increases triglycerides and has side effects that include constipation, nausea, and dyspepsia. Given its modest potency, limited clinical experience, side effects, and cost, it is neither often used nor can be recommended as a main therapy for DM.

Dopamine Agonist—Bromocriptine

Bromocriptine is a dopamine agonist that has been used for decades in the treatment of prolactin-secreting pituitary adenomas and Parkinson's disease. It was noted to have glucose-lowering effects but the mechanism of action remains unknown. A rapid-acting form of bromocriptine (cycloset) was approved by the FDA in the spring of 2009 for the treatment of DM. In a short-term trial, it lowered A1c by 0.4–0.5%, about half as effective as metformin. It also had very frequent gastrointestinal side effects. Given bromocriptine's modest potency, limited clinical experience, side effects and cost, it is neither often used nor can be recommended as a main therapy for DM.

Glucagon-Like Peptide-1 Agonists—Exenatide and Liraglutide

The GLP-1 agonists are incretin mimetics that increase meal-associated glucose-dependent insulin secretion, decrease glucagon secretion, delay gastric emptying, and reduce appetite and liver fat content. Their main advantages are potency similar to metformin and moderate weight loss. Their main disadvantages are the need for injections, very frequent gastrointestinal side effects, and lack of long-term clinical outcome data. They are not for use in those with type 1 DM.

Exenatide was approved by the FDA in 2005 and is primarily used in combination with oral agents—metformin, sulfonylurea, or pioglitazone. It was also approved for use with basal insulin in 2011. The main side effects are gastrointestinal in nature—acid stomach, nausea, vomiting, and diarrhea. The FDA has expressed concern for possible association with medullary thyroid cancer because liraglutide has been associated with this tumor in rodents. A once-weekly injectable form was approved by the FDA in 2012. It has similar association with weight loss and less gastrointestinal side effects than the twice daily form. Exenatide should be injected within 60 minutes before the first and last meal each day. It must be stored in the refrigerator between 2°C (36°F) and 8°C (46°F) prior to first use and then between 2°C (36°) and 25°C (77°F).

Starting dose is 5 μg twice a day. After 1 month, it can be increased to 10 μg twice a day if needed.

Liraglutide is a longer-acting GLP-1 agonist that was approved in Europe in 2009 and by the FDA in 2010. It is stable against normal metabolic degradation by endogenous peptidases, including DDP-4. It has a black box warning from the FDA: "because of the uncertain relevance of the rodent thyroid C-cell tumor finding to humans, prescribe liraglutide only to patients for whom the potential benefits are considered to outweigh the potential risk". Serum calcitonin is elevated in some patients using liraglutide, and the FDA is requiring a cancer registry to monitor it for 15 years. It must be stored in the refrigerator between 2°C (36°F) and 8°C (46°F) prior to first use and then between 15°C (59°F) and 30°C (86°F). Starting dose is 0.6 mg once daily for 1 week to decrease incidence of gastrointestinal side effects, then 1.2 mg once daily. If glucose-lowering effects need to be increased, one can increase the dose to 1.8 mg daily.

PREVENTION OF DIABETES MELLITUS

Lifestyle modifications of eliminating excess caloric intake and getting adequate exercise have been demonstrated to prevent diabetes in studies performed in the US, Finland, China, and India.[18-21] When lifestyle goals are achieved, they are remarkably successful. Indeed in the Finnish trial,[19] when subjects with prediabetes in either the invention or control group achieved at least 4 of 5 of the lifestyle goals, DM was 100% prevented. Unfortunately, many people are unwilling or unable to adopt a healthy calorie intake or maintain adequate exercise levels to achieve lifestyle goals. Thus, there is great interest in the role of oral diabetes medications for the prevention of diabetes. Metformin,[18,21] acarbose,[16,22] and pioglitazone[23] have been studied for the prevention of DM. None has been approved by the FDA for the prevention of DM. A consensus panel of the ADA endorsed metformin as the only medication that should be considered for diabetes prevention.[24] Other medications have less long-term safety and outcome data, more side effects, and are more expensive.

The Diabetes Prevention Project (DPP) was done in the US and studied the effect of lifestyle modification or metformin on the progression from "prediabetes", defined as patients with elevated fasting and post-load glucose, to diabetes.[18] It was found that a lifestyle intervention decreased the incidence of new DM by 58% at 3 years and by 34% at the 10-year follow-up.[25] Metformin was less successful than the lifestyle intervention in the DPP, with 34% less DM at 3 years and only 18% less DM than the control group at the 10-year follow-up. More benefit was seen in overweight subjects and those less than 60 years old. An analysis of total health care cost in the DPP study over the 10-year follow-up was recently presented.[26] It showed that both the metformin and lifestyle groups had a decrease in total health care costs compared to the placebo group. Metformin actually saved overall costs because the intervention was so inexpensive. The intervention for the lifestyle group included relatively expensive supervised exercise sessions and did not save money overall but was associated with a reasonable cost for a quality-adjusted life year (QALY).[26] It can be difficult to know whom to treat with metformin to prevent DM because current methods do not allow precise identification of people that will actually progress to DM. Some practitioners use metformin to prevent DM in people with "prediabetes" defined by glucose intolerance, impaired fasting glucose or A1c of 5.7–6.4%.[1]

Modest changes in lifestyle can give excellent results.[18,19] The ADA suggested that weight loss of 7% of total body weight and 150 minutes per week of moderate exercise like walking, often gives good results. Major efforts to prevent DM should continue to focus on lifestyle intervention and how to increase the rate people reach lifestyle goals. Although metformin has not been clearly established to prevent DM, partially because defining those at very high risk to develop DM is imprecise,[24] some providers will continue to prescribe it to prevent or delay the onset of type 2 DM.

ORAL AGENTS DURING HOSPITALIZATION

Oral diabetes medications should be discontinued for the majority of patients with DM who are admitted to the hospital with an acute illness.[27] There are no data on the safety and usefulness of oral diabetes medications in the hospital.[1] The main glucose goals in hospitalized patients are to avoid severe hypoglycemia and severe hyperglycemia. All patients with a risk for hyperglycemia should have glucose estimated at the time of admission. If glucose is greater than 7.8 mmol/L (140 mg/dL) then glucose levels should be monitored. For those with persistent glucose levels from 7.8 mmol/L to 10 mmol/L (140 to 180 mg/dL) or higher, insulin is the preferred therapy, usually intensive basal and mealtime bolus insulin. For those with known DM, an A1c should also be measured if it has not been done in the 3 months prior to admission. For patients with hyperglycemia and no history of DM, an A1c should be measured. If the A1c is greater than or equal to 6.5% then it is likely diabetes was present prior to hospitalization. The diagnosis of DM is often first made upon admission to the hospital.

Continuation of oral diabetes medications could be considered in the rare patient admitted to the hospital in stable condition, who consumes meals at regular intervals, and is at little risk for use of corticosteroid use, renal insufficiency, acute illness, or use of imaging contrast material. Caution should be used in those continued on metformin as it should be stopped in those receiving contrast materials for imaging studies or those with conditions that predispose toward lactic acidosis: renal insufficiency, heart failure, and conditions associated with poor tissue perfusion.

ORAL AGENTS DURING PREGNANCY

Careful treatment of patients with childbearing potential and DM is required because congenital malformations increase in those with poorly controlled glucose and several medications are either not recommended or contraindicated during pregnancy.[28] The global epidemic of obesity and inadequate exercise includes an increasing number of young women with childbearing potential. Two-thirds of all pregnancies that occur in those with DM are unplanned. These factors contribute to the persistence of DM and gestational diabetes mellitus (GDM) associated congenital malformations. Providers taking care of diabetic women of childbearing potential need to carefully weigh the risks and benefits of any medication. Statins and angiotensin-converting enzyme (ACE) inhibitors are FDA category X (contraindicated), angiotensin II receptor blockers (ARBs) are FDA category C (risk cannot be ruled out) during the first trimester and category D (positive evidence of risk) during the last two trimesters. Women with childbearing potential need to understand the risk and benefits of these medications and have effective, ongoing family planning counseling before using these medications.

Of all the noninsulin antidiabetic agents, metformin and acarbose are classified as FDA category B—no evidence of risk in humans.[1,28] If women become pregnant on these medications, many practitioners would consider stopping them and changing to insulin. Only some insulins are FDA approved for treatment of DM or GDM in pregnancy. Intensive insulin therapies give the best results. Patients using detemir or glargine insulin should be changed to NPH and rapid-acting regular, lispro or aspart, or continuous subcutaneous insulin infusion (CSII). Details of treatment of DM during pregnancy are given in chapter "Care of Pregnant Diabetic Patient" and in the ADA consensus statement.[28]

ORAL AGENTS AS PART OF OVERALL TREATMENT OF DM

Oral agents have an essential but only partial role in the overall care needed to obtain optimal results in patients with DM. It is important for practitioners and patients not to be too "glucocentric", to just focus on and treat glucose while neglecting many other important factors.[5,12] DM is a constellation of pathological disturbances brought on by chronic excess calorie consumption and inadequate exercise, and hyperglycemia is only one of them. Hypertension and lipid problems are common treatable conditions often associated with DM. Thus when considering starting an oral agent, patients often need to be evaluated and concurrently treated for hypertension and lipid problems. Combinations of risk factors predict poor clinical outcomes much better than the presence of a single risk factor, including elevated glucose. A recent evaluation of the effects of DM, hypertension, cholesterol, and smoking showed that the combination of these risk factors has a marked effect on the lifetime risk of dying from heart disease, the major problem of those with DM.[29] The study showed that the presence of a single risk factor conferred only a modest increased risk for premature death. The presence of several risk factors markedly increased mortality at younger ages. This suggests that there is potential for greater benefit for the treatment of the combination of risk factors rather than just a single risk factor like elevated glucose.

The STENO-2 trial confirmed this potential and clearly demonstrated a marked decrease in mortality for treating the combination of risk factors: DM, hypertension, hypercholesterolemia, and smoking.[30] Studies comparing the effects glucose treatment alone have shown much less effect. Indeed, in several trials, hypertension and hypercholesterolemia were carefully treated[31-33] which may have made it more difficult to show much difference for treatment of glucose as the remaining single risk factor.

CONCLUSION

It is very important that use and reliance on oral diabetes medications not distract from other important factors for the prevention and treatment of DM. This is particularly important because there is still uncertainty if any oral diabetes medication truly has favorable effects on key patient important outcomes: morbidity, mortality and quality of life.[5] Simple medications may divert attention from the real solution: effective research and implementation of strategies to prevent diabetes. Many practitioners have seen this up close with testimonials from patients asking, "Why should I do the difficult tasks of eliminating excess calories and getting adequate exercise when I can take my medication and make my diabetes go away"? To paraphrase a recent *Lancet* editorial on DM, medicalization disempowers individuals and excludes communities, schools and urban planners who have the potential to reduce diabetes incidence. The fact that DM, a preventable disease, has reached epidemic proportion is a public health humiliation.[12]

REFERENCES

1. American Diabetes Association. Standards of medical care in diabetes—2012. *Diabetes Care*. 2012;35(Suppl 1):S11-63.
2. Bennett WL, Maruthur NM, Singh S, Segal JB, Wilson LM, Chatterjee R, et al. Comparative effectiveness and safety of medications for type 2 diabetes: an update including new drugs and 2-drug combinations. *Ann Intern Med*. 2011;154:602-13.
3. Qaseem A, Humphrey LL, Sweet DE, Starkey M, Shekelle P; Clinical Guidelines Committee of the American College of Physicians. Oral pharmacologic treatment of type 2 diabetes mellitus: a clinical practice guideline from the American College of Physicians. *Ann Intern Med*. 2012;156:218-31.
4. Saenz A, Fernandez-Esteban I, Mataix A, Ausejo-M, Roque M, Moher D. Metformin monotherapy for type 2 diabetes mellitus. *Cochrane Database Syst Rev*. 2005;3:CD002966.
5. Montori VM, Gandhi GY, Guyatt GH. Patient-important outcomes in diabetes—time for consensus. *Lancet*. 2007;370:1104-6.
6. US Department of Health and Human Services Food and Drug Administration; Center for Drug Evaluation and Research (CDER). Guidance for industry: diabetes mellitus—evaluating cardiovascular risk in new antidiabetic therapies to treat type 2 diabetes. [online] FDA website. Available from www.fda.gov/downloads/Drugs/Guidance ComplianceRegulatoryInformation/Guidances/UCM071627.pdf [Accessed May, 2013].

7. Zhang P, Zhang X, Brown J, Vistisen D, Sicree R, Shaw J, et al. Global healthcare expenditure on diabetes for 2010 and 2030. *Diabetes Res Clin Pract*. 2010;87:293-301.

8. Nathan DM, Holman RR, Buse JB, Sherwin R, Davidson MB, Zinman B, et al. Medical management of hyperglycemia in type 2 diabetes: a consensus algorithm for the initiation and adjustment of therapy: a consensus statement of the American Diabetes Association and the European Association for the Study of Diabetes. *Diabetes Care*. 2009;32:193-203.

9. Goudswaard AN, Furlong NJ, Valk GD, Stolk RP, Rutten GE. Insulin monotherapy versus combinations of insulin with oral hypoglycaemia agents in patients with type 2 diabetes mellitus. *Cochrane Database Syst Rev*. 2004;4:CD003418.

10. UK Prospective Diabetes Study (UKPDS) Group: Effect of intensive blood-glucose control with metformin on complications in overweight patients with type 2 diabetes (UKPDS 34). *Lancet*. 1998;352:854-65.

11. Davidson MB. Successful treatment of markedly symptomatic patients with type ii diabetes mellitus using high doses of sulfonylurea agents. *West J Med*. 1992;157:199-200.

12. Lancet editorial. Type 2 diabetes—time to change our approach. *Lancet*. 2010;375:2193.

13. Dormandy JA, Charbonnel B, Eckland DJ, Erdmann E, Massi-Benedetti M, Moules IK, et al. Secondary prevention of macrovascular events in patients with type 2 diabetes in the PROactive Study (PROspective pioglitAzone Clinical Trial in macroVascular Events): a randomised controlled trial. *Lancet*. 2005;366:1279-89.

14. US Food and Drug Administration. (2011). FDA drug safety communication: update to ongoing safety review of Actos (pioglitazone) and increased risk of bladder cancer. [online] FDA website. Available from www.fda.gov/Drugs/DrugSafety/ucm259150.htm [Accessed May, 2013].

15. Rodbard HW, Jellinger PS, Davidson JA, Einhorn D, Garber AJ, Grunberger G, et al. Statement by an American Association of Clinical Endocrinologists/American College of Endocrinology consensus panel on type 2 diabetes mellitus: an algorithm for glycemic control. *Endocr Pract*. 2009;15:540-59.

16. Chiasson JL, Josse RG, Gomis R, Hanefeld M, Karasik A, Laakso M, et al. Acarbose treatment and the risk of cardiovascular disease and hypertension in patients with impaired glucose tolerance: the STOP-NIDDM trial. *JAMA*. 2003;290:486-94.

17. van de Laar FA, Lucassen PL, Akkermans RP, van de Lisdonk EH, Rutten GE, van Weel C. Alpha-glucosidase inhibitors for patients with type 2 diabetes: results from a Cochrane systematic review and meta-analysis. *Diabetes Care*. 2005;28:154-63.

18. Knowler WC, Barrett-Connor E, Fowler SE, Hamman RF, Lachin JM, Walker EA, et al. Reduction in the incidence of type 2 diabetes with lifestyle intervention or metformin. *N Engl J Med*. 2002;346:393-403.

19. Tuomilehto J, Lindström J, Eriksson JG, Valle TT, Hämäläinen H, Ilanne-Parikka P, et al. Prevention of type 2 diabetes mellitus by changes in lifestyle among subjects with impaired glucose tolerance. *N Engl J Med*. 2001;344:1343-50.

20. Pan XR, Li GW, Hu YH, Jiang XG, Wang JX, Jiang YY, et al. Effects of diet and exercise in preventing NIDDM in people with impaired glucose tolerance. The Da Qing IGT and Diabetes Study. *Diabetes Care*. 1997;20:537-44.

21. Ramachandran A, Snehalatha C, Mary S, Mukesh B, Bhaskar AD, Vijay V, et al. The Indian Diabetes Prevention Programme shows that lifestyle modification and metformin prevent type 2 diabetes in Asian Indian subjects with impaired glucose tolerance (IDPP-1). *Diabetologia*. 2006;49:289-97.

22. Chiasson JL, Josse RG, Gomis R, Hanefeld M, Karasik A, Laakso M, et al. Acarbose for prevention of type 2 diabetes mellitus: the STOP-NIDDM randomised trial. *Lancet.* 2002;359:2072-7.

23. DeFronzo RA, Tripathy D, Schwenke DC, Banerji M, Bray GA, Buchanan TA, et al. Pioglitazone for diabetes prevention in impaired glucose tolerance. *N Engl J Med.* 2011; 364:1104-15.

24. Nathan DM, Davidson MB, DeFronzo RA, Heine RJ, Henry RR, Pratley R, et al. Impaired fasting glucose and impaired glucose tolerance: implications for care. *Diabetes Care.* 2007;30:753-9.

25. Knowler WC, Fowler SE, Hamman RF, Christophi CA, Hoffman HJ, Brenneman AT, et al. 10-year follow-up of diabetes incidence and weight loss in the Diabetes Prevention Program Outcomes Study. *Lancet.* 2009;374:1677-86.

26. Diabetes Prevention Program Research Group. The 10-year cost-effectiveness of lifestyle intervention or metformin for diabetes prevention: an intent-to-treat analysis of the DPP/DPPOS. *Diabetes Care.* 2012;35(4):723-30.

27. Umpierrez GE, Hellman R, Korytkowski MT, Kosiborod M, Maynard GA, Montori VM, et al. Management of hyperglycemia in hospitalized patients in non-critical care setting: an endocrine society clinical practice guideline. *J Clin Endocrinol Metab.* 2012;97:16-38.

28. Kitzmiller JL, Block JM, Brown FM, Catalano PM, Conway DL, Coustan DR, et al. Managing preexisting diabetes for pregnancy: summary of evidence and consensus recommendations for care. *Diabetes Care.* 2008;31:1060-79.

29. Berry JD, Dyer A, Cai X, Garside DB, Ning H, Thomas A, et al. Lifetime risks of cardiovascular disease. *N Engl J Med.* 2012;366:321-9.

30. Gaede P, Lund-Andersen H, Parving HH, Pedersen O. Effect of a multifactorial intervention on mortality in type 2 diabetes. *N Engl J Med.* 2008;358:580-91.

31. Gerstein HC, Miller ME, Byington RP, Goff DC, Bigger JT, Buse JB, et al. Effects of intensive glucose lowering in type 2 diabetes. *N Engl J Med.* 2008;358:2545-59.

32. ADVANCE Collaborative Group, Patel A, MacMahon S, Chalmers J, Neal B, Billot L, et al. Intensive blood glucose control and vascular outcomes in patients with type 2 diabetes. *N Engl J Med.* 2008;358:2560-72.

33. Duckworth W, Abraira C, Moritz T, Reda D, Emanuele N, Reaven PD, et al. Glucose control and vascular complications in veterans with type 2 diabetes. *N Engl J Med.* 2009; 360:129-39.

Insulin Therapy in Diabetic Patients

8
Chapter

Shubh P Kaur, Craig S Stump

ABSTRACT

It is only within the last century that people with type 1 diabetes have had available to them the life-saving therapy of exogenous insulin. While early insulin therapy used relatively crude animal pancreatic extracts, today recombinant DNA technologies provide a large array of insulin and insulin analogues with differing pharmacodynamic properties that allow more physiologic insulin replacement. Despite recent advancements in insulin options and delivery (insulin pens and pumps), challenges remain. Among these is the need to: (1) further minimize the risk of hypoglycemia caused by insulin, (2) determine which patients will benefit most from tight glycemic control using rigorous multiple dose insulin and continuous subcutaneous insulin infusion protocols, (3) develop an array of more potent insulin formulations to treat the increasing number of severely insulin resistant patients, and (4) safely close the loop in glycemic detection-delivery for a true artificial pancreas. Finally, it is important to keep in mind that although insulin is the most potent tool available for treating hyperglycemia, the initiation of insulin therapy is often delayed in type 2 diabetic patients. Such delays can expose patients to unnecessary hyperglycemic burden and risk for complications.

INTRODUCTION

The isolation of insulin, and its subsequent purification, large scale production, and use for treating diabetes remains one of the major achievements of medical science. Before the availability of insulin, treatment of diabetes was limited to severely restricting carbohydrate intake and imposing periods of fasting upon patients which achieved only modest benefits. Indeed, for patients with type 1 diabetes profound emaciation, ketoacidosis and death were unavoidable.

Our understanding of the role of the pancreas in the development of diabetes dates back to the latter part of the 18th century.[1] During this time, it was observed that injury to the pancreas could cause diabetes, and that the serum and urine from diabetic patients was sweet to the taste. Subsequent experiments demonstrated that pancreatectomy caused diabetes in dogs, but that blocking the pancreatic duct did not lead to diabetes even though the exocrine tissue atrophied. These observations led investigators to speculate that the substance regulating blood sugar was secreted internally from the preserved islets of Langerhans. That substance, initially termed "isletin", was isolated by Banting and Best in 1921 earning the former a Nobel Prize. Today, rather than having to rely on insulin extracted from animal pancreas glands, human "regular" insulin can be manufactured in large quantities using recombinant DNA technology. Moreover, these techniques are being utilized to produce an expanding array of insulin analogs with differing pharmacokinetic and pharmacodynamic properties. This versatile armamentarium of insulins has allowed patients the ability to more closely match insulin delivery to specific insulin needs during fasting and postprandial conditions (i.e., "physiological insulin replacement"). This has resulted in better overall glycemic control with less occurrence of hypoglycemia.

The physiological roles for insulin are numerous and varied. Insulin helps maintain euglycemia by stimulating glucose uptake and utilization into the skeletal muscle, heart, and adipose tissue, and by suppressing glucose production by the liver. Insulin also has important functions in suppressing lipolysis and ketogenesis, putting patients who cannot produce insulin (i.e., type 1 diabetes) at risk for ketoacidosis. The physiological effects of insulin for controlling blood glucose and ketosis are summarized in figure 1.

WHEN TO CONSIDER INSULIN?

Insulin therapy is initiated when insulin needs exceed the secretory capacity of the pancreatic beta cells. This can be very early in the course of the disease such as in type 1 diabetes or after many years of treatment with lifestyle interventions, oral antidiabetic (OAD) medications, or both. Regrettably, the initiation of insulin therapy is often delayed exposing patients to years of unnecessary hyperglycemia.[2] Delays can arise from a variety of causes and concerns including patient reservation or fear of insulin, under ascertainment of poor glycemic control, and lack of time or resources needed to educate and train patients to administer insulin. Since insulin therapy is the most effective approach to lowering blood glucose, it should be considered whenever patients present with HbA1c values greater than 9.0% (average blood glucose 11.8 mmol/L or 212 mg/dL) and/or are experiencing symptoms of hyperglycemia, such as polyuria, polydipsia, blurred vision or weight loss. Moreover, insulin therapy should not be delayed when individualized HbA1c targets can no longer be maintained by oral hypoglycemic agents (OHAs) and lifestyle efforts.

A variety of insulins are now at the disposal of the health care practitioner caring for diabetic patients (Table 1). These are generally categorized as basal insulin, bolus or prandial insulin, and combination or premixed insulin. When converting a diabetes

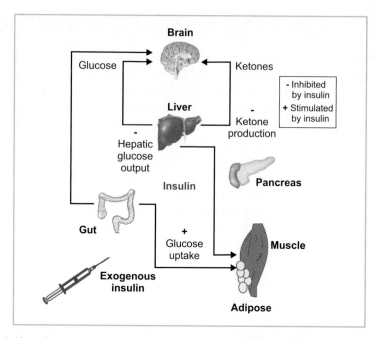

FIGURE 1 Physiological effects of insulin. Diabetes is diagnosed when endogenous insulin production is inadequate to maintain fasting glucose to less than 7 mmol/L (<126 mg/dL) and/ or postprandial glucose less than 11.1 mmol/L (<200 mg/dL). The brain consumes greater than 60% of the body's glucose during resting conditions, and always requires some glucose. Insulin is the principal regulator of blood glucose which must be maintained in order to preserve the brain. Insulin regulates glucose homeostasis directly by promoting its uptake into skeletal muscle and adipose tissue, and by suppressing hepatic glucose production. Insulin also suppresses lipolysis and ketone formation. While glucose is usually the sole source of energy for the brain, starvation causes the brain to adapt so as to utilize ketone bodies. Moreover, since insulin levels are low during starvation, ketone formation is permitted. Alternatively, the absence of insulin (i.e., type 1 diabetes) not only results in severe hyperglycemia but can also lead to ketoacidosis which is life threatening.

treatment program from oral medications to insulin, it is common to discontinue one or more of the oral agents. Sulfonylureas and glinides should be discontinued if prandial insulin is initiated to avoid redundancy in treatment, and more importantly to minimize confusion when interpreting the self-monitoring of blood glucose (SMBG) values, particularly when hypoglycemia occurs. Moreover, glucagon-like peptide-1 (GLP-1) agonists and dipeptidyl peptidase-4 (DPP-4) inhibitors have not been approved in the United States in combination with insulin. Thiazolidinediones (TZDs) can be used with insulin but at high risk for weight gain and fluid retention. These authors prefer to continue the use of metformin as long as there are no other contraindications, such as stage 3 or greater chronic kidney disease [estimated glomerular filtration rate (eGFR) < 60 mL/minute per 1.73 m^2].[3]

TABLE 1: Pharmacokinetic Properties of Insulin Preparations			
Insulin type	**Onset**	**Peak (hours)**	**Duration (hours)**
Rapid-acting			
Insulin aspart Insulin glulisine Insulin lispro	10–30 minutes	0.5–3	3–5
Short-acting			
Regular insulin	30 minutes	1–5	6–8
Intermediate-acting			
Neutral protamine Hagedorn (NPH) insulin	1–4 hours	6–8	12–16
Long-acting ("basal")			
Insulin detemir	1–2 hours	3–9	6–23
Insulin glargine	1–2 hours	Minimal peak	11–24

TYPES OF INSULIN

Bovine and porcine derived insulins were the only preparations available until the 1980s when recombinant DNA technology was introduced, allowing the production of human insulin. A variety of additives have been incorporated into animal and human insulin preparations over the years to alter the absorption characteristics, most notably protamine and zinc. In addition, over the past two decades, numerous insulin analogs have been developed that enable physicians to provide insulin in a basal-bolus fashion better able to accommodate the fasting, postabsorptive and postprandial states.

Short-Acting Insulin

Short-acting insulin or "regular" insulin has been, until recently, the mainstay mealtime insulin. Its onset of action is approximately 30 minutes and usually peaks between 2 hours and 4 hours after injection, after the expected postprandial rise in blood glucose. This has required patients to anticipate the timing and content of their meals for dose selection well before eating, usually 30 minutes. While this practice generally does not allow for the same insulin dosing precision as newer insulin analogs, regular insulin still has an important role in combination (premixed) formulations and in patients with gastroparesis for which a delay in insulin action may be desirable. When regular insulin (or a rapid insulin preparation) is selected for postprandial glycemic control, the goal should be to time the insulin injection in such a way to insure that the peak physiological effect anticipates the postprandial glucose rise. Moreover, since the effects of regular insulin can last 6 hours or longer the time between doses (meals) is important since the next dose of regular insulin can become additive creating a phenomenon often referred to as "stacking". Similar to the problems associated with combining sulfonylureas with prandial insulin, insulin stacking puts the patient at higher risk of hypoglycemia, and makes the interpretation of glycemic fluctuations and subsequent dose adjustments difficult. As a result of these and other limitations that render regular insulin less able to mimic physiologic insulin secretion, newer insulin analogs are becoming the preferred choices for prandial insulin.

Regular insulin is also available in a U-500 formulation which is 5 times as concentrated as its U-100 counterpart. Its use is reserved for patients with severe insulin resistance, usually patients requiring greater than 300 units of total insulin daily. Even in resistant patients, U-500 must be used with caution. Physicians and educators must be absolutely clear in their dosing instructions, and confirm that the patient understands the exact volume to be drawn up and delivered at each dose. Interestingly, U-500 has a delayed pharmacodynamic profile resembling intermediate-acting insulins (see below and Table 1) and, therefore, is not used in conjunction with a long- or intermediate-acting basal preparation. Injections are usually given 2 or 3 times per day with meals, beginning with prebreakfast and predinner.

Rapid-Acting Insulin

The rapid-acting insulin analogs presently available include insulin aspart, insulin glulisine, and insulin lispro. Their prompt onset of action (10–30 minutes) can be attributed to slight amino acid structure alterations in the insulin molecules which, while not significantly altering receptor binding, prevent the spontaneous formation of dimers and hexamers in solution. Dissociation is particularly marked when the solution is further diluted by the subcutaneous interstitial fluid after injection, thereby allowing a greater number of monomeric insulin molecules to be absorbed immediately. Consequently, these insulin analogs more closely mimic the physiological rise of endogenous insulin during a postprandial blood glucose spike in terms of onset, peak, and duration. The relatively fast onset and offset of action of these agents make them well suited for mealtime coverage. Thus, they tend to offer improved postprandial control of hyperglycemia while reducing subsequent hypoglycemia.[4]

An additional benefit of rapid-acting insulin analogs is that they can be administered the moment before (or after) eating, offering more flexibility in meal timing and content which is attractive to many patients who cannot commit to a predictable routine. Nevertheless, the pharmacokinetic properties of rapid-acting insulins also have several disadvantages. Since the duration of action is only about 3 hours, there can be a "gap" in insulin coverage between doses making the addition of uninterrupted basal insulin during the day necessary. Moreover, since these insulins begin to circulate quickly, they should not be administered more than 15 minutes before eating. This is a problem commonly encountered when patients are eating away from home where the exact timing of the food is unpredictable. In such situations, it is recommended that the prandial insulin be injected as the meal is presented or immediately after the meal has been consumed. Likewise, caution should be exercised when using rapid-acting insulin for treatment of hyperglycemia at a time when food is not being served or not readily available. In such cases, hypoglycemia is more likely to occur with rapid-acting insulin than short-acting regular insulin. Despite these concerns, rapid-acting insulin analogs with meals (in combination with a long-acting basal insulin) are now the preferred approach to implementing a multiple dose injection (MDI) program for most type 1, and many type 2 diabetic patients because of improved postprandial hypoglycemia profile and the increased flexibility of meals and activities it allows.

Intermediate-Acting Insulin

Intermediate neutral protamine Hagedorn (NPH) insulin has been used by diabetic patients for many years. Its onset is 1–4 hours and the duration of action is 12–16 hours. However, its considerable peak at 6–8 hours can be problematic in that hypoglycemia can occur if this peak does not match up with a meal. Other intermediate-acting insulins which are used in premixed preparations (below) include insulin lispro protamine and insulin aspart protamine. Although intermediate-acting insulins can be used for basal insulin requirements by injecting 2 to 3 times per day, this role has been largely supplanted by the longer acting agents, insulin glargine, and insulin detemir, which often require only a single injection per day and produce considerably smaller peaks. Another concern when using protamine containing products, albeit rarely, is hypersensitivity reactions since protamine is antigenic. Nevertheless, intermediate-acting insulins do offer some advantage over longer acting agents. First, these insulins can be mixed in the same syringe or vial with short- or rapid-acting insulin. Therefore, they are integral to premixed insulin preparations (discussed below) or can be drawn up sequentially and mixed in the same syringe by the patient in a "split-mixed" regimen. Moreover, an intermediate-acting insulin is sometimes an option for patients who exhibit nocturnal hyperglycemia despite good daytime control, and for whom the long-acting insulins glargine or detemir put them at risk for hypoglycemia during the day.

Long-Acting Insulin

Ultralente was the only long-acting insulin available until the advent of insulin glargine and insulin detemir. With the development of these longer acting basal insulins, the use of ultralente decreased dramatically and is no longer available. Glargine differs from native human insulin by 3 amino acid modifications that allow the molecule to be soluble in mildly acidic conditions (vial solution pH 4.0), while forming microprecipitates in the neutral pH of subcutaneous tissues. As a result, the absorption of glargine is gradual and fairly constant supplying insulin with minimal peak for approximately 24 hours.[5] This relatively flat profile is comparable to what can be achieved with continuous subcutaneous infusion (i.e., insulin pump). It is particularly useful for preventing fasting and between meal hyperglycemia with minimal nocturnal hypoglycemia.[4]

Insulin detemir is a soluble long-acting insulin preparation composed of human insulin bound to a fatty acid moiety which allows it to bind reversibly to albumin. This property provides for the slow absorption of insulin detemir over 20–24 hours in most patients. Detemir can be administered once or twice a day providing a relatively flat activity profile with lower risk of hypoglycemia than NPH insulin. Moreover, there is some clinical trial evidence suggesting there is less weight gain[6] and less intrapatient variability[7] with detemir than either NPH or glargine insulin.

Fixed Insulin Mixtures (Premixed)

Insulin is available in premixed solutions of short- or rapid-acting insulin and NPH or NPH-like insulin. The available products are:

- 50% NPH; 50% regular
- 70% NPH; 30% regular
- 50% lispro protamine suspension [neutral protamine lispro (NPL)]; 50% lispro
- 75% lispro protamine suspension (NPL); 25% lispro
- 70% Insulin aspart protamine suspension; 30% aspart.

These preparations can be an attractive option for type 2 diabetic patients who eat three predictable meals per day (Figure 2). The advantages of limiting insulin injections to twice daily and decreasing the number of finger sticks for SMBG can outweigh the restraints of meal and physical activity consistency for many people.

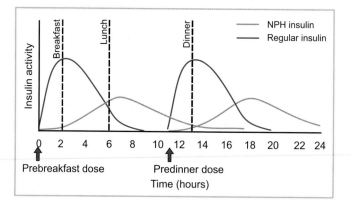

FIGURE 2 Premixed 70/30 insulin activity profile. Premixed 70/30 insulin administered twice daily before breakfast and dinner can provide a convenient and effective approach to insulin therapy in many patients with type 2 diabetes. It is most effective in patients who can maintain a fairly consistent pattern of eating and physical activity.

Moreover, premixed insulins are an option for type 2 diabetic patients who have difficulty drawing up and mixing insulins due to limitations in vision or dexterity. However, as these insulin mixtures are in fixed proportions, the inflexibility of dose adjustments can limit the usefulness of these products, since it is not possible to change either the intermediate-acting insulin or the rapid/short-acting insulin dose without changing the other. This rigidity can be overcome by allowing the patient to mix the intermediate-acting insulin and the shorter acting component to the desired proportion in the syringe before injecting. Nevertheless, many patients will not be able to attain adequate glycemic control without dangerous hypoglycemia with a premixed or split-mixed program and, therefore, will need to be transitioned to a multiple dose of insulin regimen. Due to the acidic medium required to maintain insulin glargine in a soluble form, it cannot be mixed with any other insulins. Whether mixing detemir with rapid-acting analog insulin is appropriate remains questionable.[8]

INITIATING AND ADJUSTING INSULIN THERAPY

Initial Dose

In most cases, starting an insulin program will differ for patients with type 1 and type 2 diabetes. Type 2 diabetic patients usually advance insulin therapy gradually, from the addition of basal insulin to existing OHA medications early, to a more complicated MDI routine at later stages. These patients might also do well by beginning with a premixed or split-mixed insulin program if prandial insulin is deemed necessary, and meal and activity habits are sufficiently stable and predictable. Alternatively, since patients with type 1 diabetes make very little or no insulin they will likely require basal and prandial insulin immediately upon diagnosis, advancing to a lifetime MDI or insulin pump program with flexible mealtime dosing. Occasionally, a type 1 diabetic patient may do well for several months on a simpler insulin program such as a small dose of basal insulin daily if they are still in the early "honeymoon period" of the disease.

When starting an MDI program in a type 1 diabetic patient the total daily dose (TDD) of insulin can be estimated from the body weight, usually 0.2–0.4 units per kg per day. This is generally an underestimation, with a built in safety margin, of what will likely be required for optimum glycemic control. Factors that will influence the TDD include habitual physical activity, body fatness, medications, and puberty. At the onset, approximately one half of the TDD should be given as basal insulin, either a long- or intermediate-acting insulin injected once or twice a day, respectively. The long-acting insulin can be administered either at bedtime or first thing in the morning. If NPH insulin twice a day is initiated for the basal requirements, the two doses do not need to be identical. Indeed, two-thirds of the total basal dose is generally recommended for the morning and one-third at bedtime, although this will eventually be adjusted to the individual glycemic excursion patterns.

Prandial insulin (rapid- or short-acting) will usually be administered two or more times per day with meals. As noted above, the injections are usually timed immediately (rapid-acting) or about 30 minutes (short-acting) before meals. The starting total dose of prandial insulin (one-half TDD) can be equally distributed to each meal if all meals are of similar size and composition, or distributed proportionally to the content of the respective meals. With appropriate patient education, flexibility can be added to an MDI program by making the mealtime dose dependent on the grams of carbohydrate consumed (carbohydrate counting) and an adjustment either adding or subtracting insulin from the calculated dose depending on the SMBG value measured at the time of the injection. It should be emphasized that in order for the MDI program to be successful the patient must be capable of understanding the instructions provided, and committed to frequent injections and self-testing. If this cannot be assured, a twice a day premixed or split-mixed program might be a better option.

A consensus statement for initiating and adjusting insulin in type 2 diabetes was published jointly by the American Diabetes Association (ADA) and the European Association for the Study of Diabetes (EASD) in 2009.[9,10] As noted above, the initial step often involves adding either a long- or intermediate-acting insulin at bedtime. The initial dose is usually an arbitrary low dose such as 10 units or by weight based calculation (or 0.2 units/kg) that is subsequently titrated up to a desired morning fasting target range (described below). To this end, type 2 diabetic patients often require greater insulin TDDs (>1 unit/kg) than required for type 1 diabetes in order to overcome insulin resistance. Some or all the OHA medications can be continued with this bedtime insulin dose depending on the need for postprandial coverage, adequate renal function, and risk of hypoglycemia and other side effects. It goes without saying that optimization of lifestyle interventions should also be pursued if they have not already been enacted by the patient. These efforts will help minimize the amount of insulin required to meet glycemic control targets and provide other tangible benefits.

An alternative approach for many type 2 diabetic patients is to discontinue oral medications, with the exception of metformin if appropriate, and begin a premixed insulin (Figure 2). As previously noted a premixed regimen requires 3 meals per day, and assurance of consistency in diet and physical activity. A 70/30% preparation of NPH (or NPH-like) insulin with either regular insulin or analog rapid-acting insulin would be initiated twice daily with breakfast and dinner. The intermediate-acting insulin component (70%) is designed to cover the midday, including lunch, as well as overnight. The short- or rapid-acting insulin (30%) targets the glycemic excursions after breakfast and dinner. Again, the starting TDD can be an intentionally low dose, such as 10 units or weight based 0.2 units/kg divided into two doses. Traditionally, doses have been divided two-thirds with breakfast and one-third with dinner, however, there is evidence that a 1:1 ratio is effective.[11]

Dose Adjustments

Adjusting doses after initiating insulin therapy is an ongoing process that is guided by the physician but is often implemented by the patient, or a diabetes nurse or educator. Adjustments will depend on the type and timing of insulin and on SMBG measurements. The goal is to achieve the patient's individualized HbA1c target in a safe and efficient manner. Adjustment of the basal insulin dose should be based upon SMBG levels that occur when short- or rapid-acting insulin is not exerting a significant effect, and when the patient is in a fasting or postabsorptive state. The most convenient period that usually fits these criteria is overnight. It is recommended that the bedtime dose of long- or intermediate-acting insulin be titrated up 2 units every 3 days until the fasting glucoses are within the target range (3.9–7.2 mmol/L or 70–130 mg/dL). The titration can be accelerated to 4 units every 3 days if fasting glucoses remain greater than 10 mmol/L (180 mg/dL). Alternatively, if hypoglycemia (<3.9 mmol/L or 70 mg/dL) occurs the bedtime dose should be decreased 4 units or 10% whichever is greater.[9,10] The change in SMBG from the bedtime value to morning fasting value should also be considered when adjusting the basal dose. A consistent increase or decrease in SMBG greater than 2.5 mmol/L (45 mg/dL) overnight should alert the physician, educator, and/or patient that the basal dose is either inadequate or excessive.

Prandial insulin, usually approximately 4 units, can be added to one or more meals in type 2 diabetic patients that do not meet individualized HbA1c targets with basal insulin alone. Each dose can be adjusted up in small increments every 3 days (i.e., 2 units, or up to 10% increments at higher doses) depending on the SMBG value before the next meal (i.e., prelunch value for the breakfast dose; predinner value for the lunch dose; bedtime value for the dinner dose). Preprandial SMBG targets are usually between 4.4 mmol/L and 8.3 mmol/L (80–150 mg/dL) depending on each patient's individual glycemic target and risk for hypoglycemia. OHA medications, with the possible exception of metformin, should be discontinued as prandial insulin is added.

Many patients can add significant flexibility to an MDI program by assigning a specific amount of prandial insulin for every gram of carbohydrate consumed (carbohydrate ratio) in the meal. In addition, an adjustment in dose for the SMBG value, either above or below the target blood glucose range, is often calculated. This approach, while liberating for many patients in terms of lifestyle, requires an added degree of commitment to disease education, self-monitoring, and dose computing.

Injecting Insulin

Drawing up insulin from a vial into a syringe and injecting into the subcutaneous fat is the most common delivery method. However, insulin pen devices are gaining popularity due to their convenience and portability. Insulin pens also offer some advantage for delivering very small doses, and may be helpful to patients with poor vision or dexterity. In addition, magnifying lenses and other devices are available

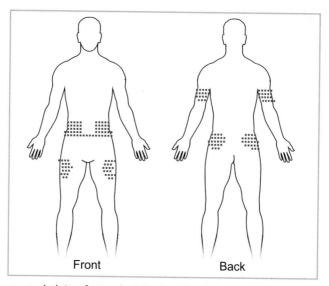

Front   Back

FIGURE 3 Recommended sites for insulin injection. The abdominal subcutaneous adipose tissue is the preferred site for injecting insulin. However, triceps, thigh, hip, and buttock adipose depots are also options.

to patients with these limitations. Insulin is most rapidly and consistently absorbed when injected into the abdominal subcutaneous fat. Other adipose depots located at the anterior thighs, triceps, hips, and buttocks can also be utilized (Figure 3). It is recommended that insulin be injected into the same general region each day to optimize consistent absorption, while altering or rotating the exact location to prevent lipodystrophy.

COMPLICATIONS OF INSULIN THERAPY

Hypoglycemia

Hypoglycemia is the most common complication of insulin therapy. It can be a consequence of a delayed meal, increased physical activity, or an attempt toward more intensive glucose control.[12] Severe hypoglycemia provokes a sympathetic adrenal counter-regulatory response that can increase the risk for morbidities and mortality. This risk increases with age, duration of diabetes and insulin therapy, hypoglycemia unawareness, and in patients with type 1 diabetes.[13,14] Hypoglycemia unawareness also increases the risk for neurological complications (neuroglycopenia). In patients with altered awareness, glycemic targets may need to be adjusted in order to minimize the risk of severe incapacitating hypoglycemia. The risk of hypoglycemia can be reduced with patient education to improve recognition of symptoms and to ensure that measures to reverse the drop in glucose are employed when symptoms begin.

Weight Gain

Weight gain is commonly seen with the initiation of insulin therapy. Indeed, with improved glycemic control glycosuria is reduced and more calories are retained for anabolic processes. In addition, when insulin doses are excessive, particularly basal insulin, a tendency toward hypoglycemia can provoke increases in caloric consumption. Weight gain can be minimized with adequate physical activity and attention to dietary intake, and by insuring that insulin doses are appropriate for both basal to postprandial glycemic requirements.

Insulin Allergy

Allergic reactions have become rare with the advent of recombinant human insulins and analogs. Yet allergic reactions can occur against insulin itself or to an additive, such as protamine. Minor reactions include wheal and flare at the injection site or more diffuse rash. Fortunately, these are the most common allergic manifestations to insulin therapy. Rarely, a severe generalized or anaphylactic reaction may develop that requires hospitalization. Specific immunotherapy has been effective in allowing patients to continue insulin therapy.[15]

Worsening Retinopathy

The Diabetes Control and Complications Trial (DCCT) revealed some evidence of worsening retinopathy during the first 6 months of intensive insulin therapy in type 1 diabetic patients.[5] The most important risk factors for worsening of retinopathy after the initiation of intensive treatment were severity of retinopathy and poorer glycemic control. It is suggested that patients with significant retinopathy undergo treatments, such as photocoagulation prior to initiation of intensive insulin treatments that would cause an abrupt drop in blood glucose.

Risk of Malignancy

In addition to its typical metabolic effects, insulin acts as a growth factor acting via the insulin-like growth factor-1 (IGF-1) receptor which provides at least a theoretical concern for malignancy. Moreover, different insulin analog structures can lead to slightly different interactions with IGF-1 receptor. This has raised concern over the mitogenic potential of these analogs. However, most of the studies looking at the risk of malignancy in patients on insulin therapy have been either small, retrospective,[16,17] or in vitro.[18] One of the largest retrospective studies, to date, performed on a United Kingdom cohort of 63,000 patients, showed no difference in cancer risk among insulin analog compared with human insulin users.[19] Given the general lack of clinical evidence linking insulin use to cancer risk, no restriction on insulin use for treatment of diabetes is warranted at this time.

Injection Site Lipodystrophy

Lipoatrophy, lipohypertrophy, or scarring can occur within the adipose tissue at the insulin injection site. Lipohypertrophy remains a relatively common side effect of insulin therapy irrespective of the type of insulin or whether it is administered by injection or continuous subcutaneous infusion. Lipoatrophy, thought to be immune mediated, has become rare at insulin injection sites since the advent of human insulins. Rotation of injection sites can help prevent these complications.

INSULIN PUMP

Since its introduction in the late 1970s, the insulin pump has made great technological leaps in form and function. Today's insulin pumps represent a midway point in the quest for an artificial pancreas in that they are able to deliver insulin and track glucose changes in the interstitial fluid. However, a closed feedback loop of glycemic detection and insulin delivery has not been achieved since advances in reliability and safety have not reached a point that would preclude operator input. Nevertheless, current insulin pumps are light, compact, and easy to carry, while offering greater functionality than their predecessors. Therefore, they can represent a significant improvement in convenience and glycemic control for many patients.

Presently, insulin pumps are worn externally being kept in a pocket or on a belt. They store insulin within cartridges or reservoirs which is delivered through a soft plastic catheter that connects to a subcutaneous insertion device (Teflon or stainless steel). Generally, the catheter will be inserted into the abdominal wall. The catheter insertion set should be changed every 3 days and rotated to a different site to avoid complications of catheter obstruction and infection. Only short-acting insulin or rapid-acting insulin analogs are approved for pump use, although concentrated human insulin U-500 has been used in special cases of severe insulin resistance. Nevertheless, rapid-acting insulins are the preferred preparation for insulin pumps since they offer desirable pharmacodynamic properties, namely, prompt and consistent absorption during the basal infusion, as well rapid onset of action and decline with meal boluses.

Patient Selection for Insulin Pump Therapy

Continuous subcutaneous insulin infusion (CSII) is useful in patients with type 1 diabetes mellitus (DM) and certain insulinopenic patients with type 2 diabetes who are unable to achieve optimal glucose control with multiple daily insulin injections.[20] Insulin deficiency can be identified by low or absent C-peptide levels concurrent with an elevated postprandial blood glucose. The patients selected for CSII should be highly motivated for optimal blood glucose control and perform SMBG at least four times a day to allow for appropriate insulin adjustments to basal and bolus doses. A certain level of education and aptitude is required to effectively calculate the appropriate insulin dose for meals (carbohydrate counting), while making adjustments for unexpected hypo- or hyperglycemia, effects of physical activity, and the impact of illness and/or fasting, and to decide when and how much to alter basal insulin infusion rates as circumstances dictate. Moreover, patients using an insulin pump should be willing to work closely with their health care practitioner, and assume responsibility and accountability for their day-to-day glycemic management. Finally, they should demonstrate a level of comfort with the technology, be able to trouble shoot minor problems and be aware of the possibility of device failure.

Intensive Insulin Therapy Using Insulin Pumps

Continuous subcutaneous insulin infusion therapy provides, to date, the best approximation of physiologic insulin release at our disposal when using exogenous insulin. Another advantage of CSII has over long-acting insulin analogs is the flexibility in basal rates throughout the day. Modern pumps can be programmed to deliver a constant basal insulin infusion rate, or more commonly, increase or decrease the rate of delivery at certain times of the day to counter anticipated fluctuations in blood glucose. Newer pumps allow multiple basal rate infusion profiles that can accommodate periodic alterations in glucose metabolism that accompany situations such as exercise, weekend activities, menstruation, and illness. Moreover, CSII offers advantages to patients who commonly experience prebreakfast hyperglycemia due to "dawn phenomenon" or waning of overnight basal insulin. Dawn phenomenon is attributed to reduced insulin sensitivity in tissues around the prewaking hours of 3 AM to 6 AM due to physiologic surge of counter regulatory hormones. In these situations, stepping up the basal rate during this time can resolve the fasting hyperglycemia, an option not available to long-acting basal insulin users.

Studies comparing intensive insulin therapy using CSII and MDI programs have revealed only modest improvement in HbA1C on the order of 0.2–0.3% in type 1 DM using CSII.[21] In type 2 DM, CSII has not shown a significant benefit in glycemic control over MDI. Moreover, while there is evidence that severe hypoglycemic episodes may be reduced in type 1 diabetic patients on an insulin pump compared to an MDI regimen,[22] a meta-analysis in 2009 failed to demonstrate a statistically significant benefit in severe hypoglycemic episodes or nocturnal hypoglycemia when comparing CSII to MDI, in patients with either type 1 or type 2 diabetes.[23]

To date, studies comparing sensor augmented pump therapy to MDI in type 1 diabetic patients have shown a modest improvement in glycemic control, documenting an average drop in HbA1c of 0.6%.[24] However, these investigators did not find any difference in hypoglycemic episodes between the two groups. Moreover, this study did not do a subgroup analysis of patients who are at high risk for hypoglycemia. Also, there are no studies comparing head-to-head sensor-augmented insulin pumps to CSII without sensors. The two modalities do seem to affect a similar amount of weight gain. Alternatively, there is data showing an improvement in quality of life for both type 1 and type 2 diabetic patients utilizing CSII by pump when compared to those on an MDI program.[21,25] Patients often reveal that they experience less social limitation, endure less pain and have greater flexibility and satisfaction on when using CSII. Finally, there is no evidence to date indicating that CSII offers any benefit in mortality or reductions in complications. While any improvements in mortality or morbidity would be difficult to document with the modest improvements in HbA1c observed with CSII compared to MDI, reduction in residual risk not captured by HbA1c is possible. These questions will need to be answered with large scale, randomized, controlled trials examining these specific primary outcomes.

Initiating Insulin Pump Therapy

Insulin pump therapy should be started under the supervision of a trained physician specialist (usually an endocrinologist) and a diabetes educator trained in pump initiation. Moreover, the patient should be comfortable and proficient in using an MDI program before converting to CSII since many of the underlying principles and assumptions are the same.

To estimate the initial doses for CSII, it is best to use the TDD of injected insulin utilized by the patient prior to the transition. The pump TDD can be estimated by calculating 80% of the injected TDD. From this value, the initial basal insulin infusion rate can be determined by dividing half the pump TDD by 24 hours. Therefore, if a patient is receiving a total of 45 units of injectable insulin per day he or she would begin with a basal infusion rate of 1.5 units per hour (45 × 0.8 units/24 hours = 1.5 units/hour). This basal insulin infusion would be initiated as a single rate for the entire 24 hours, thereby replacing the long- or intermediate-acting insulin used in an MDI program. However, the insulin pump has the advantage of being able to match individual diurnal variations in basal insulin requirements, and thus can be adjusted to more than one daily rate at a later time.

Like MDI programs, premeal insulin boluses are determined according to the size and composition of the meals, and individualized patient factors. Most pumps will calculate a bolus dose using a carbohydrate ratio(s) for the patient (units of insulin per gram of carbohydrate), and a correction dose that is dependent on the SMBG at the time of the bolus. The correction dose will adjust for glucose levels above or below a predetermined range and will be a function of an insulin sensitivity factor determined for the patient. Formulas estimating carbohydrate ratios and insulin sensitivities have been described.[26]

Disadvantages of Insulin Pump Therapy

As with any therapeutic modality CSII comes with several disadvantages. One of the most common is site infection or failure. The incidence of infections is once per year per patient. These can occur in even in the most compliant patient, although most can be treated with oral antibiotics and changing the insertion site. Surgical drainage may be required if an abscess develops, but this is rare. As only rapid- or short-acting insulin may be used in pumps, any interruption in insulin administration, either intentional or unintentional can lead to a swift development of hyperglycemia and ketoacidosis in the insulinopenic patient. Although most pumps have a built-in warning system to alert patients of battery failure or catheter obstruction preparation for these occurrences remains crucial. With adequate patient training insulin interruptions can be minimized, and if they do occur, substitution with injectable insulin can be implemented. Certainly, one of the biggest disadvantages of insulin pump therapy is the cost. At present the initial cost of the pump is approximately $6,000, with an additional $1,500 in the annual costs for disposable parts and supplies. Therefore, the cost presents a barrier to many patients and unattractive to many payers, particularly with the modest outcome benefits documented to date. Unfortunately, there has yet to be a comprehensive cost-benefit analysis of CSII use.

Sensor Augmented Insulin Pump Therapy

Real-time continuous glucose monitoring (RT-CGM) is a recent major advance in diabetes technology paving the way toward a much anticipated and sought after closed loop insulin delivery system (i.e., artificial pancreas). Currently, patients use sensor glucose levels for retrospective glycemic pattern assessment for insulin dose adjustments, and to warn patients of glycemic excursions outside a predetermined safety zone. Recent developments in sensor technology can not only alert patients to impending danger for hypo- or hyperglycemia in terms of absolute levels (e.g., < 3.9 mmol/L or 70 mg/dL) but can assess rates of change in glucose that might exceed an upper limit. Indeed, another step in closing the detection-delivery loop is a recent advance in automatically pausing insulin delivery altogether when a certain low glucose threshold is breached. Therefore, the patients thought to benefit the most from sensor augmented pump therapy are those with who experience wide fluctuations, nocturnal hypoglycemia, and hypoglycemia unawareness.

CONCLUSION

It is only within the last century that people with type 1 diabetes have had available to them the life-saving therapy of exogenous insulin. While early insulin therapy used relatively crude animal pancreatic extracts, today recombinant DNA technologies provide a large array of insulins and insulin analogs with differing pharmacodynamic properties that allow more physiologic insulin replacement. Despite recent advancements in insulin options and delivery (insulin pens and pumps), challenges remain. Among these is the need to (1) further minimize the risk of hypoglycemia caused by insulin, (2) determine which patients will benefit most from tight glycemic control using rigorous MDI and CSII protocols, (3) develop an array of more potent insulin formulations to treat the increasing number of severely insulin resistant patients, and (4) safely close the loop in glycemic detection-delivery for a true artificial pancreas. Finally, it is important to keep in mind that although insulin is the most potent tool available for treating hyperglycemia, the initiation of insulin therapy is often delayed in type 2 diabetic patients. Such delays can expose patients to unnecessary hyperglycemic burden and risk for complications.

REFERENCES

1. Medvei VC. A History of Endocrinology, 1st edition. Lancaster, England: MTP Press Limited; 1982.
2. Brown JB, Nichols GA, Perry A. The burden of treatment failure in type 2 diabetes. *Diabetes Care*. 2004;27(7):1535-40.
3. Lipska KJ, Bailey CJ, Inzucchi SE. Use of metformin in the setting of mild-to-moderate renal insufficiency. *Diabetes Care*. 2011;34(6):1431-7.
4. Gough SC. A review of human and analogue insulin trials. *Diabetes Res Clin Pract*. 2007;77(1):1-15.
5. Dunn CJ, Plosker GL, Keating GM, McKeage K, Scott LJ. Insulin glargine: an updated review of its use in the management of diabetes mellitus. *Drugs*. 2003;63(16):1743-78.
6. Hollander PA. Insulin detemir for the treatment of obese patients with type 2 diabetes. *Diabetes Metab Syndr Obes*. 2012;5:11-9.
7. Heise T, Nosek L, Rønn BB, Endahl L, Heinemann L, Kapitza C, et al. Lower within-subject variability of insulin detemir in comparison to NPH insulin and insulin glargine in people with type 1 diabetes. *Diabetes*. 2004;53(6):1614-20.
8. Cengiz E, Swan KL, Tamborlane WV, Sherr JL, Martin M, Weinzimer SA. The alteration of aspart insulin pharmacodynamics when mixed with detemir insulin. *Diabetes Care*. 2012;35(4):690-2.
9. Nathan DM, Buse JB, Davidson MB, Ferrannini E, Holman RR, Sherwin R, et al. Medical management of hyperglycaemia in type 2 diabetes mellitus: a consensus algorithm for the initiation and adjustment of therapy: a consensus statement from the American Diabetes Association and the European Association for the Study of Diabetes. *Diabetologia*. 2009; 52(1):17-30.
10. Nathan DM, Buse JB, Davidson MB, Ferrannini E, Holman RR, Sherwin R, et al. Medical management of hyperglycemia in type 2 diabetes: a consensus algorithm for the initiation and adjustment of therapy: a consensus statement of the American Diabetes Association and the European Association for the Study of Diabetes. *Diabetes Care*. 2009;32(1):193-203.
11. Raskin PR, Hollander PA, Lewin A, Gabbay RA, Bode B, Garber AJ, et al. Basal insulin or premix analogue therapy in type 2 diabetes patients. *Eur J Intern Med*. 2007;18(1):56-62.
12. Ray KK, Seshasai SR, Wijesuriya S, Sivakumaran R, Nethercott S, Preiss D, et al. Effect of intensive control of glucose on cardiovascular outcomes and death in patients with diabetes mellitus: a meta-analysis of randomised controlled trials. *Lancet*. 2009; 373(9677):1765-72.
13. Amiel SA, Dixon T, Mann R, Jameson K. Hypoglycaemia in Type 2 diabetes. *Diabet Med*. 2008;25(3):245-54.
14. UK Hypoglycaemia Study Group. Risk of hypoglycaemia in types 1 and 2 diabetes: effects of treatment modalities and their duration. *Diabetologia*. 2007;50(6):1140-7.
15. Heinzerling L, Raile K, Rochlitz H, Zuberbier T, Worm M. Insulin allergy: clinical manifestations and management strategies. *Allergy*. 2008;63(2):148-55.
16. Hemkens LG, Grouven U, Bender R, Günster C, Gutschmidt S, Selke GW, et al. Risk of malignancies in patients with diabetes treated with human insulin or insulin analogues: a cohort study. *Diabetologia*. 2009;52(9):1732-44.

17. Colhoun HM. Use of insulin glargine and cancer incidence in Scotland: a study from the Scottish Diabetes Research Network Epidemiology Group. *Diabetologia*. 2009;52(9): 1755-65.

18. Kurtzhals P, Schäffer L, Sørensen A, Kristensen C, Jonassen I, Schmid C, et al. Correlations of receptor binding and metabolic and mitogenic potencies of insulin analogs designed for clinical use. *Diabetes*. 2000;49(6):999-1005.

19. Currie CJ, Poole CD, Gale EA. The influence of glucose-lowering therapies on cancer risk in type 2 diabetes. *Diabetologia*. 2009;52(9):1766-77.

20. Handelsman Y, Mechanick JI, Blonde L, Grunberger G, Bloomgarden ZT, Bray GA, et al. American Association of Clinical Endocrinologists Medical Guidelines for Clinical Practice for developing a diabetes mellitus comprehensive care plan. *Endocr Pract*. 2011;17(Suppl 2):1-53.

21. Misso ML, Egberts KJ, Page M, O'Connor D, Shaw J. Continuous subcutaneous insulin infusion (CSII) versus multiple insulin injections for type 1 diabetes mellitus. *Cochrane Database Syst Rev*. 2010;(1):CD005103.

22. Pickup JC, Renard E. Long-acting insulin analogs versus insulin pump therapy for the treatment of type 1 and type 2 diabetes. *Diabetes Care*. 2008;31(Suppl 2):S140-5.

23. Fatourechi MM, Kudva YC, Murad MH, Elamin MB, Tabini CC, Montori VM. Clinical review: Hypoglycemia with intensive insulin therapy: a systematic review and meta-analyses of randomized trials of continuous subcutaneous insulin infusion versus multiple daily injections. *J Clin Endocrinol Metab*. 2009;94(3):729-40.

24. Bergenstal RM, Tamborlane WV, Ahmann A, Buse JB, Dailey G, Davis SN, et al. Effectiveness of sensor-augmented insulin-pump therapy in type 1 diabetes. *N Engl J Med*. 2010;363(4):311-20.

25. Raskin P, Bode BW, Marks JB, Hirsch IB, Weinstein RL, McGill JB, et al. Continuous subcutaneous insulin infusion and multiple daily injection therapy are equally effective in type 2 diabetes: a randomized, parallel-group, 24-week study. *Diabetes Care*. 2003; 26(9):2598-603.

26. Pickup JC. Insulin-pump therapy for type 1 diabetes mellitus. *N Engl J Med*. 2012;366(17): 1616-24.

Care of Pregnant Diabetic Patient

Michelle Cordoba-Kissee, Jayendra H Shah

ABSTRACT

Once considered a contraindication to pregnancy, diabetes is becoming an increasingly common aspect to the care of pregnant women. Gestational diabetes mellitus (GDM) occurs in approximately 7% of all pregnancies and is defined as "any degree of glucose intolerance with onset or first recognition during pregnancy". Of all patients with diabetes seen during pregnancy, 87% are GDM, and the remaining 13% are pregestational diabetes where diabetes in these patients was present prior to pregnancy. During pregnancy, several physiologic changes occur, and metabolism is altered. Normal early pregnancy is considered an anabolic state, with increases in maternal fat stores and less insulin requirements, as the body builds caloric reserves in preparation for demands later in pregnancy. In contrast, during the second and third trimesters, pregnancy is considered a state of accelerated starvation with increased glucose consumption by the fetus and the placenta, and endogenous insulin production increases while insulin sensitivity decreases as the pregnancy progresses. In summary, the profound hormonal changes during pregnancy are responsible for plasma volume changes, water retention and their effect on glucose metabolism. In pregnancy, fasting and postprandial insulin concentrations are high, whereas blood glucose levels are low; up to 20% of normal. In addition to glucose consumption by the fetus, increased peripheral glucose utilization, decreased hepatic glucose production, and increased glycogen deposition are responsible for lower glucose concentrations in pregnancy. The low blood glucose levels in combination with insulin resistance is responsible for increased lipolysis resulting in increased use of fat as free fatty acids and ketones as energy consumption in pregnant women. This makes glucose and amino acids available for fetal energy consumption. The maternal transfer of glucose, amino acids, and ketones but not of large lipids occurs through the placenta. Thus, the placenta plays a huge role in controlling the maternal and fetal metabolism by a multitude of produced hormones and selective transfer of nutrients. This chapter discusses physiological changes during pregnancy, criteria to make diagnosis of GDM and management of diabetic patients during various trimesters of the pregnancy and during labor.

INTRODUCTION

Once considered a contraindication to pregnancy, diabetes is becoming an increasingly common aspect to the care of pregnant women. Gestational diabetes mellitus (GDM) occurs in approximately 7% of all pregnancies[1] and is defined as "any degree of glucose intolerance with onset or first recognition during pregnancy".[2] Implied in this definition is the assumption that some women with previously unrecognized pregestational diabetes will be diagnosed at pregnancy as having GDM. Some authors have described this diagnosis of GDM as "detection of an underlying beta-cell defect through routine glucose screening in pregnancy".[3] Of all patients with diabetes seen during pregnancy, 87% are GDM, and the remaining 13% are pregestational diabetes where diabetes in these patients was present prior to pregnancy.[4]

During pregnancy, several physiologic changes occur, and metabolism is altered. Normal early pregnancy is considered an anabolic state, with increases in maternal fat stores and less insulin requirements, as the body builds caloric reserves in preparation for demands later in pregnancy. Insulin needs are often reduced during early pregnancy. In contrast, during the second and third trimesters, pregnancy is considered a state of accelerated starvation with increased glucose consumption by the fetus and the placenta,[5] and endogenous insulin production increases while insulin sensitivity decreases as the pregnancy progresses.[6,7] The endocrine changes during pregnancy play a big role in the physiologic and metabolic alteration. The concentrations of hypothalamic hormones, such as gonadotropin-releasing hormone (GnRH), growth hormone-releasing hormone (GHRH), corticotropin-releasing hormone (CRH), and thyrotropin-releasing hormone (TRH) are increased during pregnancy. The rise in these hormones is also attributed to their production in the placenta. The increase in these hormones leads to an ultimate increase in growth hormone, cortisol, and thyroxine during pregnancy. In addition, the placenta also produces human chorionic somatomammotropin (hCS), also known as human placental lactogen (hPL), progesterone, and chorionic gonadotropins. Increased estradiol levels during pregnancy are thought to be responsible for the steadily rising level of prolactin.[8-11] In summary, the profound hormonal changes during pregnancy are responsible for plasma volume changes, water retention, and their effect on glucose metabolism. The insulin resistance is likely multifactorial with contributions from hormones, such as human placental lactogen, prolactin and cortisol. In addition, a decrease in gastrointestinal motility from elevated progesterone levels can increase in carbohydrate absorption.[6] In pregnancy, fasting and postprandial insulin concentrations are high whereas blood glucose levels are low; up to 20% of normal. In addition to glucose consumption by the fetus, increased peripheral glucose utilization, decreased hepatic glucose production, and increased glycogen deposition are responsible for lower glucose concentrations in pregnancy. The low blood glucose levels in combination with insulin resistance are responsible for increased lipolysis resulting in increased use of fat as free fatty acids and ketones as energy sources in pregnant women. This makes glucose and amino acids available for fetal energy consumption. The maternal transfer of glucose, amino acids, and ketones, but not of large lipids, occurs through the placenta. Thus, the placenta plays a huge role in controlling the maternal and fetal metabolism by a multitude of produced hormones and selective transfer of nutrients.[12-14]

RECOMMENDATIONS FOR SCREENING AND DIAGNOSING DIABETES IN PREGNANCY

Because less than one-third of diabetic women in the United States receive preconceptional counseling, it has been recommended that a diabetic women's plans for pregnancy be reviewed at any health care visit.[15,16] Once pregnancy has occurred, women not known to be diabetic should undergo a risk assessment for GDM at the first prenatal visit, and those who are considered high risk should have glucose tolerance testing. These high-risk women who, on the initial screen, are not found to have GDM as well as those women at average risk should then undergo glucose testing at 24–28 weeks of pregnancy[1,17] (Figure 1).

The criteria for the diagnosis of gestational diabetes have been debated. Women who are diagnosed with diabetes on their first prenatal visit should be given the diagnosis of overt, rather than gestational, diabetes when they have a fasting plasma glucose level greater than 126 mg/dL (7.0 mmol/L) or a random plasma glucose greater than 200 mg/dL (11.1 mmol/L), if it can be confirmed on an additional day.[18]

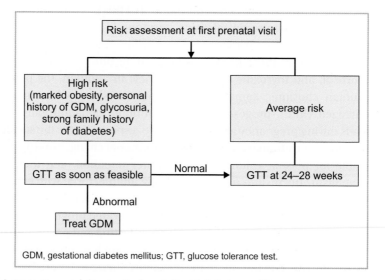

GDM, gestational diabetes mellitus; GTT, glucose tolerance test.

FIGURE 1 Detection and diagnosis of gestational diabetes mellitus.
Source: Adapted from American Diabetes Association. Gestational diabetes mellitus. *Diabetes Care*. 2004;27(Suppl 1):S88-90, and American Diabetes Association. Standards of medical care in diabetes—2012. *Diabetes Care*. 2012;35(Suppl 1):S11-63.

Patients may undergo either a one-step or two-step approach to glucose tolerance testing as described below. Whereas American Diabetes Association (ADA) previously described both approaches,[1] it now recommends that all pregnant women without previously diagnosed diabetes undergo a one-step 75 g oral glucose tolerance test (OGTT).[18] The American College of Obstetricians and Gynecologists (ACOG), however, continue to recommend a two-step approach.[19]

The one-step approach uses an OGTT to assess blood glucose response after an oral glucose load. Both 75 g and 100 g glucose loads have been used. Regardless of the glucose load amount, the test should be done after fasting 8–14 hours, and two threshold values must be met or exceeded to diagnose diabetes. The threshold values between the 75 g and the 100 g tests are the same except there is an additional 3-hour cutoff if a 100 g load is used.[1] There has been debate over these threshold values. For the 100 g glucose load, Carpenter-Coustan have suggested for fasting, 1-, 2-, and 3-hours, the lower threshold values of 95 mg/dL (5.3 mmol/L), 180 mg/dL (10 mmol/L), 155 mg/dL (8.6 mmol/L), and 140 mg/dL (7.8 mmol/L),[20] respectively, whereas the National Diabetes Data Group (NDDG) criteria recommend fasting, 1-, 2-, and 3-hour plasma glucose levels of 105 mg/dL (5.8 mmol/L), 190 mg/dL (10.5 mmol/L), 165 mg/dL (9.2 mmol/L), and 145 mg/dL (8.1 mmol/L), respectively, for diagnosis of GDM.[21] Women who met Carpenter-Coustan criteria but were not treated compared with women who were diagnosed by NDDG criteria and were treated are at more risk for hypertensive disorders of pregnancy and increased infant birth weight. Therefore, it may be warranted to implement the more inclusive GDM diagnostic criteria[22] (Tables 1 and 2).

Alternatively, the International Association of Diabetes and Pregnancy Study Groups (IADPSG) proposed using a 75 g oral glucose load with a 2-hour glucose measurement. For diagnosis of GDM, any one or more of the thresholds needs to be met or exceeded, including a fasting plasma glucose 92 mg/dL (5.1 mmol/L), a 1-hour plasma glucose 180 mg/dL (10 mmol/L), or a 2-hour plasma glucose 153 mg/dL (8.5 mmol/L).[23] However, this approach has not been endorsed by the

TABLE 1: One-step 100 g Oral Glucose Tolerance Test (Recommended by ACOG)		
	Carpenter-Coustan criteria blood glucose	NDDG criteria blood glucose
Fasting	95 mL/dL (5.3 mmol/L)	105 mg/dL (5.8 mmol/L)
1 hour	180 mg/dL (10 mmol/L)	190 mg/dL (10.5 mmol/L)
2 hour	155 mg/dL (8.6 mmol/L)	165 mg/dL (9.2 mmol/L)
3 hour	140 mg/dL (7.8 mmol/L)	145 mg/dL (8.1 mmol/L)

ACOG, American College of Obstetricians and Gynecologists; NDDG, National Diabetes Data Group.
Note: Two positive values are needed to diagnose gestational diabetes.
Source: Adapted from ACOG Committee on Obstetric Practice. Committee opinion no. 504: screening and diagnosis of gestational diabetes mellitus. *Obstet Gynecol.* 2011;118(3):751-3, and American Diabetes Association. Standards of medical care in diabetes—2012. *Diabetes Care.* 2012;35(Suppl 1):S11-63.

TABLE 2: One-step 75 g Oral Glucose Tolerance Test (Recommended by ADA and IADPSG)	
	Blood glucose
Fasting	92 mg/dL (5.1 mmol/L)
1 hour	180 mg/dL (10 mmol/L)
2 hour	153 mg/dL (8.5 mmol/L)

ADA, American Diabetes Association; IADPSG, International Association of Diabetes and Pregnancy Study Groups.
Note: One positive value is needed to diagnose gestational diabetes.
Source: Adapted from ACOG Committee on Obstetric Practice. Committee opinion no. 504: screening and diagnosis of gestational diabetes mellitus. *Obstet Gynecol.* 2011;118(3):751-3., and American Diabetes Association. Standards of medical care in diabetes—2012. *Diabetes Care.* 2012;35(Suppl 1):S11-63.

ACOG Committee on Obstetric Practice, who recommend the 100 g, 3-hour test using either the Carpenter-Coustan or NDDG criteria, citing that there has not been evidence to show improved maternal and fetal outcomes based on IADPSG.[19]

The two-step approach was used formerly but is no longer endorsed by the ADA.[1,18] The ACOG, however, continues to recommend a two-step approach.[19] The first step consists of a screen by patient history, clinical risk factors, or with a screening glucose challenge test (GCT), and those women with an elevated glucose would then proceed to a formal 100-g OGTT as the second step. The GCT includes a 50 g oral glucose load followed by a 1-hour blood glucose determination. The threshold for this screening test has also been debated, with cutoff values of both 130 mg/dL (7.2 mmol/L) and 140 mg/dL (7.8 mmol/L) considered acceptable.[24] If a woman's blood glucose is higher than the specified threshold during the screen, an OGTT would be performed for diagnosis of GDM. If the patient's blood glucose is more than 200 mg/dL (11.1 mmol/L) at 1 hour, she meets criteria for GDM at that point and does not need to be referred for OGTT.

In India, a country in which the population is at an increased risk for GDM based on ethnicity, the utility of a universal, nonfasting screen has been investigated. Pregnant women underwent a nonfasting, 75 g oral GCT with subsequent measurement of plasma glucose 2 hours later. Seventy-two hours later, they also underwent the standard fasting, 75-g OGTT with measurement of plasma glucose 2 hours later. The oral GCT had 100% specificity and sensitivity for identifying GDM when compared to the OGTT and offered the convenience of a nonfasting evaluation.[25]

Upon identification of diabetes, pregnant women are classified according to the White criteria as outlined in table 3.

It has been shown that increasing maternal blood glucose, even at values lower than those that meet criteria to be considered diabetic, is associated with increased perinatal morbidity in a continuous manner.[26] Obesity and diabetes are independently associated with increased birth weight, newborn percent body fat, increased umbilical cord blood C-peptide, primary cesarean delivery, and preeclampsia. Risk is further increased when obesity and diabetes are combined.[27]

TABLE 3: White Classification of Pregnant Diabetic Women	
Revised White classification	Status of diabetes with or without complications
A1	Diet alone, any duration or onset age
A2	Diet alone insufficient, insulin required
B	Onset age 20 years or older and duration less than 10 years
C	Onset age 10–19 years or duration 10–19 years
D	Onset age under 10 years, duration over 20 years, background retinopathy, or hypertension (not preeclampsia)
F	Nephropathy with over 500 mg/day proteinuria
R	Proliferative retinopathy or vitreous hemorrhage
H	Arteriosclerotic heart disease clinically evident
T	Prior renal transplantation

Source: Adapted from Hare JW, White P. Gestational diabetes and the White classification. Diabetes Care. 1980;3:394-6, and White P. Pregnancy complicating diabetes. *Am J Med*. 1949;7(5):609-16.

GUIDELINES FOR MANAGEMENT OF PREGNANT DIABETIC PATIENTS

It is recommended that women who have been diagnosed with GDM be seen every 1–2 weeks until 36 weeks of pregnancy and weekly thereafter.[15] Weight gain recommendations for pregnant women include 12.5–17.5 kg for women with normal weight and 5.5–10 kg in those who are obese.[28] In general, pregnant diabetic patients should avoid gaining excessive weight to prevent further insulin resistance and fetal complications such as macrosomia. Nutritional counseling by a registered dietician is recommended in all women with GDM, and the ADA recommends that women without medical or obstetrical contraindications participate in moderate exercise,[1] which helps increasing insulin sensitivity, helps reduce weight gain, and prepares the patient for needed strength during labor. Specific recommendations have also included exercise sessions of 20–30 minutes at least three to four times weekly[15] to daily.[29]

Trimester-wise evaluation of diabetes in pregnancy is prescribed in table 4.

First Trimester

As mentioned above, women presenting for prenatal care should be assessed for their risk of diabetes as well as undergo routine prenatal testing, such as Rh type and antibody screen, hemoglobin or hematocrit, cervical cytology, rubella immunity testing, urine culture, HIV, syphilis, hepatitis B, and Chlamydia testing.[30] As mentioned previously, pregnant women with diabetes are generally classified into diabetic types based on the revised White criteria (Table 3). All diabetic patients

TABLE 4: Trimester-wise Evaluation of Diabetes in Pregnancy

First trimester
- Routine labs (see text for details)
- Routine obstetric ultrasound
- Glycosylated hemoglobin (HbA1c)
- Random urinary protein to creatinine ratio*
- Thyroid-stimulating hormone (TSH) and free thyroxine (FT4)*
- Electrocardiogram*
- Retinal examination with dilated pupil*

Second trimester
- Routine screen for aneuploidy and neural tube defects
- Detailed fetal anatomy ultrasound 18–20 weeks
- Fetal echocardiogram
- HbA1c

Third trimester
- Group B beta-hemolytic streptococcus
- HbA1c

*In patients with pregestational diabetes.

should be referred for a screening retinal examination at their first prenatal visit.[15] Diabetic women with a history of microalbuminuria or those who have had diabetes for more than 10 years should be screened for nephropathy either before pregnancy or at the first prenatal visit. In most cases, a daily prenatal vitamin with iron is generally recommended as well.

Second Trimester

During the second trimester, pregnant women with diabetes are seen every 2–4 weeks or more frequently as needed. Pregnant diabetic patients should undergo screening for aneuploidy as recommended for nondiabetics. As they are at increased risk for neural tube defects, screening with ultrasound alone or in combination with maternal serum alpha-fetoprotein is recommended. A detailed fetal anatomy survey ultrasound should be performed at 18 weeks. An ultrasound with a four-chamber view of the fetal heart and outflow tracts is recommended at 18–20 weeks.[17] While some advocate dedicated fetal echocardiography for all diabetic pregnant women, others feel a more selective approach is more appropriate after initial fetal anatomic survey.[31,32]

Third Trimester

If women with GDM have hypertension or a history of stillbirth, they should be started on twice weekly nonstress tests (NSTs) at 32 weeks of gestation.[15] Additional testing including fetal movement counting, a biophysical profile (consisting of nonstress testing and sonographic assessment of fetal movement, fetal tone, fetal breathing, and amniotic fluid volume), and the contraction stress tests are usually started at 32–34 weeks of gestation.[16] Maternal surveillance should include blood pressure and urine protein monitoring to detect hypertensive disorders.[1]

MONITORING OF DIABETES IN PREGNANCY

Self-monitoring of capillary blood glucoses (SMBG) should be recorded several times daily, though there is debate over the timing and frequency. Some experts recommend every morning while fasting, before each meal, either 1 or 2 hours after each meal and at bedtime.[16] Others recommend measurements each morning while fasting and 1 or 2 hours after each meal, the frequency of which may be decreased if good glucose control is maintained.[15] Glycemic goals for pregnancy include a fasting glucose level of 95 mg/dL (5.3 mmol/L) or less, 1-hour postprandial levels of 140 mg/dL (7.8 mmol/L) or less, and 2-hour postprandial values of 120 mg/dL or less (6.7 mmol/L).[16]

The use of 1-hour versus 2-hour postprandial glucose monitoring has also been controversial. Using continuous glucose monitoring, it has been shown that the mean time to peak postprandial glucose is 90 minutes in pregnant diabetics[33] but perinatal outcome data are lacking. It has even been suggested that the timing of the glucose could be checked at different times (e.g., 1-hour versus 2-hour) postprandially depending on type and time of the meal.[34] There were no significant differences in perinatal outcome when 1-hour postprandial and 2-hour postprandial monitoring were compared, though women using 2-hour postprandial measurements had a statistically nonsignificant tendency toward increased fetal macrosomia and delivery by cesarean section.[35] When compared to preprandial glycemic monitoring, 1-hour postprandial monitoring is more predictive of fetal macrosomia[36] and has been associated with less preeclampsia and smaller neonatal triceps skinfold thickness[37] as well as improved glycemic control and decreased risk of neonatal hypoglycemia, macrosomia, and cesarean delivery.[38] A 1-hour postprandial glucose value of 130 mg/dL (7.3 mmol/L) has been suggested as the level to decrease fetal macrosomia without increasing the incidence of small-for-gestational-age infants.[39] Therefore, we recommend monitoring of 1-hour postprandial blood glucose.

Glycosylated hemoglobin (HbA1c) has been shown to have a consistent correlation with mean plasma glucose during pregnancy, although the average plasma glucose for a given HbA1c may be lower than in nonpregnant patients.[40] Various physiologic changes in the pregnancy including volume expansion and change in red cell life span cause a fall in HbA1c level during midtrimester and then a rise in the third trimester. It is also important to recognize that pregnant nondiabetic women have lower HbA1c levels than nondiabetic nonpregnant women. For planned pregnancy in pregestational diabetic patients, HbA1c is recommended to be less than 6%[16] or 6.1%[17] if safely achievable. The pregestational diabetic patients whose HbA1c is more than

10% are advised against pregnancy until desirable glycemic control (HbA1c <7.0%) is achieved.[17] Because the erythrocyte life span is shortened during pregnancy, some have suggested the utility of using HbA1c hemoglobin more frequently, even weekly, to guide management decisions during pregnancy.[41]

MANAGEMENT OF DIABETES IN PREGNANCY

If the above goals are not met in women with GDM, dietary intervention is recommended. Additionally, insulin therapy should be started if blood glucose remains elevated despite dietary adherence, though data are lacking regarding the number of glucose elevations required prior to initiating insulin.[24] The use of oral hypoglycemic medications during pregnancy remains controversial.[24] The sulfonylurea glyburide (glibenclamide) may be used for glycemic control during pregnancy,[15] though some favor its substitution with insulin.[29] In a study involving pregnant women with GDM who required treatment, those randomized to glyburide versus insulin were found to have similar incidences of complications including fetal macrosomia and large for gestational age, lung complications, hypoglycemia, anomalies and neonatal intensive care unit admissions. Additionally, glyburide was not detected in the cord serum of any infant in the glyburide group.[42]

Like glyburide, the use of metformin in pregnancy remains controversial as well.[29] When considering its use, the known risks of hyperglycemia need to outweigh the potential and admittedly unknown risks of metformin in pregnancy.[43] The argument has been made that women who were taking metformin prior to conception continue it through the first 8–12 weeks of pregnancy, with the rationale that the anticipated hyperglycemia as a result of metformin discontinuation poses a greater risk to the fetus during embryogenesis than do the potential risks of the medication itself.[43] Additional potential uses of metformin during pregnancy include cases where either the mother refuses insulin or it is otherwise unavailable for use or where metformin could enhance glycemic control in addition to insulin in women with severe insulin resistance.[43] We prefer the use of insulin to control hyperglycemia in pregnant diabetic patients.

Insulin analogs are most often the treatment of choice in pregnant diabetic patients. Traditionally, treatment has included an intermediate insulin, such as neutral protamine Hagedorn (NPH) insulin given before breakfast and again either before dinner or before bedtime, with a preference for bedtime dosing. Additionally, either short- or rapid-acting insulin should be given with meals. Options include short-acting regular insulin given 30 minutes prior to meals or rapid-acting insulins, such as lispro or aspart given right before eating.[16] A small study which randomized women with GDM to insulin lispro, insulin aspart, or regular human insulin has suggested that both lispro and aspart are associated with less fetal macrosomia and improved postprandial blood sugars when compared to regular human insulin.[44] Another study in which women with type 1 diabetes who were pregnant or planning pregnancy were randomized to insulin lispro or human regular insulin in addition to NPH found that women receiving insulin lispro had less hypoglycemia, less postprandial hyperglycemic excursions, and achieved comparable HbA1c's while maintaining similar safety profiles and pregnancy outcomes.[45] The rapid-acting analog insulin aspart has also been shown to have no difference in fetal loss, perinatal mortality, congenital malformation, and neonatal short-term complications.[46] Others have found no difference between lispro and regular insulin, in terms of glycemic control and complications. Pregnant patients with type 1 diabetes randomized to the lispro group had more hypoglycemia, and those in the regular group had more episodes of severe hypoglycemia. Women receiving lispro also had less glycemic excursions after lunch, though the remaining meals were comparable.[47] Currently, rapid-acting insulin, such as lispro or aspart is favored over regular insulin in pregnant diabetics.

The long-acting basal insulins (glargine and detemir) have not been adequately studied in pregnancy to recommend their use[6]. Although they have not been officially approved in Europe and the United States, they continue to be used off-label.[29,48] Studies have not shown an increase in adverse fetal or maternal outcomes in which glargine was used during pregnancy.[49,50] A retrospective trial of pregnant type 1 diabetic patients suggested that congenital malformation and birth weights were the same in women treated with insulin glargine and in those who used NPH.[51] A retrospective cohort study found that infant and mother morbidity and mortality were not increased with glargine when compared to NPH. In addition, infants of mothers with pregestational diabetes treated with glargine had less fetal macrosomia and neonatal hypoglycemia when compared to those infants whose mothers used NPH. The authors recommended that pregestational diabetics may stay on glargine during pregnancy.[52]

A case control study involving pregnant women with type 1 diabetes demonstrated that there were no differences between treatment with glargine versus NPH in regards to complications and hypoglycemia, but glargine use was associated with better fasting and 2-hour postprandial glucose at breakfast in the first and second trimesters. Fetuses of mothers taking glargine were, however, noted to have a higher incidence of femoral length at less than 50th percentile.[53] Another case control study also found that pregnant women with both GDM and type 1 diabetes who used glargine, when compared to those using intermediate-acting human insulin, had no difference in neonatal morbidity or birth weights.[54] We feel intermediate-acting insulin can be used safely in the management of pregnant diabetic patient.

An alternative to basal and multiple bolus daily insulin injection regimens, a continuous subcutaneous insulin infusion (CSII) via an insulin pump is also recommended in some difficult to control pregnant diabetic patients. Maternal and perinatal outcomes were comparable in women using CSII—mostly with regular insulin—versus those using multiple daily injections of regular and intermediate insulins.[55] Similarly, there was no difference in outcome between patients using CSII with rapid-acting insulin analogs versus those using multiple daily injections of glargine plus rapid-acting analogs.[56] Several studies have reported similar pregnancy outcomes for women using CSII versus those using multiple daily injections.[48,56-61]

Finally, in women with insulin resistance who require more than 200 units of insulin daily, the use of concentrated (U-500) is an option.[15,62] Because U-500 is regular insulin that is concentrated five times more than regular U-100 and has unique pharmacokinetics, it should be used with caution.

MANAGEMENT OF DIABETES IN LABOR AND DELIVERY

Elective delivery may be considered in poorly controlled patients at 38–39 weeks of gestation.[15] If they have reassuring antenatal testing, patients with well-controlled diabetes can progress to their due date, but expectant management after the expected date of delivery is not recommended.[1] Given the risk of fetal macrosomia, delivery during the 38th week is generally recommended, but fetal macrosomia itself is not an indication for labor induction.[16] Women who have a macrosomic fetus should be counseled on the risks and benefits of vaginal birth, induction of labor, and cesarean section,[17] and cesarean delivery should be considered if the fetal weight is estimated to be 4,500 g or more.[15]

During labor, patients who have required pharmacological treatment of their diabetes should undergo capillary glucose monitoring every 1-2 hours.[15,17] It is important to recognize that some women may not need insulin during active labor.[16] A regular insulin intravenous (IV) infusion with IV dextrose solution as needed can be titrated to maintain capillary blood glucose less than 110 mg/dL (6.1 mmol/L)[15,16] or between 72 mg/dL (4 mmol/L) and 126 mg/dL (7 mmol/L).[17] Diabetic women on subcutaneous insulin pumps may continue their basal infusion during labor.[16] After delivery, insulin requirements sharply decrease, and it is prudent to decrease the insulin dose to 25–40% of the predelivery dose to prevent hypoglycemia.[48] Infants of diabetic mothers should be monitored for hypoglycemia, hypocalcemia, and hyperbilirubinemia.[15]

Following delivery, insulin should be reduced in women with preexisting diabetes and discontinued in women who were diagnosed with gestational diabetes.[17] Women with GDM should test their blood sugar postpartum and undergo a fasting plasma glucose measurement 6 weeks after delivery.[17] Breastfeeding can lead to even lower insulin needs, and insulin may need to be lowered in the lactating patient. Finally, insulin analogs can be safely used in lactation.[48]

MANAGEMENT OF DIABETES DURING POSTPARTUM PERIOD

In patients diagnosed with GDM, recommendations include reassessment of diabetes status at 6[1,63] to 6–12[64] weeks postpartum. The ADA recommends screening at 6–12 weeks after delivery with a 75 g OGTT.[1] Those women who return to normal glucose levels should be reassessed for diabetes at least every 3 years.[1] The children of diabetic mothers should also be monitored for of obesity and diabetes.[1] The majority of cases of gestational diabetes resolve during postpartum period,[63] although approximately 15% will remain glucose intolerant or become overtly diabetic.[15]

CONCLUSION

Several areas regarding diabetes in pregnancy remain to be explored. The development of GDM screening recommendations from an international perspective is needed to identify in a cost-effective manner those women who would benefit from intervention. It is important to achieve normoglycemia in the pregnant diabetic patients to obviate abnormal maternal and fetal outcomes, such as fetal death, fetal overweight, macrosomia, and other congenital anomalies. More data are needed to support using oral hypoglycemic agents during pregnancy. Similarly, the use of the long-acting insulin analogs, such as glargine and detemir during pregnancy appears to be a promising therapeutic tool, but limited safety and pregnancy outcome data preclude its use at the present time. A randomized controlled trial comparing NPH versus insulin detemir, both with insulin aspart, in type 1 diabetic pregnant women has been completed, the results of which are anticipated in near future.[65]

REFERENCES

1. American Diabetes Association. Gestational diabetes mellitus. *Diabetes Care.* 2004; 27(Suppl 1):S88-90.
2. Metzger BE, Coustan DR. Summary and recommendations of the Fourth International Workshop-Conference on gestational diabetes mellitus. The Organizing Committee. *Diabetes Care.* 1998;21(Suppl 2):B161-7.
3. Buchanan TA, Page KA. Approach to the patient with gestational diabetes after delivery. *J Clin Endocrinol Metab.* 2011;96(12):3592-8.
4. Wier LM, Witt E, Burgess J, Elixhauser A. Hospitalization Related to Diabetes in Pregnancy, 2008: Statistical Brief #102.
5. Kamalakannan D, Baskar V, Barton DM, Abdu TA. Diabetic ketoacidosis in pregnancy. *Postgrad Med J.* 2013; 79:454-7.
6. Landon MB, Catalano PM, Gabbe SG. Diabetes mellitus complicating pregnancy. In: Gabbe SG, Niebyl JR, Galan HL, Jauniaux ER, Landon MB, Simpson JL, Driscoll DA (Eds). Obstetrics: Normal and Problem Pregnancies, 6th edition. Philadelphia, PA: Elsevier; 2012. pp. 888-921.
7. Catalano PM, Tyzbir ED, Roman NM, Amini SB, Sims EA. Longitudinal changes in insulin release and insulin resistance in nonobese pregnant women. *Am J Obstet Gynecol.* 1991;165:1667-72.
8. Petraglia F, Sawchenko PE, Rivier J, Vale W. Evidence for local stimulation of ACTH secretion by corticotropin-releasing factor in human placenta. *Nature.* 1987;328:717-9.
9. Mazlan M, Spence-Jones C, Chard T, Landon J, McLean C. Circulating levels of GH-releasing hormone and GH during human pregnancy. *J Endocrinol.* 1990;125:161-7.
10. Bajoria R, Babawale M. Ontogeny of endogenous secretion of immunoreactive-thyrotropin releasing hormone by human placenta. *J Clin Endocrinol Metab.* 1998;83:4148-55.

11. Tyson JE, Hwang P, Guyda H, Friesen HG. Studies of prolactin secretion in human pregnancy. *Am J Obstet Gynecol.* 1972;113:14-20.

12. Hernandez TL, Friedman JE, Van Pelt RE, Barbour LA. Patterns of glycemia in normal pregnancy: should the current therapeutic targets be challenged? *Diabetes Care.* 2011; 34:1660-8.

13. Herrera E. Metabolic adaptations in pregnancy and their implications for the availability of substrates to the fetus. *Eur J Clin Nutr.* 2000;54(Suppl 1):S47-51.

14. McIntyre HD, Chang AM, Callaway LK, Cowley DM, Dyer AR, Radaelli T, et al. Hormonal and metabolic factors accociated with variation in insulin sensitivity in human pregnancy. *Diabetes Care.* 2010;33:356-60.

15. Gabbe SG, Graves CR. Management of diabetes mellitus complicating pregnancy. *Obstet Gynecol.* 2003;102:857-68.

16. ACOG Committee on Practice Bulletins. ACOG Practice Bulletin. Clinical Management Guidelines for Obstetrician-Gynecologists. Number 60, March 2005. Pregestational diabetes mellitus. *Obstet Gynecol.* 2005;105(3):675-85.

17. Guideline Development Group. Management of diabetes from preconception to the postnatal period: summary of NICE guidance. *BMJ.* 2008;336(7646):714-7.

18. American Diabetes Association. Standards of medical care in diabetes—2012. *Diabetes Care.* 2012;35(Suppl 1):S11-63.

19. ACOG Committee on Obstetric Practice. Committee opinion no. 504: screening and diagnosis of gestational diabetes mellitus. *Obstet Gynecol.* 2011;118(3):751-3.

20. Carpenter MW, Coustan DR. Criteria for screening tests for gestational diabetes. *Am J Obstet Gynecol.* 1982;144(7):768-73.

21. National Diabetes Data Group. Classification and diagnosis of diabetes mellitus and other categories of glucose intolerance. *Diabetes.* 1979;28(12):1039-57.

22. Berggren EK, Boggess KA, Stuebe AM, Jonsson Funk M. National Diabetes Data Group vs Carpenter-Coustan criteria to diagnose gestational diabetes. *Am J Obstet Gynecol.* 2011; 205(3):253.e1-7.

23. Coustan DR, Lowe LP, Metzger BE, Dyer AR, International Association of Diabetes and Pregnancy Study Groups. The Hyperglycemia and Adverse Pregnancy Outcome (HAPO) study: paving the way for new diagnostic criteria for gestational diabetes mellitus. *Am J Obstet Gynecol.* 2010;202(6):654.e1-6.

24. American College of Obstetricians and Gynecologists Committee on Practice Bulletins— Obstetrics. ACOG Practice Bulletin. Clinical management guidelines for obstetrician-gynecologists. Number 30, September 2001 (replaces Technical Bulletin Number 200, December 1994). Gestational diabetes. *Obstet Gynecol.* 2001;98(3):525-38.

25. Anjalakshi C, Balaji V, Balaji MS, Ashalata S, Suganthi S, Arthi T, et al. A single test procedure to diagnose gestational diabetes mellitus. *Acta Diabetol.* 2009;46(1):51-4.

26. HAPO Study Cooperative Research Group, Metzger BE, Lowe LP, Dyer AR, Trimble ER, Chaovarindr U, et al. Hyperglycemia and adverse pregnancy outcomes. *N Engl J Med.* 2008;358(19):1991-2002.

27. Catalano PM, McIntyre HD, Cruickshank JK, McCance DR, Dyer AR, Metzger BE, et al. The hyperglycemia and adverse pregnancy outcome study: associations of GDM and obesity with pregnancy outcomes. *Diabetes Care.* 2012;35:780-6.

28. Rasmussen KM, Yaktine AL (Eds). Weight Gain During Pregnancy. Washington, DC. National Academies Press (US); 2009.

29. Mathiesen ER, Ringholm L, Damm P. Pregnancy management of women with pregestational diabetes. *Endocrinol Metab Clin North Am.* 2011;40(4):727-38.

30. American Academy of Pediatrics, American College of Obstetricians and Gynecologists. Guidelines for Perinatal Care, 6th edition. Elk Grove Village, Illinois: AAP; Washington, DC: ACOG; 2007.

31. Odibo AO, Coassolo KM, Stamilio DM, Ural SH, Macones GA. Should all pregnant diabetic women undergo a fetal echocardiography? A cost-effectiveness analysis comparing four screening strategies. *Prenat Diagn.* 2006;26(1):39-44.

32. Sekhavat S, Kishore N, Levine JC. Screening fetal echocardiography in diabetic mothers with normal findings on detailed anatomic survey. *Ultrasound Obstet Gynecol.* 2010;35(2):178-82.

33. Ben-Haroush A, Yogev Y, Chen R, Rosenn B, Hod M, Langer O. The postprandial glucose profile in the diabetic pregnancy. *Am J Obstet Gynecol.* 2004;191(2):576-81.

34. Sivan E, Weisz B, Homko CJ, Reece EA, Schiff E. One or two hours postprandial glucose measurements: are they the same? *Am J Obstet Gynecol.* 2001;185(3):604-7.

35. Weisz B, Shrim A, Homko CJ, Schiff E, Epstein GS, Sivan E. One hour versus two hours postprandial glucose measurement in gestational diabetes: a prospective study. *J Perinatol.* 2005;25(4):241-4.

36. Jovanovic-Peterson L, Peterson CM, Reed GF, Metzger BE, Mills JL, Knopp RH, et al. Maternal postprandial glucose levels and infant birth weight: the Diabetes in Early Pregnancy Study. *Am J Obstet Gynecol.* 1991;164(1 Pt 1):103-11.

37. Manderson JG, Patterson CC, Hadden DR, Traub AI, Ennis C, McCance DR. Preprandial versus postprandial blood glucose monitoring in type 1 diabetic pregnancy: a randomized controlled clinical trial. *Am J Obstet Gynecol.* 2003;189(2):507-12.

38. de Veciana M, Major CA, Morgan MA, Asrat T, Toohey JS, Lien JM, et al. Postprandial versus preprandial blood glucose monitoring in women with gestational diabetes mellitus requiring insulin therapy. *N Engl J Med.* 1995;333(19):1237-41.

39. Combs CA, Gunderson E, Kitzmiller JL, Gavin LA, Main EK. Relationship of fetal macrosomia to maternal postprandial glucose control during pregnancy. *Diabetes Care.* 1992;15(10):1251-7.

40. Gandhi RA, Brown J, Simm A, Page RC, Idris I. HbA1c during pregnancy: its relationship to meal related glycaemia and neonatal birth weight in patients with diabetes. *Eur J Obstet Gynecol Reprod Biol.* 2008;138(1):45-8.

41. Jovanovic L, Savas H, Mehta M, Trujillo A, Pettitt DJ. Frequent monitoring of A1C during pregnancy as a treatment tool to guide therapy. *Diabetes Care.* 2011;34(1):53-4.

42. Langer O, Conway DL, Berkus MD, Xenakis EM, Gonzales O. A comparison of glyburide and insulin in women with gestational diabetes mellitus. *N Engl J Med.* 2000;343(16):1134-8.

43. Simmons D. Metformin treatment for type 2 diabetes in pregnancy? *Best Pract Res Clin Endocrinol Metab.* 2010;24(4):625-34.

44. Di Cianni G, Volpe L, Ghio A, Lencioni C, Cuccuru I, Benzi L, et al. Maternal metabolic control and perinatal outcome in women with gestational diabetes mellitus treated with lispro or aspart insulin. *Diabetes Care.* 2007;30(4):e11.

45. Mathiesen ER, Kinsley B, Amiel SA, Heller S, McCance D, Duran S, et al. Maternal glycemic control and hypoglycemia in type 1 diabetic pregnancy: a randomized trial of insulin aspart versus human insulin in 322 pregnant women. *Diabetes Care.* 2007;30(4):771-6.

46. Hod M, Damm P, Kaaja R, Visser GH, Dunne F, Demidova I, et al. Fetal and perinatal outcomes in type 1 diabetes pregnancy: a randomized study comparing insulin aspart with human insulin in 322 subjects. *Am J Obstet Gynecol.* 2008;198(2):186.e1-7.

47. Persson B, Swahn ML, Hjertberg R, Hanson U, Nord E, Nordlander E, et al. Insulin lispro therapy in pregnancies complicated by type 1 diabetes mellitus. *Diabetes Res Clin Pract.* 2002;58(2):115-21.

48. de Valk HW, Visser GH. Insulin during pregnancy, labour and delivery. *Best Pract Res Clin Obstet Gynaecol.* 2011;25(1):65-76.

49. Gallen IW, Jaap A, Roland JM, Chirayath HH. Survey of glargine use in 115 pregnant women with type 1 diabetes. *Diabet Med.* 2008;25(2):165-9.

50. Egerman RS, Ramsey RD, Kao LW, Bringman JJ, Haerian H, Kao JL, et al. Perinatal outcomes in pregnancies managed with antenatal insulin glargine. *Am J Perinatol.* 2009; 26(8):591-5.

51. Di Cianni G, Torlone E, Lencioni C, Bonomo M, Di Benedetto A, Napoli A, et al. Perinatal outcomes associated with the use of glargine during pregnancy. *Diabet Med.* 2008; 25(8):993-6.

52. Fang YM, MacKeen D, Egan JF, Zelop CM. Insulin glargine compared with neutral protamine Hagedorn insulin in the treatment of pregnant diabetics. *J Matern Fetal Neonatal Med.* 2009;22(3):249-53.

53. Imbergamo MP, Amato MC, Sciortino G, Gambina M, Accidenti M, Criscimanna A, et al. Use of glargine in pregnant women with type 1 diabetes mellitus: a case-control study. *Clin Ther.* 2008;30(8):1476-84.

54. Price N, Bartlett C, Gillmer M. Use of insulin glargine during pregnancy: a case-control pilot study. *BJOG.* 2007;114(4):453-7.

55. Lapolla A, Dalfrà MG, Masin M, Bruttomesso D, Piva I, Crepaldi C, et al. Analysis of outcome of pregnancy in type 1 diabetics treated with insulin pump or conventional insulin therapy. *Acta Diabetol.* 2003;40(3):143-9.

56. Bruttomesso D, Bonomo M, Costa S, Dal Pos M, Di Cianni G, Pellicano F, et al. Type 1 diabetes control and pregnancy outcomes in women treated with continuous subcutaneous insulin infusion (CSII) or with insulin glargine and multiple daily injections of rapid-acting insulin analogues (glargine-MDI). *Diabetes Metab.* 2011;37(5):426-31.

57. Volpe L, Pancani F, Aragona M, Lencioni C, Battini L, Ghio A, et al. Continuous subcutaneous insulin infusion and multiple dose insulin injections in type 1 diabetic pregnant women: a case-control study. *Gynecol Endocrinol.* 2010;26(3):193-6.

58. González-Romero S, González-Molero I, Fernández-Abellán M, Domínguez-López ME, Ruiz-de-Adana S, Olveira G, et al. Continuous subcutaneous insulin infusion versus multiple daily injections in pregnant women with type 1 diabetes. *Diabetes Technol Ther.* 2010;12(4):263-9.

59. Cypryk K, Kosiński M, Kamińska P, Kozdraj T, Lewiński A. Diabetes control and pregnancy outcomes in women with type 1 diabetes treated during pregnancy with continuous subcutaneous insulin infusion or multiple daily insulin injections. *Pol Arch Med Wewn.* 2008;118(6):339-44.

60. Kernaghan D, Farrell T, Hammond P, Owen P. Fetal growth in women managed with insulin pump therapy compared to conventional insulin. *Eur J Obstet Gynecol Reprod Biol.* 2008;137(1):47-9.

61. Chen R, Ben-Haroush A, Weismann-Brenner A, Melamed N, Hod M, Yogev Y. Level of glycemic control and pregnancy outcome in type 1 diabetes: a comparison between multiple daily insulin injections and continuous subcutaneous insulin infusions. *Am J Obstet Gynecol.* 2007;197(4):404.e1-5.

62. Hatipoglu B, Soni S, Espinosa V. Glycemic control with continuous subcutaneous insulin infusion with use of U-500 insulin in a pregnant patient. *Endocr Pract.* 2006;12(5):542-4.

63. Expert Committee on the Diagnosis and Classification of Diabetes Mellitus. Report of the expert committee on the diagnosis and classification of diabetes mellitus. *Diabetes Care.* 2003;26(Suppl 1):S5-20.

64. ACOG Committee on Obstetric Practice. ACOG Committee opinion no. 435: postpartum screening for abnormal glucose tolerance in women who had gestational diabetes mellitus. *Obstet Gynecol.* 2009;113(6):1419-21.

65. Mathiesen ER, Damm P, Jovanovic L, McCance DR, Thyregod C, Jensen AB, et al. Basal insulin analogues in diabetic pregnancy: a literature review and baseline results of a randomised, controlled trial in type 1 diabetes. *Diabetes Metab Res Rev.* 2011;27(6):543-51.

Type 2 Diabetes in Youth

10
Chapter

Jayendra H Shah

ABSTRACT

This chapter describes that the incidence of type 2 diabetes in youth has dramatically increased globally in recent years. In the United States, ethnic minorities of Native American, African-American, Hispanic, Pacific Islanders, and Asian-American have experienced marked increase of type 2 diabetes in youth than general population. The global rise in obesity in youth appears to be responsible for the increased incidence of type 2 diabetes in youth. Positive family history of diabetes in 1st and 2nd degree relatives and low birth weight with overweight during puberty are strong predictor of type 2 diabetes in youth. Many youth are diagnosed with type 2 diabetes during screening or routine clinical and laboratory examination. The identification of type 2 diabetes in youth can be done clinically in most patients. However, in some youth, differentiation between type 1 and type 2 may be difficult even after determination of islet cell autoantibodies. The chapter discusses the differences in the presentation and pathophysiology of type 1 and type 2 diabetes in youth and further explores the treatment for optimal glycemic control, weight reduction and maintenance, nutritional counseling according to daily activities, and exercise planning. The author contends that involvement of all family members with youth in planning of nutritional treatment and exercise program is essential. Glycemic control can be achieved with metformin, if nutritional management, exercise, and weight reduction are not effective. In some youth with type 2 diabetes, especially the one with characteristics of both type 1 and 2 diabetes, insulin treatment may be needed for glycemic control.

INTRODUCTION

In recent years, increased incidence of type 2 diabetes has been observed in the youth. This increased incidence of type 2 diabetes is associated with increased incidence of obesity in the youth. The rise in type 2 diabetes in youth has been universal and several countries have reported increased incidence of both obesity and type 2 diabetes. For example, in the United States, a study reported that the incidence of diabetes in youth between the ages of 10 and 19 was increased from 0.7 per 100,000 in 1982 to 7.2 per 100,000 in 1994.[1] Other studies have also reported increased incidence of diabetes and obesity in youth.[2,3] In Thailand, the incidence of diabetes in youth was reported to be increased between periods of 1986 and 1999 from 5% to 18% with increase in obesity between 1990 and 1996 from 5.8% to 13.3%.[4] A study from Japan reported that after year 1981, the incidence of type 2 diabetes in youth aged 13–15 was increased to 6.43 per 100,000 with associated rise in obesity.[5] A study from Argentina reported that from 1992 to 2001, new cases of type 2 diabetes in youth increased from 0% to 4.3%.[6] In the United States, the incidence and prevalence of type 2 diabetes in various ethnic groups is on the rise compared to general population (Figures 1A and B). It was estimated in 2001 the prevalence of type 2 diabetes among youth 10–19 years old to be 1.45 per 1,000 in Navajo Indians, 1.06 per 1,000 in African-American, 0.52 per 1,000 in Asian-Pacific Islander, 0.46 in Hispanic, and 0.18 per 1,000 in non-Hispanic White (Figure 1B).[7-11]

Although obesity is most important risk factor for developing type 2 diabetes in youth by causing insulin resistance, other conditions causing insulin resistance, positive family history of diabetes and ethnicity may also play a role. Puberty[12] due to increase growth hormone secretion and polycystic ovary syndrome is also known to cause insulin resistance and, therefore, play a role in the development of type 2 diabetes in youth. Also, it appears that subjects with highest prepubertal body weight and lowest birth weight have highest risk for insulin resistance and, therefore, developing type 2 diabetes.[13] It has been reported that over 40% of youth with type 2 diabetes have positive family history of diabetes in one parent, grandparent, or first-

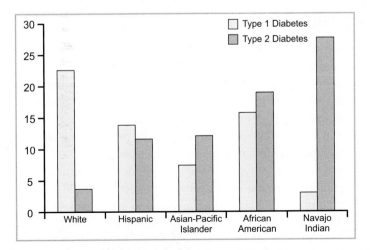

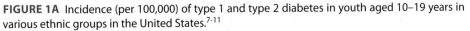

FIGURE 1A Incidence (per 100,000) of type 1 and type 2 diabetes in youth aged 10–19 years in various ethnic groups in the United States.[7-11]

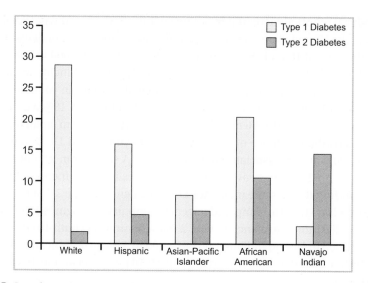

FIGURE 1B Prevalence (per 1,000) of type 1 and type 2 diabetes in youth aged 10–19 years in various ethnic groups in the United States.[7-11]

degree relative.[14,15] The risk of type 2 diabetes in youth is increased if both parents are diabetic and a second-degree relative is diabetic. As outlined above, the prevalence of type 2 diabetes is higher in Navajo and African-American compared to other groups and general population.[7-11] Type 2 diabetes is also 1.3–1.7 times more common in female than male youth.[2,3] This increased risk may be related to female youth having a risk of developing polycystic ovary syndrome.

CLINICAL PRESENTATION AND DIAGNOSIS

Many youths are diagnosed with type 2 diabetes during routine physical examination and routine laboratory test for urine and blood glucose determination. Polyuria and polydipsia due to hyperglycemia can be presenting symptoms. It is important to recognize that youth with type 2 diabetes can present with diabetic ketoacidosis (DKA) or hyperglycemic hyperosmolar state. Initial presentation of DKA is variable, 5–25% of cases in youth with type 2 diabetes.[2,16] The presentation with ketonuria and DKA is more common in African-American and Hispanic youths.[2,17]

The diagnostic criteria for type 2 diabetes in youth are same as in adults with type 2 diabetes. Fasting plasma glucose of greater than or equal to 126 mg/dL (7 mmol/L), random plasma glucose of greater than or equal to 200 mg/dL (11.1 mmol/L) with symptoms of hyperglycemia, or glycosylated hemoglobin (HbA1c) greater than or equal to 6.5%; one of these criteria when confirmed by repeat test on another day is diagnostic of type 2 diabetes. It is important to make diagnosis of type 2 diabetes in youth compared to type 1 diabetes as treatment options and long-term implication

TABLE 1: Differences Between Type 2 and Type 1 Diabetes in Youth		
	Type 2 diabetes in youth	**Type 1 diabetes in youth**
Presentation	Asymptomatic-insidious to severe	Acute
Age at onset	Usually at puberty	Bimodal (4–6 and 10–14 years of age)
Ketosis/ketoacidosis	Less common	Common
Female:Male ratio	1.7:1	1:1
Family history of first- and second-degree relatives with diabetes	>80%	<10%
Ethnicity in USA	Common in ethnic minorities (Figures 1A and B)	Common in non-Hispanic white
Overweight or obese	>80%	<25%
Insulin resistance	Present	Absent
Other insulin resistance conditions (acanthosis nigricans, polycystic ovary syndrome, hypertension, hyperlipidemia)	Common	Rare
C-peptide (presence of endogenous insulin)	Usually present	Reduced to absent
Islet cell antibodies (IAA, GAD, ICA, ZnT8, IA-2)*	Rarely present	Present

*Autoantibodies: IAA—to insulin; GAD—to glutamic acid decarboxylase; ICA—to islet cell cytoplasm; ZnT8—beta cell-specific autoantibody to zinc transporter; IA-2—to tyrosine phosphatase.

are different (Table 1). The onset of type 2 diabetes in youth is usually after onset of puberty whereas type 1 diabetes in youth has bimodal distribution, one peak at 4-6 years of age and another at the ages of 10–14 years, early pubertal age. The youth with type 2 diabetes is generally overweight or obese with insulin resistance. Other conditions causing insulin resistance, such as polycystic ovary syndrome, acanthosis nigricans, hyperlipidemia, and hypertension are present in youth with type 2 diabetes. Because obesity in youth is more common in recent years, as many as 25% of type 1 diabetic youth may be overweight or obese. However, causes of insulin resistance are rare in youth with type 1 diabetes. Positive family history of diabetes is more common in youth with type 2 diabetes. Presentation with DKA is more common in youth with type 1 diabetes than type 2 diabetes. Ethnic minority group youth (i.e., Native American, African-American, Hispanic, Pacific Islander, or Asian American) is more likely to present with type 2 diabetes. In difficult cases, low serum C-peptide levels and presence of islet cell autoantibodies will suggest type 1 diabetes.[18] Sometimes even with the specific laboratory tests, the differentiation between type 1 and type 2 diabetes in youth is difficult. Some of the youths diagnosed with type 2 diabetes were tested positive with some of the islet cell autoantibodies. Some of the youths present with clinical characteristics of both type 1 and type 2 diabetes and with mixed test findings it becomes very difficult to classify such diabetic youth in type I or type 2 diabetes category.

In youth coexisting Cushing's syndrome, pheochromocytoma, glucagonoma, cystic fibrosis, chronic pancreatitis, and hemochromatosis may be responsible for glucose intolerance or frank diabetes. A careful clinical examination and appropriate tests should help in the differential diagnosis. Fasting plasma glucose or HbA1c determination is recommended by American Diabetes Association (ADA)[19] every 3 years after the age 10 in obese youths who have two or more of following risk factors:

- Family history of diabetes (first- or second-degree relative)
- History of gestational diabetes in mother when pregnant with youth
- Youth belonging to high-risk ethnic group (Native American, African-American, Hispanic, Asian American, or Pacific Islander)
- Coexisting conditions indicative of insulin resistance (polycystic ovary syndrome, acanthosis nigricans, hyperlipidemia and hypertension).

TREATMENT

Overall management of youth with type 2 diabetes is very similar to the management of type 2 diabetes in adults. The objective for the treatment is to maintain optimal glycemic control to prevent long-term microvascular and macrovascular complications and treat associated conditions like hyperlipidemia and hypertension. Every effort should be made to decrease insulin resistance which will help in achieving optimal glycemic control. Weight reduction and maintenance with increase activities and exercise planning which will help in reducing insulin resistance are crucial aspect of the management of type 2 diabetes in youth. The lifestyle modification in the youth is difficult and therefore, involvement of parents and other family members as well as multidisciplinary help from nurse educator, nutritionist, and psychologist is essential. In nutritional therapy, counseling the diabetic youth for ethnically appropriate diet and education for entire family about the diet, increasing activities, and exercise is important. Furthermore, it is most effective when entire family is included in the discussion and planning of dietary and weight loss goal.[20] The input from the family and youth and understanding of their likes and dislikes of food are essential in making adherence to the nutritional therapy successful. Nutritional therapy should also consider growth needs for youth around puberty. The calorie composition of daily diet is similar to that recommended in the adult diabetic patient. For example, total calories should be comprised of carbohydrates 45–65%, fat 30% (less than 10% from saturated fat, cholesterol less than 300 mg), and protein 15% in daily diet. Although very low calorie diet has been shown to be successful in the treatment of type 2 diabetes in youth,[21] we feel that long-term adherence to it by these young patients may be difficult. The overweight and obese youth with type 2 diabetes should be encouraged to participate in regular walking, field sports, running games, dancing, cycling, swimming, and strength training.

Pharmacologic therapy should be considered in the asymptomatic patients with mild to moderate hyperglycemia who are unable to achieve glycemic goal by nutritional and exercise therapy after 3 months trial or in the symptomatic patients with moderate to severe hyperglycemia. Although US Food and Drug Administration has only approved metformin and insulin for the treatment of diabetes in youth (children), clinicians have successfully used other oral agents. A multicenter trial has showed efficacy of sulfonylurea drug (glimepiride) in type 2 diabetic youth.[22] The Treatment Options for Type 2 Diabetes in Adolescents and Youth (TODAY) study[14,23] examined the efficacy of metformin alone, metformin plus intensive lifestyle changes, and metformin plus rosiglitazone therapy in youth with type 2 diabetes. The study's primary outcome of treatment failure showed 51.7% treatment failure in metformin alone, 46.6% treatment failure in metformin plus intensive lifestyle changes, and 38.6% failure in metformin plus rosiglitazone group. The study defined the weight loss target as 7 percentage point decrease in percent overweight. Six months after initiation of treatment, the weight loss target was reached as follows: 24.3% of youth in metformin alone, 31.2% in metformin plus intensive lifestyle changes, and 16.7% in metformin plus rosiglitazone group. We recommend that initial pharmacologic treatment in patients with moderate hyperglycemia should be metformin. In symptomatic patients with moderate to severe hyperglycemia, insulin therapy should be instituted with self-monitoring of blood glucose. Metformin may be added once target glycemic control is achieved. We prefer the long-acting insulin and, if needed, preprandial fast-acting insulin bolus treatment.

CONCLUSION

The incidence of type 2 diabetes in youth has dramatically increased globally in recent years. In the United States, ethnic minorities of Native American, African-American, Hispanic, Pacific Islanders, and Asian American have experienced marked increase of type 2 diabetes in youth than general population. The global rise in obesity in youth appears to be responsible for the increased incidence of type 2 diabetes in youth. Positive family history of diabetes in first- and second-degree relatives and low birth weight with overweight during puberty are strong predictor of type 2 diabetes in youth. Many youths are diagnosed with type 2 diabetes during screening or routine clinical and laboratory examination. The identification of type 2 diabetes in youth can be done clinically in most patients. However, in some youths differentiation between type 1 and type 2 diabetes may be difficult even after determination of islet cell autoantibodies. The presentation of type 2 diabetes in youth may be asymptomatic or with symptoms of hyperglycemia. Some youths with type 2 diabetes may present with DKA or hyperosmolar state. The treatment should be geared for optimal glycemic control, weight reduction and maintenance, nutritional counseling according to daily activities, and exercise planning. Involvement of all family members with youth in planning of nutritional treatment and exercise program is essential. Glycemic control can be achieved with metformin, if nutritional management, exercise and weight reduction are not effective. In some youths with type 2 diabetes, especially the one with characteristics of both type 1 and type 2 diabetes, insulin treatment may be needed for glycemic control.

REFERENCES

1. Pinhas-Hamiel O, Dolan LM, Daniels SR, Standiford D, Khoury PR, Zeitler P. Increased incidence of non-insulin-dependent diabetes mellitus among adolescents. *J Pediatr.* 1996;128:608-15.

2. Silverstein JH, Rosenbloom AL. Treatment of type 2 diabetes mellitus in children and adolescents. *J Pediatr Endocrinol Metab.* 2000;13(Suppl 6):1403-9.

3. Scott CR, Smith JM, Cradock MM, Pihoker C. Characteristics of youth-onset noninsulin-dependent diabetes mellitus and insulin-dependent diabetes mellitus at diagnosis. *Pediatrics.* 1997;100:84-91.

4. Likitmaskul S, Kiattisathavee P, Chaichanwatanakul K, Punnakanta L, Angsusingha K, Tuchinda C. Increasing prevalence of type 2 diabetes mellitus in Thai children and adolescents associated with increasing prevalence of obesity. *J Pediatr Endocrinol Metab.* 2003;16:71-7.

5. Urakami T, Kubota S, Nitadori Y, Harada K, Owada M, Kitagawa T. Annual incidence and clinical characteristics of type 2 diabetes in children as detected by urine glucose screening in the Tokyo metropolitan area. *Diabetes Care.* 2005;28:1876-81.

6. Pinhas-Hamiel O, Zeitler P. The global spread of type 2 diabetes mellitus in children and adolescents. *J Pediatr.* 2005;146:693-700.

7. Dabelea D, DeGroat J, Sorrelman C, Glass M, Percy CA, Avery C, et al. Diabetes in Navajo youth: prevalence, incidence, and clinical characteristics: the SEARCH for Diabetes in Youth Study. *Diabetes Care.* 2009;32(Suppl 2):S141-7.

8. Mayer-Davis EJ, Beyer J, Bell RA, Dabelea D, D'Agostino R, Imperatore G, et al. Diabetes in African American youth: prevalence, incidence, and clinical characteristics: the SEARCH for Diabetes in Youth Study. *Diabetes Care.* 2009;32(Suppl 2):S112-22.

9. Lawrence JM, Mayer-Davis EJ, Reynolds K, Beyer J, Pettitt DJ, D'Agostino RB, et al. Diabetes in Hispanic American youth: prevalence, incidence, demographics, and clinical characteristics: the SEARCH for Diabetes in Youth Study. *Diabetes Care.* 2009; 32(Suppl 2):S123-32.

10. Liu LL, Yi JP, Beyer J, Mayer-Davis EJ, Dolan LM, Dabelea DM, et al. Type 1 and type 2 diabetes in Asian and Pacific Islander U.S. youth: the SEARCH for Diabetes in Youth Study. *Diabetes Care.* 2009;32(Suppl 2):S133-40.

11. Bell RA, Mayer-Davis EJ, Beyer JW, D'Agostino RB, Lawrence JM, Linder B, et al. Diabetes in non-Hispanic white youth: prevalence, incidence, and clinical characteristics: the SEARCH for Diabetes in Youth Study. *Diabetes Care.* 2009;32(Suppl 2):S102-11.

12. Ball GD, Huang TT, Gower BA, Cruz ML, Shaibi GQ, Weigensberg MJ, et al. Longitudinal changes in insulin sensitivity, insulin secretion, and beta-cell function during puberty. *J Pediatr.* 2006;148:16-22.

13. Amiel SA, Sherwin RS, Simonson DC, Lauritano AA, Tamborlane WV. Impaired insulin action in puberty. A contributing factor to poor glycemic control in adolescents with diabetes. *N Engl J Med.* 1986;315:215-9.

14. Copeland KC, Zeitler P, Geffner M, Guandalini C, Higgins J, Hirst K, et al. Characteristics of adolescents and youth with recent-onset type 2 diabetes: the TODAY cohort at baseline. *J Clin Endocrinol Metab*. 2011;96:159-67.

15. Tattersal RB, Fajans SS. Prevalence of diabetes and glucose intolerance in 199 offspring of thirty-seven conjugal diabetic parents. *Diabetes*. 1975;24:452-62.

16. Pinhas-Hamiel O, Dolan LM, Zeitler PS. Diabetic ketoacidosis among obese African-American adolescents with NIDDM. *Diabetes Care*. 1997;20:484-6.

17. Neufeld ND, Raffel LJ, Landon C, Chen YD, Vadheim CM. Early presentation of type 2 diabetes in Mexican-American youth. *Diabetes Care*. 1998;21:80-6.

18. Klingensmith GJ, Pyle L, Arslanian S, Copeland KC, Cuttler L, Kaufman F, et al. The presence of GAD and IA-2 antibodies in youth with a type 2 diabetes phenotype: results from the TODAY study. *Diabetes Care*. 2010;33:1970-5.

19. Basevi V, Di Mario S, Morciano C, Nonino F, Magrini N. Comment on: American Diabetes Association. Standards of medical care in diabetes—2011. *Diabetes Care*. 2011; 34(Suppl 1):S11-61.

20. Wrotniak BH, Epstein LH, Paluch RA, Roemmich JN. The relationship between parent and child self-reported adherence and weight loss. *Obes Res*. 2005;13:1089-96.

21. Willi SM, Martin K, Datko FM, Brant BP. Treatment of type 2 diabetes in childhood using a very-low-calorie diet. *Diabetes Care*. 2004;27:348-53.

22. Gottschalk M, Danne T, Vlajnic A, Cara JF. Glimepiride versus metformin as monotherapy in pediatric patients with type 2 diabetes: a randomized, single-blind comparative study. *Diabetes Care*. 2007;30:790-4.

23. TODAY Study Group, Zeitler P, Epstein L, Grey M, Hirst K, Kaufman F, et al. Treatment options for type 2 diabetes in adolescents and youth: a study of the comparative efficacy of metformin alone or in combination with rosiglitazone or lifestyle intervention in adolescents with type 2 diabetes. *Pediatr Diabetes*. 2007;8:74-87.

Management of Hyperlipidemia in Diabetic Patients

Hussein Yassine

ABSTRACT

All diabetics should be counseled on the appropriate lifestyles that include physical activity and a balanced diet. Patients with diabetes who are obese should be counseled on caloric restriction with an emphasis on appropriate carbohydrate intake. In this chapter, the author focuses on pharmacotherapy for hyperlipidemia in patients with both type 1 and type 2 diabetes. He reviews the classification of diabetes as a cardiovascular risk equivalent pointing out to newer evidence that not all diabetics are at the same risk of cardiovascular disease. The clinical outcomes in diabetic patients on statins, niacin, fibrates, fish oil, bile acid sequestrants, and ezetimibe are reviewed. The chapter provides evidence that a therapy tailored to patient's risk may outweigh the current treat-to-target low-density lipoprotein goals as recommended by the Adult Treatment Panel III guideline. This review reflects the author's analysis of the literature pertinent to the pharmacologic treatment of hyperlipidemia in diabetes.

INTRODUCTION

All diabetics should be counseled on the appropriate lifestyles that include physical activity and a balanced diet. Patients with diabetes, who are obese, should be counseled on caloric restriction with an emphasis on appropriate carbohydrate intake. In this chapter, we focus on pharmacotherapy for hyperlipidemia in patients with both type 1 and type 2 diabetes. We review the classification of diabetes as a cardiovascular risk equivalent pointing out to newer evidence that not all diabetics are at the same risk of cardiovascular disease (CVD). We review the clinical outcomes in diabetic patients on statins, niacin, fibrates, fish oil, bile acid sequestrants, and ezetimibe. We recommend that all diabetic patients at high risk of CVD should be started on a statin therapy. We provide evidence that a therapy tailored to patient's risk may outweigh the current treat-to-target low-density lipoproteins (LDL) goals as recommended by the adult treatment panel III (ATP III) guideline. This review reflects the authors analysis of the literature pertinent to the pharmacologic treatment of hyperlipidemia in diabetes. It may or may not reflect the standard of care set by current guidelines. We ask the reader to refer to the guidelines set forth by the American Diabetes Association (ADA)[1] and/ or the ATP III[2] for more information on the guidelines.

TREATMENT OF HYPERLIPIDEMIA IS PROBABLY THE MOST IMPORTANT DRIVING FACTOR FOR DECREASING THE CARDIOVASCULAR RISK IN DIABETES

The STENO-2 study found that a multifactorial intervention with therapies directed toward modifying lifestyle, reducing total cholesterol, lowering blood pressure, and improving glycemic control had a dramatic benefit in reducing the risk of the primary composite end-point and microalbuminuria in patients with type 2 diabetes and when compared to patients who received conventional therapy. This study demonstrated the greatest absolute reduction in the risk for cardiovascular events when compared to other studies that are specifically targeted to only one cardiovascular risk factor.[3] A subsequent analysis of those factors that could be responsible for the dramatic reduction in cardiovascular events in the STENO-2 study showed that reduction in total cholesterol accounted for approximately 70% of the overall benefit, with less of the overall benefit attributable to either improvement in glycemic control or reduction of systolic blood pressure.[4] STENO-2 and several other trials [Action to Control Cardiovascular Risk in Diabetes (ACCORD), Anglo-Scandinavian Cardiac Outcomes Trial (ASCOT), and Collaborative AtoRvastatin Diabetes Study (CARDS)][5,6] suggest that treatment of hyperlipidemia in type 2 diabetes leads to improved mortality and lower CVD. For the most part, the benefit is derived from statin use in patients at high risk for CVD.

IDENTIFYING RISK FACTORS FOR CARDIOVASCULAR DISEASE IN DIABETES

Emerging evidence suggests that benefit for treating diabetic patients with statins is related to the risk of CVD. In general, patients at a very low risk for CVD will not likely benefit from statin treatment.[7] Although diabetes is considered a CVD equivalent, not all diabetics are at the same risk of having CVD events. Hence, the choice and treatment goals are contingent on the risk of CVD. The most commonly used algorithm for risk stratification for CVD is Framingham risk score. The first Framingham risk score (1998) incorporated age, gender LDL-cholesterol (LDL-C), high-density lipoproteins (HDL)-cholesterol, blood pressure (including whether the patient is treated or not), diabetes, and smoking to derive an estimated risk of developing coronary heart disease (CHD) (myocardial infarction, coronary artery disease death, and angina) within 10 years. The Framingham risk score was modified (2002) by

TABLE 1: Adult Treatment Panel III (ATP-III) Risk Classifiers and Proportion of Patients in Each Risk

High risk (2%)	Established CHD and CHD equivalents. Any of the following: • Established CHD • Diabetes • Established noncardiac vascular disease—peripheral arterial disease, abdominal aortic • Aneurysm, carotid artery disease (symptomatic, e.g. transient ischemic attack or stroke of carotid origin, or >50% stenosis on angiography or ultrasound) • A 10-year risk of CHD events >20% using Framingham scoring
Intermediate risk (16%)	Multiple (2+) risk factors (cigarette smoking, hypertension, HDL <40 mg/dL, family history of premature CHD, age >45 in men, >55 in women)
Low risk (82%)	0–1 risk factors

CHD, coronary heart disease; HDL, high-density lipoproteins.

ATP III for use in the recommendations for screening and treatment of dyslipidemia.[2] The modifications include elimination of diabetes from the algorithm (since it was considered to be a CVD equivalent), broadening of the age range, and inclusion of hypertension treatment and age-specific points for smoking and total cholesterol. The Framingham/ATP III criteria (Table 1) were used to estimate the distribution of CHD risk in the United States in an analysis of data from National Health and Nutrition Examination Survey (NHANES III) among 11,611 patients (age 20–79 years) without self-reported CHD, stroke, peripheral artery disease, or diabetes.[8] The 10-year CHD risk results and the proportion of patients in each category are listed in table 1.

Is the CVD Risk for all Diabetics Similar to Having a Prior CVD Event: Role for Coronary Calcium Screening

Recent evidence questions the labeling of all diabetes patients as a CHD equivalent. In the Multi-Ethnic Study of Atherosclerosis (MESA) study,[9] 38% of 6,841 diabetic study participants had no coronary artery calcium (CAC) detected and their annual event rate was less than 1% during the 6-year follow-up. In general, a CAC score greater than 400 is highly predictive of CAD events and a score of 0 is highly predictive of event-free survival in the typical 5-year follow-up for several studies.[10] It might be prudent to reclassify diabetic patients who appear at a lower rate of events using CAC screening, given the recent concerns on statin use and possible adverse effects that could include memory loss[11] or muscle pains. The low-risk subjects might be younger (<40) or with recent onset diabetes, but no evidence of increased triglycerides, low HDL or the markers of insulin resistance syndromes. We need a prospective outcome study that allocates patients on treatments with or without statins, based on CAC score before a broader recommendation of CAC use for statin therapy is recommended.

LOW-DENSITY LIPOPROTEIN CHOLESTEROL LEVELS DO NOT ACCURATELY REPRESENT ATHEROGENIC CHOLESTEROL IN DIABETES

Although LDL-C is a powerful predictor of CVD in the general population, its use as a marker of CVD in diabetes could be problematic. LDL consists of a heterogenous set of particles and it is likely that small dense LDL (also reflected by increased LDL particle numbers) represent atherogenic LDL.[12] Small dense LDL or increased LDL particle numbers are not often measured in patients, unless a vertical auto profile (VAP) or nuclear magnetic resonance (NMR) tests are ordered for subfractions or particles, respectively. There is considerable evidence to suggest that small dense LDL participates in the process of atherogenesis[12] and the small dense LDL particle reduction by statins reduces CVD events in patients at risk of CVD. The odds ratio for events was much higher when LDL and HDL particle numbers were used instead of routine HDL and LDL-C measures in the Veterans Affairs High-Density Lipoprotein Intervention Trial (VA-HIT) study.[13] An example of how LDL-C places a biomarker role is exemplified by the use of fish oil. Fish oil (omega-3 fatty acids) has favorable anti-atherogenic effects, but it increases LDL-C.[14] The mechanism of LDL increase reveals an increase in the fluffy and buoyant less dense LDL, not affecting small dense LDL. Several recent analyses suggest that LDL-C is not a good measure of small dense LDL in the setting of diabetes and metabolic syndrome characterized by low HDL-C and elevated trigylcerides.[15] In the Framingham study, patients with low LDL-C and elevated LDL particle numbers had a CVD risk equivalent to patients with elevated LDL-C. Conversely, patients with elevated LDL-C and low LDL particle numbers had a decreased risk of CVD equivalent to patients with lower LDL-C.[16] These patients comprise of 20% of the Framingham population. Subsequent validation in the MESA trial suggested that patients with low HDL and elevated triglycerides had elevated LDL particle numbers.[17] An analysis of VA-HIT trial revealed that patients with in the upper quartile of the LDL/HDL particle ratio had a 71 odds ratio of having a CVD event, and substantial predictive capacity compared to LDL/HDL cholesterol capacity that had an odds ratio of 7.[13] Till date, however, no trials have been completed on using LDL or HDL particles as targets of therapy.

STATINS ARE FIRST-LINE AGENTS IN TREATING DIABETIC PATIENTS AT INCREASED RISK FOR CARDIOVASCULAR DISEASE

Several prospective randomized control trials have shown that statin use in diabetes prevents CVD events and decreases overall mortality. The cholesterol and recurrent events (CARE) trial[18] and the Heart Protection Study[19] found significant improvement in outcomes with statin therapy even at LDL-C values below 116 mg/dL. The CARDS study found similar benefits of statin therapy in patients with an LDL-C above or below 120 mg/dL.[6] A meta-analysis of patients with diabetes in 14 randomized trials of statins (n = 18,686) also found that relative benefits appeared unrelated to the baseline LDL-C.[20]

The author recommends using a risk-based (tailored) approach in using statins. In high-risk patients, we recommend using atorvastatin 80 mg or rosuvastatin 40 mg/day. Since 2012 atorvastatin is generic, it is the preferred choice of therapy. In diabetic patients at medium risk for CVD, we recommend atorvastatin at doses of 10–40 mg/day. This contrasts to ATP III guidelines[2] that targets LDL-C levels to less than 70 mg/dL in high-risk patients and less than 100 mg/dL in all diabetics. A recent study on a simulated population comparing tailored approach versus treat to target concluded that a tailored treatment strategy prevents more CHD events while treating fewer persons with high-dose statins than LDL-C-based target approaches.[21]

Statin Intolerant Patient

Myopathy is the main reason for statin discontinuation. We do not recommend routine measurement of creatine kinase (CK) in patients taking statin therapy. Asymptomatic CK elevations up to 3–5 times upper limit of normal (ULN) are not uncommon, and the statin can be continued and CK reevaluated in 2–4 weeks to establish stability or decline in CK levels. Care should be taken to establish that the patient is truly asymptomatic and muscle weakness does not exist. In 2012, the Food and Drug Administration (FDA) eliminated the recommendation that patients on statins undergo periodic monitoring of liver enzymes, because this approach is ineffective in detecting and preventing the "rare and unpredictable" serious liver injuries related to statins. Statin therapy should be interrupted if the patient shows signs of serious liver injury, hyperbilirubinemia, or jaundice. The statin therapy should not be restarted if the drugs cannot be ruled out as a cause of the problems.

Management of Statin-induced Myopathy

After muscle symptoms resolve and patients are rechallenged, many will tolerate a lower dose of the same or another statin. In general, a lower dose of a statin of similar efficacy would be the next choice. Approximate comparable efficacy can be obtained from 5 mg of rosuvastatin, 10 mg of atorvastatin, 20 mg of simvastatin, 40 mg of pravastatin or lovastatin, and 80 mg of fluvastatin.[22] Fluvastatin, although less efficacious per milligram than other statins, has been recommended by some experts because of its relatively low incidence of myalgia compared with other statins.[22] In addition to decreasing statin dose, less frequent dosing intervals can also be effective. For example, 2.5–20 mg of rosuvastatin once a week has been shown to decrease LDL-C by 25% and be tolerated by up to 70% in statin-intolerant patients.[23] Twice and alternate-day regimens of rosuvastatin and atorvastatin alone or with ezetimibe have also been well tolerated in patients with muscle symptoms as well as transaminase elevations.[24]

USE OF NIACIN IN PATIENTS WITH DIABETES

Niacin is probably the oldest lipid medication with outcome data. The coronary drug project showed that long-term immediate niacin use at doses greater than 1,500 mg/day leads to reduced CVD events and decreased overall mortality to 15 years after the trial ended.[25,26] It is believed that the benefit of niacin is related to its HDL raising ability (niacin raises HDL by 20–50%). But niacin also lowers LDL up to 40%. Niacin in higher doses produces flushing as a side effect that can be burden to a significant number of patients. Although flushing could be reduced by gradually increasing niacin dose taken with food and/or 30 minutes preceded by small dose of aspirin, flushing has limited niacin use in larger population with CVD. There are recent studies which question the use of niacin treatment as a first-line agent. These studies include AIM-HIGH[27] and HPS-2 thrive.[28] AIM-HIGH selected patients above 45 years of age with established, stable CHD, cerebrovascular or carotid arterial disease, or peripheral arterial disease. They also had low levels of HDL-C (<40 mg/dL in men, <50 mg/dL in women), elevated triglycerides (150–400 mg/dL), and LDL-C levels lower than 180 mg/dL if they were not taking a statin at entry. After a median follow-up of only 3 years, the data and safety monitoring board recommended to stop the study early because the boundary for futility had been crossed and unexpectedly, the rate of ischemic stroke was higher in the niacin-treated patients than in those receiving placebo. AIM-HIGH was not simply a direct comparison of niacin versus placebo on top of standard medical practice. The investigators recognized that niacin has additional effects, in particular, lowering levels of atherogenic lipids, and they attempted to control these effects by titrating the other LDL-C-lowering therapies during the study. As a result, the trial was actually a comparison between niacin plus low-dose simvastatin on the one hand and placebo plus high-dose simvastatin (and, more often, also ezetimibe) on the other.

In the AIM-HIGH,[27] HPS-2 thrive,[28] and the JUPITER trial[29] (Justification for the Use of Statins in Primary Prevention: An Intervention Trial Evaluating Rosuvastatin). This suggests that raising HDL-C by conventional therapies might not be the elixir promised to reduce the increase residual risk of CVD in diabetes in the setting of lower LDL-C levels. HDL-C contains a heterogeneous subset of particles that has both atherogenic and antiatherogenic effects. There are certain species of HDL that have a favorable impact on both the size and structure of experimental plaques in animal models. Until we develop such targeted therapies; the prevention of CVD by solely raising of HDL-C is not currently supported. In 2012, niacin is a second-line agent if statins are not tolerated or if aggressive LDL reduction is needed on top of statin therapy.

USE OF FIBRATES IN PATIENTS WITH DIABETES

Fibrates are second-line agents in statin intolerant patients. Fibrates available in the United States include gemfiborzil and fenofibrate. Gemfibrozil has been shown to prevent CVD outcomes in both Helsinki trial[30] and VA-HIT. Gemfibrozil is least effective in patients without diabetes or metabolic syndrome. Thus, they are of particular interest when non-HDL-C is elevated despite statin therapy in patients with elevated triglycerides and low HDL-C. The mechanism of benefit for gemfibrozil is not clear but might be related to LDL lowering and HDL raising effects. It must be noted that gemfibrozil should not be used in combination with statin metabolized by liver cytochrome enzyme CYP3A4 (as simvastatin and atrovastatin) due to reports of rhabdomyolysis resulting from decreased metabolism of the drug in the liver. There is less data in support of the use of fenofibrates. In fact, both the fenofibrate intervention and event lowering in diabetes (FIELD)[31] trial and ACCORD failed to show an incremental benefit in CVD prevention on top of statin use. The ACCORD-Lipid trial[32] tested the hypothesis that the addition of a fibrate to lower plasma triglycerides and increase plasma HDL cholesterol levels in statin-treated patients with type 2 diabetes mellitus would provide benefit as compared to the use of statin alone to lower LDL-C. The overall result of ACCORD-Lipid trial was negative; the combination of fenofibrate and simvastatin did not lower the rate of the primary composite end-point of cardiovascular death, nonfatal myocardial infarction, and nonfatal stroke compared to treatment with simvastatin plus placebo. A prespecified subgroup analysis indicated that participants with triglyceride levels in the upper third and HDL-C levels in the lower third at baseline (dyslipidemic group) had a much higher rate for the primary outcome than all other individuals, and fenofibrate treatment reduced the primary outcome by 32% in this group. There is a need to do more trials focusing on this particular group before a generalized recommendation is made. As we mentioned earlier, this subgroup did not benefit from the addition of niacin in the AIM-HIGH study when aggressive LDL lowering therapy was pursued. It is of interest to study the effect of fibrates on CVD risk in patients aggressively treated by statins. Gemfibrozil dose is 600 mg to be taken 30 minutes before breakfast and dinner for better absorption. The typical dose for fenofibrates (Tricor) is 145 mg/day. The dose should be reduced to 48 mg/day in patients with renal disease.

Use of Fish Oil in the Management of Diabetic Hyperlipidemia

The main indication of using fish oil or omega-3s in diabetes is for the purpose of lowering triglyceride in subjects with very elevated trigylceride levels (>1,000 mg/dL) to prevent pancreatitis. There is good evidence from GISSI-P[33] and Japan eicosapentaenoic acid (EPA) lipid intervention study (JELIS)[34] that omega-3 intake prevents sudden death in secondary prevention trial. Their use in primary prevention of CVD is less certain[35] as there are no clinical trials to date that favor the use of omega-3s in the primary prevention of CVD or sudden death. Diabetic patients at high risk for CVD may warrant a different approach and it might be prudent to add 1 g/day of omega-3 to prevent sudden death; however, a randomized control trial in this population is needed before making strong recommendation.

USE OF EZETIMIBE IN THE MANAGEMENT OF HYPERLIPIDEMIA

The use of ezetimibe has fallen out of favor in recent years due to its lack of efficacy in preventing CVD events in the ENHANCE trial when combined to statins as compared to statin alone.[36] Ezetimibe lowers LDL-C by preventing its absorption at the Neimann-Pick intestinal receptor NPC1L1 at the brush border of the small intestine. It could be argued that ezetimibe is a reasonable choice of treatment in patients who are severely intolerant to all other hyperlipidemic agents. Ezetimibe is not absorbed and has minimal side effects, and is well tolerated in statin intolerant patients. There is an uncommon disease of sistosterolemia where plant cholesterol is absorbed leading to increased CVD and ezetimibe represents a unique drug in this situation to prevent plant sterol absorption and CVD in this population.

USE OF BILE ACID RESINS

Bile acid sequestrants are third-line agents in the management of hyperlipidemia. They have prominent gastrointestinal side effects. Among bile acid resins, colesevelam is the most tolerated. Colesevelam induces moderate but significant improvements in HbA1c and LDL-C.[37] Outcome data are needed to determine whether or not colesevelam confers long-term protection against micro- and macrovascular complications. Although colesevelam does not induce weight gain, triglyceride levels tend to increase ~15%, the implications of which are unknown.[37] The mechanisms by which colesevelam improves glycemia are not yet understood.

TREATMENT OF HYPERTRIGLYCERIDEMIA IN DIABETES

The clinical benefits of lowering elevated plasma triglyceride levels by any pharmacologic means have not yet been convincingly demonstrated. In diabetic patients with triglycerides less than 700 mg/dL, non-HDL-C serves as a good marker of atherogenic small dense LDL and becomes the target of treatment with statins as first-line agents in accordance with ATP III guidelines. However, we recommend the tailored approach over the non-HDL target approach due to the factors described herein. The two main lines of treatment for elevated triglycerides in diabetes to prevent pancreatitis are fibrates and fish oil. We recommend the use of gemfibrozil 600 mg BID with meals and 4 g of fish oil per day. Fish oil doses required to lower triglycerides are several fold higher than the doses that may reduce coronary mortality or sudden death. At least 4 g of the active fish oil (DHA and EPA) are needed to significantly lower triglycerides by 30–40%. If the patient has a high risk for CVD or had prior CVD events, then fenofibrate can substitute gemfibrozil to allow the addition of statins. Recall that gemfibrozil increases the risk of myopathy when used with most statins, in particular simvastatin, lovastatin, and atorvastatin.

HYPERLIPIDEMIA IN TYPE 1 VERSUS TYPE 2 DIABETES

For the most part, the management of hyperlipidemia in type 1 and type 2 diabetes is same. Patients with type 1 diabetes have an insulin deficiency state and can have very elevated triglycerides if noncompliant with insulin therapies. Younger type 1 diabetics who have excellent control of their diabetes may not need lipid therapy until age of 40, unless they have an increased CVD risk (Table 1).

CONCLUSION

We conclude that statin therapy is cornerstone in reducing heart disease in patients with diabetes and an increased risk for CVD. There is no sufficient evidence to favor statin use in patients with diabetes but at low risk for CVD. Coronary calcium scanning might assist in reclassifying low to medium risk patients. For statin intolerant patients, several options exist that include reducing the dose or frequency of statin use, or using less potent statins. Gemfibrozil is beneficial alternative to statins in patients with low HDL cholesterol and elevated triglycerides. Fish oil at lower doses prevents sudden cardiac death in high risk diabetes patients, but evidence for its use in low risk populations are lacking. Higher doses of fish are useful for lowering triglycerides, in particular for the prevention of pancreatitis. Recent studies suggest that niacin or ezetimibe treatments are falling out of favor and should be a second line treatment in patients with diabetes who do not tolerate statins.

REFERENCES

1. American Diabetes Association. Standards of medical care in diabetes—2012. *Diabetes Care.* 2012;35 Suppl 1:S11-63.
2. Third Report of the National Cholesterol Education Program (NCEP) Expert Panel on Detection, Evaluation, and Treatment of High Blood Cholesterol in Adults (Adult Treatment Panel III) final report. *Circulation.* 2002;106(25):3143-421.
3. Gaede P, Vedel P, Larsen N, Jensen GV, Parving HH, Pedersen O. Multifactorial intervention and cardiovascular disease in patients with type 2 diabetes. *N Engl J Med.* 2003; 348(5):383-93.
4. Gaede P, Pedersen O. Intensive integrated therapy of type 2 diabetes: implications for long-term prognosis. *Diabetes.* 2004;53 Suppl 3:S39-47.
5. Sever PS, Dahlöf B, Poulter NR, Wedel H, Beevers G, Caulfield M, et al. Prevention of coronary and stroke events with atorvastatin in hypertensive patients who have average or lower-than-average cholesterol concentrations, in the Anglo-Scandinavian Cardiac Outcomes Trial—Lipid Lowering Arm (ASCOT-LLA): a multicentre randomised controlled trial. *Lancet.* 2003;361(9364):1149-58.
6. Colhoun HM, Betteridge DJ, Durrington PN, Hitman GA, Neil HA, Livingstone SJ, et al. Primary prevention of cardiovascular disease with atorvastatin in type 2 diabetes in the Collaborative Atorvastatin Diabetes Study (CARDS): multicentre randomised placebo-controlled trial. *Lancet.* 2004;364(9435):685-96.

7. Taylor F, Ward K, Moore TH, Burke M, Davey Smith G, Casas JP, et al. Statins for the primary prevention of cardiovascular disease. *Cochrane Database Syst Rev.* 2011;(1):CD004816.

8. Ford ES, Giles WH, Mokdad AH. The distribution of 10-Year risk for coronary heart disease among US adults: findings from the National Health and Nutrition Examination Survey III. *J Am Coll Cardiol.* 2004;43(10):1791-6.

9. Malik S, Budoff MJ, Katz R, Blumenthal RS, Bertoni AG, Nasir K, et al. Impact of sub-clinical atherosclerosis on cardiovascular disease events in individuals with metabolic syndrome and diabetes: the multi-ethnic study of atherosclerosis. *Diabetes Care.* 2011; 34(10):2285-90.

10. Pletcher MJ, Tice JA, Pignone M, Browner WS. Using the coronary artery calcium score to predict coronary heart disease events: a systematic review and meta-analysis. *Arch Intern Med.* 2004;164(12):1285-92.

11. Muldoon MF, Barger SD, Ryan CM, Flory JD, Lehoczky JP, Matthews KA, et al. Effects of lovastatin on cognitive function and psychological well-being. *Am J Med.* 2000;108(7):538-46.

12. Packard C, Caslake M, Shepherd J. The role of small, dense low density lipoprotein (LDL): a new look. *Int J Cardiol.* 2000;74 Suppl 1:S17-22.

13. Otvos JD, Collins D, Freedman DS, Shalaurova I, Schaefer EJ, McNamara JR, et al. Low-density lipoprotein and high-density lipoprotein particle subclasses predict coronary events and are favorably changed by gemfibrozil therapy in the Veterans Affairs High-Density Lipoprotein Intervention Trial. *Circulation.* 2006;113(12):1556-63.

14. Petersen M, Pedersen H, Major-Pedersen A, Jensen T, Marckmann P. Effect of fish oil versus corn oil supplementation on LDL and HDL subclasses in type 2 diabetic patients. *Diabetes Care.* 2002;25(10):1704-8.

15. Kathiresan S, Otvos JD, Sullivan LM, Keyes MJ, Schaefer EJ, Wilson PW, et al. Increased small low-density lipoprotein particle number: a prominent feature of the metabolic syndrome in the Framingham Heart Study. *Circulation.* 2006;113(1):20-9.

16. Cromwell WC, Otvos JD, Keyes MJ, Pencina MJ, Sullivan L, Vasan RS, et al. LDL Particle Number and Risk of Future Cardiovascular Disease in the Framingham Offspring Study - Implications for LDL Management. *J Clin Lipidol.* 2007;1(6):583-92.

17. Mora S, Szklo M, Otvos JD, Greenland P, Psaty BM, Goff DC Jr, et al. LDL particle subclasses, LDL particle size, and carotid atherosclerosis in the Multi-Ethnic Study of Atherosclerosis (MESA). *Atherosclerosis.* 2007;192(1):211-7.

18. Sacks FM, Tonkin AM, Craven T, Pfeffer MA, Shepherd J, Keech A, et al. Coronary heart disease in patients with low LDL-cholesterol: benefit of pravastatin in diabetics and enhanced role for HDL-cholesterol and triglycerides as risk factors. *Circulation.* 2002;105(12):1424-8.

19. Collins R, Armitage J, Parish S, Sleigh P, Peto R; Heart Protection Study Collaborative Group. MRC/BHF Heart Protection Study of cholesterol-lowering with simvastatin in 5963 people with diabetes: a randomised placebo-controlled trial. *Lancet.* 2003; 361(9374):2005-16.

20. Kearney PM, Blackwell L, Collins R, Keech A, Simes J, Peto R, et al. Efficacy of cholesterol-lowering therapy in 18,686 people with diabetes in 14 randomised trials of statins: a meta-analysis. *Lancet.* 2008;371(9607):117-25.

21. Hayward RA, Krumholz HM, Zulman DM, Timbie JW, Vijan S. Optimizing statin treatment for primary prevention of coronary artery disease. *Ann Intern Med.* 2010;152(2):69-77.

22. Jacobson TA. Toward "pain-free" statin prescribing: clinical algorithm for diagnosis and management of myalgia. *Mayo Clin Proc.* 2008;83(6):687-700.

23. Ruisinger JF, Backes JM, Gibson CA, Moriarty PM. Once-a-week rosuvastatin (2.5 to 20 mg) in patients with a previous statin intolerance. *Am J Cardiol.* 2009;103(3):393-4.

24. Gadarla M, Kearns AK, Thompson PD. Efficacy of rosuvastatin (5 mg and 10 mg) twice a week in patients intolerant to daily statins. *Am J Cardiol.* 2008;101(12):1747-8.

25. Clofibrate and niacin in coronary heart disease. *JAMA.* 1975;231(4):360-81.

26. Canner PL, Berge KG, Wenger NK, Stamler J, Friedman L, Prineas RJ, et al. Fifteen year mortality in Coronary Drug Project patients: long-term benefit with niacin. *J Am Coll Cardiol.* 1986;8(6):1245-55.

27. Boden WE, Probstfield JL, Anderson T, Chaitman BR, Desvignes-Nickens P, Koprowicz K, et al. Niacin in patients with low HDL cholesterol levels receiving intensive statin therapy. *N Engl J Med.* 2011;365(24):2255-67.

28. High patient compliance with nicacin/laropiprant in large clinical trial: interim safety and tolerability results from HPS-2 THRIVE study released at 2012 ESC congress: drug trends in cardiology. *Cardiovasc J Afr.* 2012;23(8):471.

29. Ridker PM, Genest J, Boekholdt SM, Libby P, Gotto AM, Nordestgaard BG, et al. HDL cholesterol and residual risk of first cardiovascular events after treatment with potent statin therapy: an analysis from the JUPITER trial. *Lancet.* 2010;376(9738):333-9.

30. Frick MH, Elo O, Haapa K, Heinonen OP, Heinsalmi P, Helo P, et al. Helsinki Heart Study: primary-prevention trial with gemfibrozil in middle-aged men with dyslipidemia. Safety of treatment, changes in risk factors, and incidence of coronary heart disease. *N Engl J Med.* 1987;317(20):1237-45.

31. Keech AC, Mitchell P, Summanen PA, O'Day J, Davis TM, Moffitt MS, et al. Effect of fenofibrate on the need for laser treatment for diabetic retinopathy (FIELD study): a randomised controlled trial. *Lancet.* 2007;370(9600):1687-97.

32. Ginsberg HN, Elam MB, Lovato LC, Crouse JR 3rd, Leiter LA, Linz P, et al. Effects of combination lipid therapy in type 2 diabetes mellitus. *N Engl J Med.* 2010;362(17):1563-74.

33. Marchioli R, Barzi F, Bomba E, Chieffo C, Di Gregorio D, Di Mascio R, et al. Early protection against sudden death by n-3 polyunsaturated fatty acids after myocardial infarction: time-course analysis of the results of the Gruppo Italiano per lo Studio della Sopravvivenza nell'Infarto Miocardico (GISSI)-Prevenzione. *Circulation.* 2002;105(16):1897-903.

34. Yokoyama M, Origasa H, Matsuzaki M, Matsuzawa Y, Saito Y, Ishikawa Y, et al. Effects of eicosapentaenoic acid on major coronary events in hypercholesterolaemic patients (JELIS): a randomised open-label, blinded endpoint analysis. *Lancet.* 2007;369(9567):1090-8.

35. Hooper L, Thompson RL, Harrison RA, Summerbell CD, Moore H, Worthington HV, et al. Omega 3 fatty acids for prevention and treatment of cardiovascular disease. *Cochrane Database Syst Rev.* 2004;(4):CD003177.

36. Kastelein JJ, Akdim F, Stroes ES, Zwinderman AH, Bots ML, Stalenhoef AF, et al. Simvastatin with or without ezetimibe in familial hypercholesterolemia. *N Engl J Med.* 2008;358(14):1431-43.

37. Younk LM, Davis SN. Evaluation of colesevelam hydrochloride for the treatment of type 2 diabetes. *Expert Opin Drug Metab Toxicol.* 2012;8(4):515-25.

Management of Hypertension in Diabetic Patients

Venkateswara K Rao

ABSTRACT

Epidemiological surveys have shown that more than 70% of the United States adults with diabetes also have hypertension. Co-existence of diabetes and hypertension is associated with greater degree of arterial stiffness and accelerated arterial aging. Presence of hypertension in either type 1 or type 2 diabetes increases the risk of atherosclerotic cardiovascular disease including stroke. The microvascular complications of diabetes are also accelerated by hypertension, particularly the retinopathy. These high risks associated with hypertension in diabetic patients mandate earlier and more intensive therapy. The current recommendation from expert committees is that all diabetics with hypertension should receive appropriate therapy to accomplish a goal blood pressure of 130/80 mmHg. In this chapter, the author has presented a comprehensive review of various modalities of treatment of hypertension in diabetic patients.

INTRODUCTION

The incidence of type 2 diabetes is rapidly increasing with a life-time risk in the United States estimated to be 33% for men and 39% for women.[1] Epidemiological surveys have shown that more than 70% of adults in the United States with diabetes also have hypertension.[2] Coexistence of diabetes and hypertension is associated with greater degree of arterial stiffness and accelerated arterial aging.[3] Presence of hypertension in either type 1[4] or type 2[5] diabetes increases the risk of atherosclerotic cardiovascular disease including stroke.[6] The microvascular complications of diabetes are also accelerated by hypertension, particularly the retinopathy.[7] These high risks associated with hypertension in diabetic patients mandate earlier and more intensive therapy. The current recommendation from expert committees (American Diabetes Association, European Society of Hypertension, and the Joint National Committee 7) is that all diabetics with hypertension should receive appropriate therapy to accomplish a goal blood pressure (BP) of 130/80 mmHg.[8-10]

PATHOGENESIS OF HYPERTENSION IN DIABETIC PATIENTS

A Finnish diabetologist in a 1999 lecture has stated provocatively that "diabetes is a cardiovascular disease which you diagnose by measuring the blood glucose". In type 1 diabetic patients, the hypertension is usually caused by the underlying diabetic nephropathy and typically manifest at the onset of microalbuminuria. In type 2 diabetics, hypertension is already present in one-third of patients at the time of the diagnosis of diabetes. The hypertension in these patients may be related to underlying diabetic nephropathy or concurrent essential hypertension or possibly due to secondary hypertension with an underlying curable cause.[11] The association between hypertension and kidney disease is closely linked. Increased BP markedly accelerates the progression of diabetic nephropathy, and microalbuminuria is a known risk factor for progression of cardiovascular disease.[12] Many randomized clinical trials have shown that aggressive BP control reduces the rate of decline in renal function [estimated glomerular filtration rate (GFR)] and delays the progression to end-stage renal failure.[13-15] Similarly, the relationship between diabetes and ischemic heart disease is also tight. Diabetic patients carry the same risk of cardiovascular mortality as nondiabetic patients who suffered a previous myocardial infarction.[16] In the multiple risk factor intervention trial, over a 12-year follow-up period, in the hypertensive subjects (systolic BP >200 mmHg), diabetes increased the cardiovascular risk by 1.89 folds.[16] Thus, the cardiovascular risk from hypertension and diabetes is additive. In diabetic patients, an increase in diastolic or systolic BP of 5 mmHg is associated with 20–30% increase in cardiovascular complications.[17]

The precise mechanisms underlying hypertension and accelerated cardio-vascular disease in the diabetic subjects are unknown. However, based on animal experiments, clinical associations, and response to therapy, the following pathogenetic mechanisms have been proposed in the scientific literature.

Activation of Renin-Angiotensin System

Angiotensin II plays a fundamental role in controlling the functional and structural integrity of arterial wall and contributes to the pathological mechanisms underlying vascular complications of diabetes.[18,19] Angiotensin II exerts its action via two receptor subtypes. Angiotensin II receptor type 1 (AT1 receptor) activation causes vasoconstriction, increased release of aldosterone and vasopressin. It also promotes myocyte hypertrophy, mediated by excess production of endothelin 1, cyclooxygenase, and lipoxygenase products of arachidonic acid metabolism. On the contrary, activation of angiotensin II receptor type 2 (AT2 receptor) causes vasodilatation and inhibits myocyte cell proliferation. The vasodilator effects are mediated via local production of nitric oxide, prostaglandin E2 and I2. An imbalance in the activation of these opposing receptors leads to excess production of vasoconstrictor molecules, which in turn promotes the progression of occlusive vascular disease in the diabetic subjects.[20] AT1 receptors mediate most of the angiotensin II effects on the vessel wall and the cardiac muscle.

Oxidative Stress

Hyperglycemia/hypertension increases protein glycation and generation of oxidative products of glucose metabolism and accumulation of reactive oxygen species [nicotinamide adenine dinucleotide phosphate-oxidases (NADP-H), cyclooxygenase and lipooxygenases, xanthine oxidase, etc.]. Oxidative stress on the vascular endothelium causes inhibition of nitric oxide synthesis and promotes Ca^{2+} entry into the vascular smooth muscle cells. The above factors working in synergy contribute to vascular occlusion and tissue hypoxia and lead to the long-term microvascular (retinopathy, nephropathy, and neuropathy) as well as macrovascular (coronary, cerebral, and peripheral) complications of diabetes.[21,22]

Activation of Calcium Channels

Extracellular influx of calcium into the vascular smooth muscle cells via the L type of calcium channels causes intense and sustained vasoconstriction. Angiotensin II is intimately involved in promoting Ca^{2+} entry via the L type calcium channels. Enhanced activity and density of dihydropyridine calcium channels (DCC) has been reported in streptozocin-induced diabetic rats.[23] Ca^{2+} entry through the DCC is negatively influenced by nitric oxide. The reduced nitric oxide in diabetics (due to endothelial dysfunction) may also promote Ca^{2+} entry into the vascular smooth muscle cells. The activation of AT1 receptors and DCCs together may contribute to structural alterations in the vessel walls (endothelial cells and smooth muscle cells) and reduce the blood flow to vital organs.

Insulin Resistance and Hyperinsulinemia

In patients with type 2 diabetes/obesity and metabolic syndrome, hyperinsulinemia is very prevalent. A few earlier studies have suggested that insulin by itself may increase BP by (i) promoting distal tubular reabsorption of sodium and subsequent expansion of plasma volume[24] and (ii) enhancing the pressor responsiveness to circulating norepinephrine in those who have intact autonomic function.[25]

Salt Sensitivity

In salt sensitive diabetic patients who have normal renal function and are on high sodium diet, the exaggerated vascular responsiveness to angiotensin II may promote vasoconstriction. When there is renal damage, malfunction of renal tubular epithelial cells result in their inability to reabsorb filtered sodium. As a result, excess sodium losses in urine occur leading to hypovolemia and further drop in GFR. Since, sodium restriction does not reduce vascular reactivity to angiotensin II, salt restricted diets may be less effective in BP control in hypertensive type 2 diabetic patients.[26]

THERAPEUTIC INTERVENTIONS TO CONTROL HYPERTENSION IN DIABETIC PATIENTS

The interventions can be divided into two categories: (i) administration of pharmacological agents and (ii) other complementary medical treatments. Based on their mode of action, the pharmacologic agents are subdivided into the following groups:

- Inhibitors or renin-angiotensin system
- Calcium antagonists
- Beta blockers
- Vasodilators
- Alpha adrenergic blockers
- Diuretics.

Inhibitors of Renin-Angiotensin System

The effector molecule angiotensin II is generated by the conversion of angiotensin I by the angiotensin converting enzyme (ACE), which then mediates its vasoconstrictor effect by activating the AT1 receptors. To reduce the peripheral vascular resistance and control the hypertension, drugs aimed at inhibiting the ACE inhibitors (ACEIs), such as the lisinopril and drugs that block the activity of AT1 receptors [angiotensin receptor blockers (ARBs)] like the losartan have been tested in experimental models and clinical studies. The results confirmed that ACEIs and ARBs are effective agents in (i) controlling hypertension and (ii) slowing the progression of both micro- and macrovascular disease in diabetic patients.

AT-1 Receptor Blockers

Mechanism of Action

They blocks the AT1 receptor-mediated vasoconstrictor effects of angiotensin II, which contributes to a drop in peripheral vascular resistance and consequently a reduction in BP. The ARBs routinely used in clinical practice and their prescribed doses are shown in table 1.

Adverse Effects

- Initial drop in glomerular filtration rate: in the kidney, AT1 receptors cause efferent arteriolar vasoconstriction. The ARB class of drugs reverses the vasoconstrictor effects of AT1 receptors on the efferent arteriole. As a consequence, the intraglomerular pressure will decrease resulting in a small drop in GFR (<15%) which is an expected hemodynamic consequence in patients receiving ARBs

TABLE 1: Angiotensin Receptor Blockers (ARBs) Routinely Used in Clinical Practice, and Their Prescribed Doses

Drug	Trade name in the United States	Dose prescribed
Losartan	Cozaar	25–100 mg/day
Valsartan	Diovan	80–320 mg/day
Irbesartan	Avapro	150–300 mg/day
Candesartan	Atacand	8–32 mg/day
Telmisartan	Micardis	20–80 mg/day
Olmesartan	Benecar	20–40 mg/day
Eprosaran	Teveten	400–800 mg/day

or ACEIs. It is not a significant problem in clinical practice, except in situations where the blood flow into the glomerulus via the afferent arteriole is diminished. Examples of such clinical states include marked hypovolemia, hypotension, use of nonsteroidal anti-inflammatory drugs that inhibit prostaglandin-mediated renal blood flow and bilateral renal artery occlusive disease. Under these circumstances, the ARBs can contribute to further worsening of GFR by their effect on reducing the intracapillary BP

- Mild hyperkalemia: ARBs also block the effects of angiotensin II on aldosterone production. The resulting hypoaldosteronism can cause impaired excretion of potassium at the distal tubule and lead to hyperkalemia. It is recommended that clinicians monitor the patient's GFR and serum potassium levels within the first couple of weeks after initiation of treatment with ARBs or ACEIs.

Long-term Benefits

- Preservation of residual renal function and slowing the progression of diabetic nephropathy: blocking the vasoconstrictor effects of angiotensin II via AT1 receptors on the efferent arterioles leads to reduction in intraglomerular pressure. This in turn causes lesser filtration of protein at the glomerulus leading to a decrease in proteinuria. The reduction in intraglomerular hypertension also lowers the risk of segmental and global glomerulosclerosis and thereby leads to preservation of renal function irrespective of the stage in chronic kidney disease (CKD). Angiotensin II also promotes collagen deposition within the renal tubules and renal interstitium via the fibrogenic molecules, such as transforming growth factor beta. Blocking these fibrogenic effects of angiotensin II on the kidney parenchyma and by lowering the intracapillary hypertension, ARBs play a pivotal role in delaying the progression of renal failure in the CKD patients

- Favorable effect in congestive heart failure (CHF) and stroke: by blocking the AT1-mediated vasoconstriction, the ARBs reduce the afterload and improve the myocardial function in patients with congestive cardiomyopathy and have a beneficial effect in other vascular occlusive disease states. Because of their proven benefit in controlling hypertension and their favorable effect on the kidneys and cardiovascular system, with a minimal side-effect profile, ARBs are the first line of drugs used for the control of hypertension in diabetic patients. They can be used as monotherapy, or in combination with ACEIs, or calcium antagonists and other traditional agents, such as beta blockers, alpha adrenergic blockers, and diuretics.

Angiotensin Converting Enzyme Inhibitors

Mode of Action

The mode of action is similar to ARBs. This class of drugs prevent the generation of angiotensin II by blocking the enzyme that converts angiotensin I to angiotensin II. Commonly prescribed ACEIs, their trade names, and prescribed doses are shown in table 2.

Adverse Effects

- Initial small drop in glomerular filtration rate: similar mechanism as the ARBs
- Mild hyperkalemia: the underlying mechanism is similar to that of ARBs
- Anemia: ACEIs use may lead to anemia in some patients, as they can block erythropoietin-induced red cell production
- Bradykinin-mediated dry cough, hypotension, and angioedema: ACEIs prevent the degradation of bradykinin. The increased bradykinin levels may cause dry cough, angioedema affecting the face, oral cavity or bowel wall, and hypotension because of intense vasodilatation. Since ARBs have no effect on the bradykinin breakdown, such problems are not seen in patients using ARBs.

TABLE 2: Commonly Prescribed Angiotensin Converting Enzyme Inhibitors (ACEIs), Their Trade Names, and Doses		
Drug	Trade name in the United States	Prescribed dose
Lisinopril	Prinivil, Zestril	20–80 mg/day
Benazepril	Lotensin	20–80 mg/day
Fosinopril	Monopril	20–80 mg/day
Quinapril	Acupril	20–80 mg/day
Enalapril	Vasotec	10–40 mg/day
Ramipril	Altace	2.5–20 mg/day
Trandalapril	Mavik	2–8 mg/day

Long-term Benefits

- Preservation of renal function and slowing the progression of renal disease: the underlying mechanism is similar to that of ARBs
- Favorable effects in congestive heart failure and stroke: the underlying mechanism is similar to the ARBs
- Increasing the renal, coronary, and cerebrovascular blood flow: in addition to preventing the angiotensin II-mediated vasoconstriction, the elevation of bradykinin which is a potent vasodilator has an added benefit in promoting the blood flow to vital organs.

Calcium Antagonists

Calcium antagonists are very effective in lowering the BP, often used in patients with hypertension and coronary artery disease.

Mode of Action

They block Ca^{2+} entry into the vascular smooth muscle and reduce sympathetic mediated vasoconstriction. Of the two categories of calcium antagonists, the dihydropyridine group (nifedipine and amlodipine) blocks the L-type channels in the vascular smooth muscle cells leading to vasodilation and thereby lowers the BP. The nondihydropyridine group (verapamil and diltiazm) block the T-type channels in the myocardial cells leading to a negative inotropic effect and thus contribute to a lower systolic BP.

Calcium antagonists do not have the same degree of renoprotective effects or cardiovascular benefits as the ACEIs or ARBs and, therefore, used as a second line of therapeutic agents in the management of hypertension in diabetic patients.

Adverse Effects

Pedal edema: because of the precapillary arteriolar vasodilatation, transudation of fluid and salt from the vascular bed into the interstitial space would occur and this leads to a dose-dependent peripheral edema in the legs and feet

Gum hypertrophy: gum hypertrophy is another adverse effect noted with the dihydropyridine group of calcium antagonists

Reduction in cardiac output and bradycardia: more frequently seen in patients using the nondihydropyridine group of calcium antagonists. They should be used cautiously in patients who have CHF, heart block, or on other antiarrhythmic agents.

Beta Blockers
Mode of Action

Most beta blockers exert a negative inotropic and chronotropic effect on the myocardium and thus lower the BP. They cause partial blockade of renin release from the kidneys which may further contribute to the hypotensive effect of these agents. They are preferred agents when hypertension is associated with ischemic cardiomyopathy and diastolic dysfunction and in patients with tachyarrhythmias.

Adverse Effects

There are many adverse effects including worsening of the metabolic profile in the diabetic patients (insulin resistance, hyperlipidemia), unawareness of hypoglycemic symptoms, and stagnation of blood flow contributing to ischemic gangrene in patients with preexisting peripheral arterial occlusive disease. Others include worsening of bronchospasm in patients with preexisting asthma or chronic obstructive pulmonary disease, erectile dysfunction, and lethargy. Newer, more selective agents (both alpha and beta adrenergic blockers), such as carvedilol and nebivolol have a better side-effect profile. In a randomized control trial, compared to atnelol, patients who received carvedilol had significantly lower plasma glucose and insulin levels, lower triglyceride levels, increased high-density lipoprotein cholesterol, and lesser oxidative stress on vascular endothelium.[27] Further, carvedilol has renoprotective effects as shown by a reduction in proteinuria and improved renal blood flow and GFR levels and it is a preferred beta blocker in patients with diabetes, hypertension, and concurrent renal disease or other vascular occlusive diseases.[28]

Diuretics

The earlier thinking that diabetic patients have excess sodium and water retention and consequently higher plasma volumes and raised cardiac output has not been confirmed in recent years. Whether the sodium and water retention within the interstitial space of the vessel walls would lead to increased peripheral vascular resistance and contribute to hypertension is also a debatable issue. Nevertheless, diuretics have an important role in the management of hypertension in hypervolemic patients with clinical or radiological evidence of CHF. A return to the euvolemic state, following the diuretic use will reduce the cardiac afterload and lower the BP. With improved myocardial function and stroke volume in the euvolemic state, the renal blood flow will increase and the GFR may rise to the pre-CHF levels. In the CKD patients with normal cardiac function, the plasma volumes are generally on the low side because of salt wasting from underlying tubular atrophy and unresponsiveness of the tubular epithelium to the effects of circulating aldosterone. The routine use of diuretics in this CKD population with chronic hypovolemia may lead to further reduction in the GFR levels. When the hypovolemia is corrected with saline replacement, the lower GFR will often return to the baseline value.

Adverse Effects

There are multiple adverse effects from the use of thiazides and loop particularly in the elderly subjects. They include hypovolemia, prerenal azotemia, hyperuricemia and exacerbation of gout, hyperglycemia, hyperlipidemia, hypokalemia, hypocalcemia, hypomagnesemia, and symptomatic hyponatremia. Therefore, one has to carefully weigh the risk-benefit ratio when prescribing diuretics for the management of hypertension in diabetic patients.

Other Antihypertensive Drugs

Vasodilators (hydralazine and minoxidil), alpha adrenergic blockers (prazosin and doxazosin), direct renin inhibitors (aliskerin), and drugs acting through the vasomotor center (cloindine, methyldopa) have all been used in the management of hypertension in diabetic patients, but not as first-line agents. They have a role in drug-resistant hypertension or when patients have concurrent illnesses, such as benign prostatic hypertrophy or postural hypotension from diabetic autonomic neuropathy.

Combination Therapy and the Impact on Renal and Cardiovascular Outcomes

Although any of the drugs in the above categories could lower the BP; to minimize the side-effects and improve their effectiveness, most clinicians will resort to using a combination of two or more drugs. The goal here is not only to lower the BP, but to improve the cardiovascular and renal outcomes. Many clinical trials at the national and international level were conducted to see which drug combination, and what target BP level, would accomplish the above goals. The results of some of these relevant trials are shown in table 3. Due to the nature of these studies conducted on large number of patients across different continents, most of them are elderly and have concurrent illnesses, and many of them are based on intention to treat type of analysis; one has to cautiously interpret the results and use them only as guidelines in managing hypertension in individual patients.

What should be the Target BP in Diabetic Patients?

Although the opinion of the experts[8-10] based on earlier studies was to aim for tight control with a systolic BP of less than 130 mmHg and diastolic BP of less than 80 mmHg in the diabetic patients, the results published from large scale randomized clinical trials (Table 4) conducted in recent years[39-43] makes one think carefully whether the benefits of lowering the systolic BP below 130 mmHg outweigh the risks including the drug side-effects, additional medication costs, and the diminished blood flow (via stiffer vessels with narrowed lumens) to vital organs from lowering the systolic BP to less than 130 mmHg. In addition, most of the type 2 diabetics that we encounter in clinical practice are elderly subjects with pre-existing atherosclerotic vascular disease, and the lower pressures may even promote vascular thrombosis in critical segments such as the coronary arteries that bifurcate at an angle. The new evidence clearly shows that systolic BP of 140 mmHg or less provides as much benefit as 130 mmHg or less, and at a lower risk with reference to cardiovascular and renal outcomes in the elderly type 2 diabetic population.[39-43]

TABLE 3: Impact of Combination Drug Therapy on Cardiovascular and Renal Outcomes

Study	Sample size	Drugs compared	Results
ACE inhibitor and ARB combination vs. ARB alone vs. ACE inhibitor alone			
CALM[29]	197	Candesartan + lisinorpril vs. candesartan vs. lisinopril	Combination Rx group had lower blood pressure readings and greater reduction in proteinuria
ONTARGET[30]	25,620	Telmisartan + ramipril vs. telmisartan vs. ramipril	Combination Rx group had more hypotension and renal dysfunction, and there was no additional benefit in lowering the cardiovascular risk. ARB group however had lower incidence of angioedema and cough compared to the ACE inhibitor group
ACE inhibitor/ARB and Ca^{2+} channel blocker/beta blocker			
BENEDICT[31]	1,204	Tandalopril + verapamil vs. verapmil alone	Combination Rx had lower incidence of micro-albuminuria compared to verapamil alone
FACET[32]	380	Fosinopril vs. amlodipine	ACE inhibitor group had lower incidence of primary end points (stroke, MI and hospitalizations)
ABCD[33]	470	Enalapril vs. nisoldipine	ACE inhibitor group had a 5-fold reduction in fatal and nonfatal MI
VALUE[34]	15,245	Valsartan vs. amlodipine	No significant difference in the cardiovascular outcomes between the two groups
LIFE[35]	9,193	Losartan vs. atenelol	ARB group had lower incidence of cardiovascular events and lower mortality
RENAAL[36]	1,513	Losartan + conventional drugs vs. placebo + conventional drugs (ACE inhibitors were not used in either group)	ARB provided better renal protection and readmission rate for heart failure was lower. But the cardiovascular events and overall mortality was similar

ACE, angiotensin converting enzyme; ARB, angiotensin receptor blockers; MI, myocardial infarction.

Which Drugs to Use in Diabetic Patients with Concurrent Hypertension?

Many observational studies and controlled clinical trials have shown that almost all antihypertensive drugs (diuretics, beta blockers, vasodilators, calcium antagonists, direct renin inhibitors, ACEIs, and ARBs) can lower BP in diabetic patients.

TABLE 4: Impact of Tighter Blood Pressure Control (<130/80 mmHg) on Cardiovascular and Renal Outcomes

Study	Sample size	Target blood pressure	Results
HOT[14]	1,501	Target diastolic BP <80 mmHg vs. <90 mmHg	Tight control group had lower cardiovascular events and overall mortality
UKPDS[37]	1,148	Target BP 150/85 mmHg vs. 180/105 mmHg	Tight control group had lower cardiovascular events, but overall mortality was similar
INVEST[38]	6,400	Target systolic BP <130 mmHg vs. 130–139 mmHg vs. >140 mmHg	Tight control group and usual control group had similar outcomes, but the uncontrolled group had higher cardiovascular events. The risk for all cause mortality was significantly higher in the tight control group compared to usual control. Systolic BP <110 mmHg carried twice the risk of death
ACCORD[39]	4,733	Target systolic BP <120 mmHg vs. <140 mmHg	No difference in composite outcome of fatal or nonfatal cardiovascular events, but the number of agents used and the adverse events from drug Rx was higher in the tight control group

Since monotherapy is inadequate and side effects are higher, in most instances a combination drug therapy is required to accomplish the target BP readings. The principle objective of the practising physician is to select a combination that not only accomplishes BP control, but also provides better long-term outcomes by delaying the progression of cardiovascular (macrovascular) and renal (microvascular) disease. Further, the drug combination chosen should result in lesser adverse events and should be cost-effective in the current day and age. With those objectives in mind, the ACEI group of drugs is the preferred choice for initial treatment of hypertension, but in those who cannot tolerate (angioedema or dry cough), they can be replaced with ARBs, while accepting the higher cost of these drugs relative to ACEIs. The choice of the second line of agents is somewhat determined by the concurrent comorbidities, such as CHF or symptomatic coronary artery disease (angina, prior myocardial infarction).

Both calcium antagonists and selective beta blockers were shown to be very effective in this subpopulation of diabetic patients with concurrent hypertension. When patients are unable to tolerate this second line of drugs because of leg edema (Ca^{2+} antagonists) or severe bradycardia (beta blockers) or if the BP is not fully controlled with a combination of the first- and second-line agents, one can choose a vasodilator, such as hydralazine or minoxidil as the third-line agent to control hypertension.

Most nephrologists do not use diuretics in the elderly diabetic patients in the absence of a documented hypervolemia, because of the concern that their use can lead to reduced intravascular volume and acute renal failure from a prerenal cause. In the euvolemic patient, they can serve as the third-line agents with effects comparable to vasodilators. In edematous patients with CHF, diuretics can play a critical role in achieving the euvolemic state and should be used. Other agents, such as alpha adrenergic agents, either central (clonidine) or peripheral (e.g., prazosin) are chosen, if the patients have concurrent medical problems, such as postural hypotension from autonomic dysfunction or prostatic hypertrophy.

NONPHARMACOLOGICAL APPROACHES FOR THE MANAGEMENT OF HYPERTENSION IN DIABETIC PATIENTS

Both observational studies and small scale clinical trials have shown the benefit of employing other adjunctive maneuvers to achieve the goal of effective BP in the diabetic patients over the long-term. They are complementary to the pharmacologic management and not substitutes. These measures include promoting weight loss in obese subjects, correction of dyslipidemia, yoga and meditation, and use of sesame seed oil in cooking.[44] Additional methods that were shown to be effective are mobile telemonitoring,[45] proactive partnering with the patient in arriving at treatment decisions,[46] seeking the collaboration of community pharmacists and nurses,[47] and assisting the patients with financial aid to afford the copayments for prescribed drugs.[48] Thus, a multifactorial intervention[49] is almost always required that would include both pharmacological and complementary treatments for achieving adequate BP control and minimize the long-term vascular complications.

CONCLUSION

The incidence of type 2 diabetes is rapidly rising in all countries around the world. Approximately 70% of diabetic patients have concurrent hypertension. Both the glycemic environment and hypertension accelerate the progression of vascular (macro- and micro-) disease leading to disabling complications and excess mortality. In a few randomized clinical trials, controlling the hypertension had better cardiovascular and renal protection than controlling the blood sugar alone. Other risk factors for vascular occlusive disease, such as dyslipidemia, increased platelet activity (prothrombotic state), nicotine and amphetamine abuse, and obesity also need therapy to retard the progression of vascular disease in the diabetic patients.

Of the different therapeutic measures one can employ, pharmacologic therapy is the gold standard. ACEIs and ARBs are shown to be the most effective in controlling BP and in delaying the progression of cardiovascular and renal disease and should be used as the first line of therapy. In patients who are intolerant to the renin-angiotensin blocking drugs, and in those with suboptimal BP control despite taking them in adequate doses, the second line of agents, such as the calcium antagonists and selective beta blockers can be added to the treatment regimen.

Other traditional antihypertensive agents, such as vasodilators, alpha adrenergic blockers, and diuretics can be used if the BP control is suboptimal with current therapy, or if there were significant drug-related adverse events, or in the presence of other comorbidities, such as fluid overload, prostatic hypertrophy, or postural hypotension from diabetic autonomic dysfunction. Along with the pharmaceutical agents, several nonpharmacological complementary maneuvers were shown to be very effective in controlling the BP in diabetic patients. With reference to optimal BP, earlier target of less than 130/80 mmHg may need to be reevaluated in view of new data showing no additional cardiovascular protection with the lower readings compared to a target systolic BP of less than 140 mmHg. Further, recent studies have shown that in the tight control group, there were more drug-related side effects, higher overall mortality, and extra financial costs. The clinician in community practice may need to use the antihypertensive drugs and other complementary measures together to achieve the desired goals in this high-risk population of elderly diabetic patients with concurrent hypertension.

REFERENCES

1. Narayan KM, Boyle JP, Thompson TJ, Sorensen SW, Williamson DF. Life time risk for diabetes mellitus in the United States. *JAMA*. 2003;290(14):1884-90.
2. Geiss LS, Rolka DB, Engelgau MM. Elevated blood pressure among U.S. adults with diabetes, 88-1994. *Am J Prev Med*. 2002;22(1):42-8.
3. Tedesco MA, Natale F, Di Salvo G, Caputo S, Capasso M, Calabró R, et al. Effects of coexisting hypertension and type II diabetes mellitus on arterial stiffness. *J Human Hypertens*. 2004;18(7):469-73.
4. Knerr I, Dost A, Lepler R, Raile K, Schober E, Rascher W, et al. Tracking and prediction of arterial blood pressure from childhood to young adulthood in 868 patients with type I diabetes: a multicenter longitudinal survey in Germany and Austria. *Diabetes Care*. 2008;31(4):736-27.
5. Mazzone T, Chait A, Plutzky J. Cardiovascular disease risk in type 2 diabetes mellitus: insights from mechanistic studies. *Lancet*. 2008;371(9626):1800-9.
6. Stamler J, Vaccaro O, Neaton JD, Wentworth D. Diabetes, other risk factors, and 12-yr cardio vascular mortality for men screened in the Multiple Risk Factor Intervention Trial (MRFIT). *Diabetes Care*. 1993;16(2):434-44.
7. Gallego PH, Craig ME, Hing S, Donaghue KC. Role of blood pressure in the development of early retinopathy in adolescents in type I diabetes: prospective cohort study. *BMJ*. 2008;337:a918.
8. American Diabetes Association. Standards of medical care in diabetes–2009. *Diabetes Care*. 2009;32 (Suppl 1):S13-61.
9. Mancia G, DeBecker G, Domicizak A, Cifkova R, Fagard R, Germano G, et al. 2007 Guidelines for the Management of Arterial Hypertension: The Taskforce for the management of arterial hypertension of the European Society of Hypertension (ESH) and of the European Society of Cardiology (ESC). *J Hypertens*. 2007;25(6):1105-87.

10. Chobanian AV, Bakris GL, Black HR, Cushman WC, Green LA, Izzo JL, et al. The seventh report of the Joint National Committee on prevention, detection, evaluation and treatment of high blood pressure. The JNC-7 report. *JAMA*. 2003;289(19):2560-72.

11. Sowers JR, Stump CS. Insights into the biology of diabetic vascular disease: what's new? *Am J Hypertens*. 2004;17(11 Pt 2):2S-6S.

12. de Zeeuw D. Should albuminuria be a therapeutic target in patients with hypertension and diabetes? *Am J Hypertens*. 2004;17(11 Pt 2):11S-15S.

13. UK Prospective Diabetes Study (UKPDS)Group. Tight blood pressure control and risk of macrovascular and microvascular complications in type 2 diabetes: UKPDS 38. *BMJ*. 1998;317(7160):703-13.

14. Hansson L, Zanchetti A, Carruthers SG, Dahlöf B, Elmfeldt D, Julius S, et al. Effects of intensive blood-pressure lowering and low-dose aspirin in patients with hypertension: principal results of the Hypertension Optimal Treatment (HOT) randomised trial. HOT Study Group. *Lancet*. 1998;351(9118):1755-62.

15. Birkenhager WH, Staessen JH, Gasowski J, de Leeuw PW. Effects of antihypertensive treatment on endpoints in the diabetic patients randomized in the Systolic Hypertension in Europe (Syst-Eur) trial. *J Nephrol*. 2000;13(3):232-7.

16. Haffner SM, Lehto S, Rönnemaa T, Pyörälä K, Laakso M. Mortality from coronary heart disease in subjects with type 2 diabetes and in nondiabetic subjects with and without prior myocardial infarction. *N Engl J Med*. 1998;339(4):229-34.

17. MacMahon S. Antihypertensive drug treatment: the potential, expected and observed effects on vascular disease. *J Hypertens Suppl*. 1990;8(7):S239-44.

18. Carey RM, Wang ZQ, Siragy HM. Update: role of the angiotensin type-2 (AT(2)) receptor in blood pressure regulation. *Curr Hypertens Rep*. 2000;2(2):198-201.

19. Widdop RE, Jones ES, Hannan Re, Gaspari TA. Angiotensin AT2 receptors: cardiovascular hope or hype? *Br J Pharmacol*. 2003;140(5):809-24.

20. Kaschina E, Unger T. Angiotensin AT1/AT2 receptors: regulation, signalling and function. Blood Press. 2003;12(2):70-88.

21. Kumar AH, Ramarao P. Saga of renin-angiotensin system and calcium channels in hypertensive diabetics: does it have a therapeutic edge? *Cardiovasc Drug Rev*. 2005;23(2): 99-114.

22. Cai H, Harrison DG. Endothelial dysfunction in cardiovascular disease: the role of oxidant stress. *Circ Res*. 2000;87(10):840-4.

23. Wang R, Wu Y, Tang G, Wu L, Hanna ST. Altered L-type Ca(2+) channel currents in vascular smooth muscle cells from experimental diabetic rats. *Am J Physiol Heart Circ Physiol*. 2000;278(3):H714-22.

24. Saudek CD, Boulter PR, Knopp RH, Arky RA. Sodium retention accompanying insulin treatment of diabetes mellitus. *Diabetes*. 1974;23(3):240-6.

25. Beretta-Piccoli C, Weidmann P. Exaggerated pressor responsiveness to norepinephrine in nonazotemic diabetes mellitus. *Am J Med*. 1981;71(5):829-35.

26. Tuck M, Corry D, Trujillo A. Salt-sensitive blood pressure and exaggerated vascular reactivity in the hypertension of diabetes mellitus. *Am J Med*. 1990;88(3):210-6.

27. Giugliano D, Acampora R, Marfella R, De Rosa N, Ziccardi P, Ragone R, et al. Metabolic and cardiovascular effects of carvedilol and atenolol in non-insulin-dependent diabetes mellitus and hypertension. A randomized, controlled trial. *Ann Intern Med*. 1997;126(12):955-9.

28. Hart PD, Bakris GL. Should beta-blockers be used to control hypertension in people with chronic kidney disease? *Semin Nephrol*. 2007;27(5):555-64.

29. Mogensen CE, Neldam S, Tikkanen I, Oren S, Viskoper R, Watts RW, et al. Randomised controlled trial of dual blockade of renin-angiotensin system in patients with hypertension, microalbuminuria, and non-insulin dependent diabetes: the candesartan and lisinopril microalbuminuria (CALM) study. *BMJ*. 2000;321(7274):1440-4.

30. ONTARGET investigators, Yusuf S, Teo KK, Pogue J, Pogue J, Dyal L, et al. Telmisartan, Ramipril, or both in patients at high risk for vascular events. *N Engl J Med*. 2008;358:1547-59.

31. Ruggenenti P, Fassi A, Ilieva AP, Bruno S, Iliev IP, Brusegan V, et al. Preventing microalbuminuria in type 2 diabetes. *N Engl J Med*. 2004;351(19):1941-51.

32. Tatti P, Pahor M, Byington RP, Di Mauro P, Guarisco R, Strollo G, et al. Outcome results of the Fosinopril versus Amlodipine Cardiovascular Events Randomized Trial (FACET) in patients with hypertension and NIDDM. *Diabetes Care*. 1998;21(4):597-603.

33. Estacio RO, Jeffers BW, Hiatt WR, Biggerstaff SL, Gifford N, Schrier RW. The effect of nisoldipine as compared with enalapril on cardiovascular outcomes in patients with non-insulin dependent diabetes and hypertension. *N Engl J Med*. 1998;338(10):645-52.

34. Julius S, Weber MA, Kjeldsen SE, McInnes GT, Zanchetti A, Brunner HR, et al. The Valsartan Antihypertensive Long-Term Use Evaluation (VALUE): outcomes in patients receiving monotherapy. *Hypertension*. 2006;48(3):385-91.

35. Lindholm LH, Ibsen H, Dahlöf B, Devereux RB, Beevers G, de Faire U, et al. Cardiovascular morbidity and mortality in patients with diabetes in the Losartan Intervention For Endpoint reduction in hypertension study (LIFE): a randomized trial against atenolol. Lancet. 2002;359(9311):1004-10.

36. Brenner BM, Cooper ME, de Zeeuw D, Keane WF, Mitch WE, Parving HH, et al. Effects of losartan on renal and cardiovascular outcomes in patients with type 2 diabetes and nephropathy. *N Engl J Med*. 2001;345(12):861-9.

37. Adler AI, Stratton IM, Neil HA, Yudkin JS, Matthews DR, Cull CA, et al. Association of systolic blood pressure with macrovascular and microvascular complications of type 2 diabetes (UKPDS 36): prospective observational study. *BMJ*. 2000;321(7258):412-9.

38. Pepine CJ, Handberg EM, Cooper-Dehoff RM, Marks RG, Kowey P, Messerli FH, et al. A calcium antagonist vs a non-calcium antagonist hypertension treatment strategy for patients with coronary artery disease. The International Verapamil-Trandolapril Study (INVEST): a randomized controlled trial. *JAMA*. 2003;290(21):2805-16.

39. ACCORD study group, Cushman WC, Evans GW, Byington RP, Goff DC, Grimm RH, et al. Effects of intensive blood-pressure control in type 2 diabetes mellitus. *N Engl J Med*. 2010;362(17):1575-85.

40. Cooper-DeHoff RM, Gong Y, Handberg EM, Bavry AA, Denardo SJ, Bakris GL, et al. Tight blood pressure control and cardiovascular outcomes among hypertensive patients with diabetes and coronary artery disease. *JAMA*. 2010;304(1):61-8.

41. Elliott WJ. What should be the blood pressure target for diabetic patients? *Curr Opi Cardiol*. 2011;26(4):308-13.

42. van Hateren KJ, Landman GW, Kleefstra N, Groenier KH, Kamper AM, Houweling ST, et al. Lower blood pressure associated with higher mortality in elderly diabetic patients (ZODIAC-12). *Age Ageing*. 2010;39(5):603-9.

43. Mancia G, Laurent S, Agabiti-Rosei E, Ambrosioni E, Burnier M, Caulfield MJ, et al. Reappraisal of European guidelines on hypertension management: a European Society of Hypertension Task Force document. *J Hypertens*. 2009;27(11):2121-58.

44. Sankar D, Rao MR, Sambandam G, et al. A pilot study of open label sesame oil in hypertensive diabetics. *J Med Food*. 2006;9(3):408-12.

45. Earle KA, Istepanian RS, Zitouni K, Sungoor A, Tang B. Mobile telemonitoring for achieving tighter targets of blood pressure control in patients with complicated diabetes: a pilot study. *Diabetes Technol Ther*. 2010;12(7):575-9.

46. Heisler M. Actively engaging patients in treatment decision making and monitoring as a strategy to improve Hypertension outcomes in diabetes mellitus. *Circulation*. 2008; 117(11):1355-7.

47. McLean DL, McAlister FA, Johnson JA, King KM, Makowsky MJ, Jones CA, et al. A randomized trial of the effect of community pharmacist and nurse care on improving blood pressure management in patients with diabetes mellitus: study of cardiovascular risk intervention by pharmacists-hypertension (SCRIP-HTN). *Arch Intern Med*. 2008; 168(21):2355-61.

48. Yang Y, Thumula V, Pace PF, et al. Nonadherence to angiotensin-converting enzyme inhibitors and/or angiotensin II receptor blockers among high-risk patients with diabetes in Medicare Part D programs. J Am Pharm Assoc (2003). 2010;50(4):527-31.

49. Garde P, Vedel P, Larsen N, Jensen GV, Parving HH, Pedersen O. Multifactorial intervention and cardiovascular disease in patients with type 2 diabetes. *N Engl J Med*. 2003; 348(5):383-93.

Diabetic Neuropathy

Jayendra H Shah

ABSTRACT

Diabetic neuropathy is one of the most common and troubling complication of diabetes as it creates moderate to severe pain and the treatment is not uniformly effective and at times, it leads to lower extremity amputation. Sensory symmetrical peripheral neuropathy with or without pain is the most common type of neuropathy that afflicts diabetic patients. Amyotrophy or radiculopathy causes unilateral muscle weakness and pain in the lower extremity and unilateral involvement of the muscles of upper arm, thorax, or abdomen with pain and weakness. Peroneal, ulnar, or median nerve mononeuropathy in extremities cause weakness, foot drop, and pain. Mononeuropathy of cranial nerves cause ptosis, diplopia, and facial palsy. Autonomic neuropathy of the gastrointestinal tract manifests as gastroesophageal reflux disease, gastroparesis, diarrhea, steatorrhea, malabsorption syndrome, and fecal incontinence. Orthostatic hypotension, loss of diurnal variation in blood pressure, resting tachycardia, exercise intolerance, silent myocardial ischemia, and infarction are manifestations of autonomic neuropathy involving cardiovascular system. The autonomic neuropathy involving periphery manifests as trophic changes in skin and nail, non-cardiac and non-renal edema of feet, Charcot's joint, partial ptosis of upper eyelids, and disproportionate sweating with food ingestion. Genitourinary autonomic neuropathy causes mainly erectile dysfunction in male and dyspareunia in female patients. It causes urinary bladder dysfunction in both sexes. Diabetic neuropathic cachexia, a rare complication of diabetes, has acute or subacute onset of symptoms of anorexia, marked weight loss, painful sensory peripheral neuropathy, and depression. In this chapter, pathophysiology of these various diabetic neuropathy, its manifestation, and treatment are described. A stepwise approach in the management of diabetic neuropathy is also recommended in this chapter.

INTRODUCTION

Diabetic neuropathy is one of the most common complications of diabetes. Neuropathy in diabetic patients can be classified as follows (Table 1):

- Sensory symmetrical peripheral polyneuropathy
- Amyotrophy and mononeuropathy
  - Asymmetrical amyotrophy of lower and upper extremities; thoracic and abdominal muscles
  - Asymmetrical neuropathy of peroneal, ulnar, medial, and cranial nerves
- Autonomic neuropathy
  - Involving gastrointestinal (GI) tract
  - Involving cardiovascular system
  - Involving peripheral dysfunction
  - Involving genitourinary system
- Diabetic neuropathic cachexia (rare).

Of these different neuropathies, sensory symmetrical peripheral polyneuropathy is a common neurological complication of diabetes.[1] This neuropathy involves large myelinated and unmyelinated distal axons without significant involvement of motor axons.[2] The diabetic distal polyneuropathy is similar clinically and pathologically to that observed in the uremic or alcoholic neuropathy. However, there is early involvement of vasa nervosa in diabetic neuropathy suggesting both vascular and metabolic causes.[3] The diabetic neuropathy is associated with poor glycemic control.

RISK FACTORS

Several risk factors are associated with diabetic neuropathy:[4-6]

- Duration of diabetes
- Hyperglycemia
- Hyperlipidemia
- Smoking
- Hypertension
- Body mass index.

Of these risk factors in the development of neuropathy, severity of hyperglycemia and duration of diabetes play a significant role in type 1 and type 2 diabetic patients.[4,5]

Diabetes Control and Complication Trial (DCCT) in type 1 diabetes showed that tighter glycemic control was associated with improvement in the diabetic neuropathy when present and in others it prevented the occurrence of this complication.[7,8] At the conclusion of DCCT, the patients with intensive glycemic control were advised to continue the intensive regimen and the control patients were asked to start the intensive glycemic control. Eight years later, the separation of glycosylated hemoglobin (HbA1c), i.e., glycemic control was lost between the two groups yet intensive group still maintained the benefit of previous tight glycemia, which prevented development of neuropathy.

TABLE 1: Classification, Clinical Manifestations, Diagnosis, and Treatment of Diabetic Neuropathies

Type of diabetic neuropathy	Clinical manifestations	Diagnosis	Treatment	Comments
Sensory symmetrical peripheral polyneuropathy	• Loss of sensation to touch and pain, progress to loss of vibratory and proprioceptive sensations • Tingling and numbness, burning and shooting pain • Hyperesthesia	• Clinical findings • Electromyography and nerve conduction studies	• Optimal glycemic control • Amitriptyline • Duloxetine • Pregabalin • Valproic acid • Antioxidant alpha-lipoic acid • Topical capsaicin cream • Lidocaine patch • Topical isosorbide spray • TENS	Prognosis usually good as most patients improve
Amyotrophy (radiculopathy)	• Unilateral proximal groups of muscle weakness and pain in lower extremity • Unilateral involvement of thoracic and abdominal muscles and proximal muscles of upper arm	• Clinical examination • Electromyography and nerve conduction studies • Elevation of CSF proteins	• Symptomatic treatment • Optimal glycemic control • Treatment of painful neuropathy as above	• Prognosis guarded • Overall some improvement but lingering pain and weakness and atrophy of muscles persists
Mononeuropathy; peroneal and median nerve, cranial nerve (III, VI, VII nerves)	Unilateral muscle weakness and pain, foot drop, ptosis, diplopia, and facial palsy	• Clinical examination • Electromyography and nerve conduction study	• Symptomatic and supportive treatment • Optimal glycemic control • Treatment of pain if required	Good prognosis as most patients improve

Contd...

Contd...

TABLE 1: Classification, Clinical Manifestations, Diagnosis, and Treatment of Diabetic Neuropathies

Type of diabetic neuropathy	Clinical manifestations	Diagnosis	Treatment	Comments
Autonomic neuropathy of GI tract	GERD, gastroparesis, diarrhea, steatorrhea, fecal incontinence, and malabsorption syndrome	• Clinical examination • Radionuclide studies • Upper endoscopy • Lower endoscopy • Fecal examination	• Optimal glycemic control • Metoclopramide • Antiemetic drugs • Fluid and electrolyte balance • Loperamide, codeine, clonidine • Toilet training and biofeedback • Anorectal sphincter surgery	Some patients respond to treatment while others are refractory to treatment
Autonomic neuropathy of cardiovascular system	Orthostatic hypotension, resting tachycardia, exercise intolerance, silent myocardial ischemia and infarction, loss of diurnal variation in blood pressure, and supine hypertension during night	• Clinical examination • Blood pressure and pulse change during sustain handgrip test and during postural change	• Optimal glycemic control • Postural training and leg tensing • Discontinuation of drugs aggravating orthostatic hypotension • Fludrocortisone • Midodrine and pindolol in refractory cases	• Most patients are asymptomatic • Orthostatic hypotension usually responds to treatment
Autonomic neuropathy involving peripheral function	Dry itching skin, loss of nail, edema of feet, ulceration, cramps, Charcot's joint, partial ptosis of upper eyelids, and disproportionate sweating with food ingestion	• Clinical examination • Neuropad patch testing	• Optimal glycemic control • Foot care by podiatrist • No specific treatment for sweating	Early podiatric foot care may salvage foot from amputation

Contd...

Contd...

TABLE 1: Classification, Clinical Manifestations, Diagnosis, and Treatment of Diabetic Neuropathies

Type of diabetic neuropathy	Clinical manifestations	Diagnosis	Treatment	Comments
Genitourinary autonomic neuropathy	Urinary bladder dysfunction, erectile dysfunction and retrograde ejaculation in male, and dyspareunia in female	• History and clinical examination • Complete urodynamic study	• Scheduled urination training • Vaginal estrogen cream • Phosphodiesterase inhibitors • Bladder neck sphincter surgery	Many patients suffer from depression which should be treated
Diabetic neuropathic cachexia	• Sensory peripheral neuropathy with pain • Anorexia, marked weight loss and muscle wasting • Acute or subacute onset • Depression	• Clinical examination • Electromyography and nerve conduction studies	• Symptomatic and supportive treatment • Treatment of painful neuropathy and depression as above	• Good prognosis • Spontaneous improvement in most patients within 24 months

TENS, transcutaneous electrical nerve stimulation; CSF, cerebrospinal fluid; GI, gastrointestinal; GERD, gastroesophageal reflux disease.

The clear benefit of reversal of neuropathy or prevention of neuropathy by intensive glycemic control seen in type 1 diabetic patients is not clearly evident in type 2 diabetic patients. United Kingdom Prospective Diabetes Study (UKPDS) showed that the intensive glycemic treatment in type 2 diabetes significantly prevented or improved neuropathy, but the effect was not as pronounced as that was seen in type 1 diabetic patients.[9] Nevertheless, it is generally accepted that good glycemic control in type 1 and type 2 diabetes is associated with prevention as well as improvement of neuropathy.

Wiggins et al. in their clinical trial in diabetic patients with neuropathy observed that triglyceride levels were significantly higher in those patients in whom the neuropathy progressed as compared to those patients whose neuropathy was stable. The progression of neuropathy occurred irrespective of glycemic control, use of insulin or type of diabetes.[6] In another study, the incidence of neuropathy was significantly associated with hypertension, elevated triglyceride levels, smoking, and increased body mass index in addition to duration of diabetes and poor glycemic control.[10]

PATHOPHYSIOLOGY

In diabetic neuropathy, a combination of metabolic and vascular factors plays a pivotal role in pathophysiology. It is therefore important to understand the role of these factors as some of the treatments of diabetic neuropathy are geared to prevent or reverse the effects caused by metabolic or vascular effects.

Metabolic Factors

The most common and extensively studied metabolic alterations responsible in the pathogenesis of diabetic neuropathy are:
- Accumulation of advanced glycation end products (AGEs)
- Accumulation of excess sorbitol, causing damage to nervous tissues.

In chronic uncontrolled hyperglycemia, glucose combines with circulating amino acids and tissue proteins. Initially, these nonenzymatic glycosylated proteins are reversible but once AGEs are formed, due to Amadori rearrangement, the process becomes irreversible.[11-13] In proportion to uncontrolled hyperglycemia, AGE concentrations are increased in diabetic patients. The AGEs also bind to the cell surface receptor, receptor for AGE, whose activation is proinflammatory. The AGE also independently causes increased vascular permeability, monocyte influx, adhesion molecule expression, and procoagulant activity which ultimately contribute to the vascular injury.[14] Chronic hyperglycemia in diabetic patient stimulates intracellular aldose reductase pathway for glucose metabolism, which leads to intracellular accumulation of sorbitol. Excess intracellular sorbitol causes depletion of nicotinamide adenine dinucleotide phosphate (NADPH), decrease in intracellular myoinositol, and increased intracellular osmolality. These intracellular changes interfere with cell metabolism and ultimately lead to oxidative stress.[15] Other metabolic factors, such as protein kinase C activation causing vasoconstriction and hypoxia to nerve contribute to the cause of diabetic neuropathy.[16] Also, hyperglycemia induces excess activation of nuclear enzyme poly-ADP-ribose polymerase (PARP). Excess PARP leads to increase in protein kinase C activity, AGE formation, and abnormal changes in gene transcription. Thus, PARP inhibitors may be effective in the treatment of diabetic neuropathy.[17,18] Hyperglycemia has been shown to cause shunting of glycolytic intermediates into the hexosamine pathway, which results in the production of uridine diphosphonate-N-acetyl glucosamine modifying transcription factors, thus resulting in abnormal cell function and cell damage.[19] Medication which decreases hexosamine-modified protein has potential in the treatment of diabetic neuropathy.[20] As can be realized from the above discussion, a common theme of oxidative stress emerges which can provide a unifying metabolic pathogenic mechanism of nerve injury in diabetic neuropathy. No wonder that antioxidant treatment has been shown to clinically improve neuropathy in diabetic patients.[21,22]

Vascular Factors

The pathological finding of abnormal endoneural blood vessel wall thickness and vascular occlusion in diabetic patients suggested vascular ischemia of the neuron in the pathogenesis of diabetic neuropathy.[23] This theory supported the finding of reduced endoneural oxygen tension in the sural nerves with advanced neuropathy in diabetic patients.[24] It appears that vascular and metabolic factors may work in harmony in the pathological alteration of the nervous tissue in diabetic neuropathy. Hyperglycemia and insulin deficiency may potentiate vascular ischemia which may lead to profound metabolic changes in the nervous tissue in diabetic patients with neuropathy.[22,25] Although the exact mechanism of this metabolic-vascular interaction is not known, it appears that uncontrolled hyperglycemia in diabetic patients is responsible for metabolic and vascular changes in diabetic neuropathy. The maintenance of wear and tear of nerve fibers as well as repair and regeneration of fibers following injury depends on brain derived neurotrophic factor, vascular endothelial growth factors, neurotrophin-3 and insulin-like growth factors.[26] Insulin itself acts as neurotrophic growth factor and loss of which in addition with the deficiency of other growth factors in diabetes may have adverse effects on repair and viability of peripheral nerves.

SENSORY SYMMETRICAL PERIPHERAL POLYNEUROPATHY

This is the most common type of neuropathy seen in type 1 and type 2 diabetic patients. This neuropathy is mainly sensory and motor involvement is rare. It initially involves small peripheral fibers causing loss of pain and temperature sensations. This leads to local injuries in unaware diabetic patients and ulcer formation. Large fibers are involved in the later stage of the neuropathy with loss of vibration and proprioceptive sensation. In a severe form it may cause ataxia. Peripheral autonomic neuropathy frequently accompanies causing further trophic changes in the skin, cuticles, and small joints leading to Charcot's joint. The involvement of sensory fibers manifest as paresthesia and dysthesias with tingling and numbness feeling in toes. This at times progresses to sensations of pinprick and hyperesthesia of feet making the touch of bedsheets or clothing unbearable, especially during night. The neuropathy also manifests as sharp shooting pain or as constant dull ache in both legs. Rarely, these symptoms of peripheral neuropathy are associated with severe weight loss and depression (see the sectoin Diabetic Neuropathic Cachexia). The course of painful peripheral neuropathy may be self limited and spontaneous resolution of pain may occur within 6–24 months. The involvement of upper extremities is rare and occurs late in the advanced cases. It is important to note that in most diabetic patients, early symmetrical peripheral neuropathy is mild and often asymptomatic. Only careful clinical examination may identify the presence of peripheral neuropathy.

The main treatment is prevention of peripheral neuropathy by optimal glycemic control.[27] Several diabetes treatment trials have shown strong association with glycemic control and prevention or reversal of peripheral neuropathy.[4,5,7,8] The Oslo diabetes trial showed that a 1% rise in HbA1c was associated with 1.3 m/s slowing in the nerve conduction in type 1 diabetic patients.[28] The painful neuropathy can be managed with antidepressant tricyclic drugs. The drug of choice is amitriptyline 10–50 mg/day,[29] preferably given at bedtime. The effect of amitriptyline occurs within 2 weeks; however, maximum effect may take 6 week to occur. The dose required for the amelioration of pain is usually less than that required to treat depression. The mode of action of tricyclic antidepressant is by altering central perception of pain. Nortriptyline can be substituted in patients with anticholinergic side effects. Both of these drugs are contraindicated in patients with cardiac disease and substitution with duloxetine,[30] a dual serotonin and norepinephrin reuptake inhibitor, may help. The recommended dose of duloxetine is 60–120 mg/day. Most common side effect of duloxetine is nausea, somnolence, anorexia, and dizziness. The drug is better tolerated when taken with food. Anticonvulsant drug, pregabalin,[31] may be useful in the treatment of painful peripheral neuropathy. The mode of action of pregabalin is acting as a presynaptic inhibitor of release of excitatory neurotransmitters. The recommended dose of pregabalin is to start with 50 mg twice a day and to slowly increase to the effective dose of 100 mg three times a day or 150 mg twice a day. The side effects are sedation and confusion. Pregabalin may be habit forming and, therefore, is classified as Schedule V drug in the United States. Another anticonvulsant, valproic acid in the dose of 500–1,200 mg/day, has been recommended to treat painful diabetic peripheral neuropathy.[32] Due to its teratogenic effects, valproic acid is contraindicated for the use in the patients with childbearing age. The use of gabapentin in the treatment of painful neuropathy has been controversial and, therefore, it is not recommended.[33] Opioids, oxycodone controlled release have been used in the doses of 10–60 mg/day in the treatment of painful neuropathy.[34] Because of lack of evidence for long-term effect of oxycodone and potential for overdose and addiction, we do not recommend use of opioids in the treatment of painful neuropathy.[35] Antioxidant, alpha-lipoic acid has been used to decrease oxidative stress in the treatment of painful diabetic neuropathy. An optimal daily dose of 600 mg orally with meals has been recommended with beneficial effects.[20-22]

There are several topical applications which have been used to treat painful diabetic neuropathy. Capsaicin as 0.075% cream when applied topically four times a day has been effective in the treatment of painful diabetic neuropathy.[36] The analgesia is caused by local depletion of substance P by capsaicin. Some patients are unable to tolerate counter irritant properties of capsaicin causing local burning, which is aggravated by hot weather and hot water. Lidocain patch (5%) has been found to be effective in small number of patients.[37] However, a randomized trial is lacking. Similarly, isosorbide dinitrate topical spray has been tried with success in the treatment of painful neuropathy in small number of patients.[38] Transcutaneous electrical nerve stimulation (TENS) has been also used in the treatment of painful neuropathy and is recommended by the American Academy of Neurology.[39] We recommend that a stepwise treatment approach, similar to one recommended by American Diabetes Association,[27] be used. First, nondiabetic causes of the pain or neuropathy should be excluded and appropriately treated. Second, optimal glycemic control in type 1 and type 2 diabetes should be an utmost priority. The treatment with tricyclic drugs, such as amitriptyline should be used next. Anticonvulsant, pregabalin, should be tried if tricyclic drugs are not effective. The use of antioxidants (alpha-lipoic acid) should be reserved for refractory cases. Use of topical agents, such as capsaicin cream could be used alone or in combination with other pharmacologic drug therapy. In a refractory patient, TENS therapy may be tried. We recommend not to use opioids without referring patient to pain therapy experts.

AMYOTROPHY AND MONONEUROPATHY

The diabetic amyotrophy also known as diabetic radiculopathy presents itself as acute or subacute onset of weakness and pain with unilateral involvement of proximal group of muscles in lower extremity in diabetic patients with a fair glycemic control. It is often associated with weight loss. In many patients, eventual bilateral involvement occurs. Cerebrospinal fluid shows elevation of protein in the mean range of 90 mg/dL (5 mmol/L). Involvement of upper extremity and chest is manifested by weakness and pain in the muscles of forearm, chest and lumbar area, or mononeuropathy involving ulnar or median nerves.[40,41] Diagnosis is mainly clinical with electromyography aid and exclusion of other etiology. The treatment is mainly symptomatic and supportive. Pain treatment is similar to one outlined in the treatment of painful polyneuropathy. Immunosuppressive therapy with corticosteroids has been tried but controlled trials are not available.[42] Although generalized improvement occurs in most patients, overall prognosis for this condition is guarded as permanent weakness, foot drop or pain continues for months.

Mononeuropathy involving cranial nerve occurs in diabetic patients. Most common is the unilateral involvement of III, IV, and VI cranial nerves with clinical presentation of pain, diplopia, and ptosis.[43] The pupillary functions are spared. The Bell's palsy involving facial nerve also occurs in diabetic patients.[44] Peripheral mononeuropathy commonly involves median nerve in upper extremity while peroneal nerve causing foot drop is more common in the lower extremity. Sometimes multiple mononeuropathy occurs in the same patient (mononeuropathy multiplex). Treatment is supportive and symptomatic. The prognosis of cranial mononeuropathy is good and most patients improve in few months.

AUTONOMIC NEUROPATHY

The autonomic neuropathy in diabetic patient can present as asymptomatic or symptomatic condition. Although many organ systems can be involved, for the purpose of this chapter, we will consider GI, cardiovascular, peripheral, and genitourinary systems which are commonly involved.

Autonomic Neuropathy Involving Gastrointestinal Tract

Diabetic autonomic neuropathy of GI tract involves esophageal motility disorders causing gastroesophageal reflux disease, gastric motility problems causing gastroparesis, intestinal motility and absorption problem causing constipation and diarrhea, and anorectal sphincter problem causing fecal incontinence.[45] The hyperglycemia has been implicated in abnormal esophageal motility and decreased lower esophageal sphincter pressure. Even in healthy subjects, induced hyperglycemia has demonstrated functional abnormalities in the lower esophageal sphincter and gastroparesis.[46] The gastroparesis is thought to be not uncommon in diabetic patients. It is estimated that over 20% of type 1 diabetic patients with one other complication suffer from gastroparesis.[47] The autonomic dysfunction in diabetic gastroparesis is also related to hyperglycemia and insulin-induced hypoglycemia has been shown to accelerate the gastric emptying.[48,49] Diagnosis of gastroparesis is clinical but could be confirmed by upper endoscopy, barium swallow X-ray, stable isotope breath test, or radionuclide gastric emptying study. Treatment consists of dietary changes and administration of prokinetic agents such as metoclopramide (Reglan) 5–10 mg 30 minutes before each meal. Troublesome nausea and vomiting can be treated with antiemetic drugs.

Diabetic enteropathy manifested by diarrhea with or without steatorrhea may occur in patients with long-standing diabetes. The diarrhea is usually painless and watery occurring in bouts at night. Sometimes, the diarrhea may be associated with fecal incontinence and attributed to anorectal sphincter dysfunction.[50] In addition to autonomic neuropathy involving sympathetic system and vagal nerve, abnormal small bowel motility may be associated with bacterial overgrowth causing bile acid deconjugation and fat malabsorption. Sometimes associated conditions like exocrine pancreatic insufficiency or celiac sprue are responsible for diarrhea in diabetic patients. It is interesting to note that incidence of celiac sprue is increased in diabetes as high prevalence of human leukocyte antigen (HLA)-B8 and DR3 in both diseases suggested.[51] Finally, some of the artificial sweeteners, such as sorbitol has been implicated in diabetic diarrhea. In the treatment of patients with diarrhea, one should initially concentrate on correction of water and electrolyte imbalance and vitamins and nutritional supplementation. Diarrhea should be then treated according to the cause rather than an empiric treatment. Bacterial overgrowth should be treated with antibiotics. The patients with increased intestinal transit may deserve trial with loperamide 2–4 mg three to four times a day or codeine 30 mg three to four times a day. In patients who have increased intestinal motility as well as increased secretion causing diarrhea, treatment with clonidine 0.6 mg three times a day may be effective. However, adverse effects of clonidine, such as orthostatic hypotension, dry mouth, and delayed gastric emptying may limit its use. In patients with fecal incontinence treatment with loperamide is effective as it also causes increase in resting pressure of anorectal sphincter. Other treatments include toilet training and biofeedback techniques.[52] Diabetic patients who also suffer simultaneously with exocrine pancreatic deficiency should be treated with pancreatic enzyme and those with celiac disease should be treated with gluten-free diet.

Autonomic Neuropathy Involving Cardiovascular System

The cardiovascular autonomic neuropathy is manifested clinically as orthostatic hypotension, resting tachycardia, exercise intolerance, silent myocardial ischemia, and infarction.[53] The patients with cardiovascular autonomic neuropathy manifest persistent tachycardia at rest without any modulation in heart rate during such activities as Valsalva maneuver (which is known to cause increase in parasympathetic vagal tone). Inadequate sympathetic modulation fails to increase cardiac output causing exercise intolerance. In the advanced stage of cardiovascular autonomic neuropathy, cardiac denervation may occur with fixed heart rate. Silent myocardial infarction and sudden death are not uncommon in such patients. A silent ischemia was detected during cardiac radionuclide stress study in 22% of diabetic patients who had no known history of coronary artery disease.[54]

Orthostatic hypotension, defined as a fall in more than 20 mmHg systolic blood pressure after assuming erect posture, occurs in diabetic patients with peripheral and central cardiovascular sympathetic denervation preventing vasoconstriction in the splanchnic and peripheral vascular beds. Some of the characteristics of orthostatic hypotension in diabetic autonomic neuropathy are: (i) loss of diurnal variation in blood pressure, (ii) supine hypertension during night, (iii) drop in supine and standing blood pressure after meals and (iv) day to day variation in symptoms, which may be precipitated by insulin therapy.

Asymptomatic cardiovascular autonomic neuropathy is usually associated with peripheral neuropathy. The cardiac parasympathetic integrity is detected by cardiovascular reflex testing such as heart rate variability with deep breathing. The measurement of blood pressure changes during sustained handgrip or postural changes test the sympathetic cardiovascular integrity. In the treatment of cardiovascular autonomic neuropathy, a supervised exercise training program may be beneficial.[55] Discontinuation of the drugs like tranquilizers, diuretics, and antidepressants, which may exacerbate postural hypotension, may help. It is recommended a slow change in posture from supine to standing and while standing on both legs to tens the legs by crossing them. A significant increase in blood pressure and cardiac output has been reported by this maneuver.[56] Handgrip and/or foot dorsiflexion exercise before assuming standing position has also been recommended in these patients. Pharmacologic treatments are aimed at expanding the plasma volume by high salt diet and administration of mineralocorticoids, fludrocortisone (Florinef) 0.1–0.4 mg/day. In severe refractory cases of orthostatic hypotension treatment with fluoxetine, adrenoreceptor agonist like midodrine, or beta blockers with sympathomimetic activity like pindolol have been tried.[57,58] The supine hypertension during night may be treated with short-acting antihypertensive agents, such as captopril or verapamil at bedtime.

Autonomic Neuropathy Involving Peripheral Dysfunction

The autonomic dysfunction in the periphery involves skin, subcutaneous tissue, cuticles, upper eye lids, and joints. The clinical manifestations show up as dry itching skin, loss of nails, peripheral edema, sweating abnormalities, callus formation, ptosis of upper eye lids, fractures of small bones, and joint deformity (Charcot's joint). In diabetic patient, loss of sympathetic vascular tone causes increased peripheral blood flow, which is thought to be responsible for small bone fractures in feet with minimal stress. Edema of feet predisposes for ulcerations, and symptoms of aching feet, cramps, itching with dry skin are common in these patients. They are also prone to develop neuroarthopathy (Charcot's joint) with secondary ulcerations.[59] The absence of increased jugular venous pressure and other signs of congestive heart failure or chronic renal failure distinguish the neuropathic edema. Galvanic skin responses[60] and neuropad patch[61] testing have been utilized to diagnose peripheral sympathetic neuropathy. Foot care by podiatrist and judicious use of sympathomimetic drugs are important in the management of these patients. Early care by the podiatrist may salvage the foot from amputation. Disproportionate sweating in response to food may occur as peripheral sympathetic neuropathy.[62] Patients usually develop tolerance to this phenomena and no specific treatment is needed.

In our clinical experience, partial ptosis of upper eyelids is not an uncommon finding in diabetic patients with peripheral sensory neuropathy and long duration of diabetes (Figure 1A). It signifies peripheral autonomic (sympathetic) neuropathy involving muscle of Muller in upper eyelids with sympathetic innervations. It is

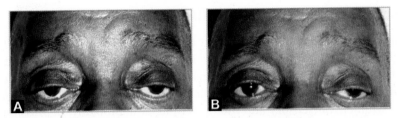

FIGURE 1 A, Bilateral ptosis of upper eyelids in a patient with peripheral autonomic (sympathetic) neuropathy. **B,** Improvement of partial ptosis in right upper eyelid after installation of a 2.5% phenylephrine eye drop in right eye.

frequently associated with other findings of peripheral autonomic neuropathy, such as trophic changes in skin, nail, and joints. The partial ptosis of upper eyelids in these patients is not associated with any cranial nerve or center nervous system abnormality. Most of the patients are asymptomatic and any specific treatment is not required. The patients compensate the partial drooping of upper eyelids with upward contraction of eyebrow and forehead muscles (Figure 1A). The sympathetic stimulation of Muller's muscle by phenylephrin eye drop corrects the partial ptosis of the eyelid (Figure 1B). The treatment with phenylephrine eye drops is not recommended as it causes dilatation of pupil and exacerbation of glaucoma (not uncommon in diabetic patients).

Also, it is not unusual for diabetic patients with peripheral autonomic neuropathy to complain about difficulty in night driving due to abnormal pupillary reflexes causing difficulties in light adaptation.

Autonomic Neuropathy Involving Genitourinary System

The autonomic neuropathy involving genitourinary system is manifested by erectile dysfunction and retrograde ejaculation in male, dyspareunia in female, and urinary bladder dysfunction. Bladder dysfunction causes infrequent urination, urine retention, and incomplete emptying of the bladder. These patients are predisposed to urinary tract infection with overflow incontinence and dribbling. The incidence of urinary bladder dysfunction and incontinence has been reported to be frequent (over 20%) in both male and female type 1 diabetic patients.[63,64] Sexual dysfunctions are also common in these patients and frequently associated with depression. Vaginal dryness is more common in diabetic women and erectile dysfunction in male diabetic patients compared to nondiabetic patients. This is discussed in detail in the chapter "Sexual Dysfunction in Diabetes". The urodynamic studies are needed to confirm bladder dysfunction in diabetic patients. The treatment consists of scheduled urination training and if needed treatment with bethanechol 10–30 mg three times a day is recommended. In more advance cases, bladder neck sphincter reconstructive surgery may be required.

DIABETIC NEUROPATHIC CACHEXIA

This rare syndrome of diabetic neuropathy has been described mainly in 60–70-year-old male patients with type 2 diabetes.[65-67] Rarely, the diabetic neuropathic cachexia is reported in female patients.[68,69] The hallmark of syndrome is that it is usually associated with mild type 2 diabetes which is easy to control but with a profound painful symmetrical sensory and motor peripheral neuropathy, depression, and anorexia. An association with malabsorption[70] and hypothyroidism[68] has been reported after anorexia and weight loss.

The diagnosis is mainly clinical with findings of painful peripheral neuropathy, weakness, depression, and cachexia with weight loss to 60% of ideal body weight. Depression and anorexia with painful neuropathy are main contributing factors for weight loss in these patients. Occasionally, associated malabsorption also contributes to weight loss. Because of the history of rapid weight loss in these patients, frequently expensive investigation for occult malignancy is initiated by unwary physician. The diabetes is usually mild and easily controllable with oral agents. The peripheral neuropathy is manifested as paresthesias, loss of sensation, and painful burning sensation to shooting pain. Generalized weakness and muscle atrophy is the motor manifestation of neuropathy. Rapid progression of neuropathy from distal to more proximal area is classic of this condition. Although uncommon, the autonomic neuropathy when present is manifested by orthostatic hypotension, tachycardia, neurogenic bladder, and erectile dysfunction.

The nerve conduction and electromyography findings show mainly lower amplitude of the motor and sensory action potentials as well as reduced nerve conduction velocity consistent with peripheral neuropathy. The biopsies of nerve and muscle of these patients have shown nonspecific neurogenic muscle fiber atrophy and axonal degeneration of small and large nerve fibers without any infiltration.

It is interesting to note that other microvascular complications, such as diabetic retinopathy or nephropathy are not present with this condition.[65-70] The prognosis for recovery is usually good. Most of the patients have been reported to spontaneously improve within 24 months as the condition is self limited.[65-70] Once neuropathic pain is resolved and depression is abated, appetite returns and weight gain occurs. During the active state of the neuropathic cachexia, strong reassurance to the patients and family members is important part of the treatment. Symptomatic treatment for pain and depression with analgesics and antidepressant agents is recommended. Also, other coexisting condition such as hypothyroidism, if present needs to be appropriately treated.

CONCLUSION

Diabetic neuropathy is one of the most common and troubling complication of diabetes as it creates moderate to severe pain and the treatment is not uniformly effective and at times it leads to lower extremity amputation. Sensory symmetrical peripheral neuropathy, with or without pain, is the most common type of neuropathy that afflicts diabetic patients. Amyotrophy or radiculopathy causes unilateral muscle weakness and pain in the lower extremity and unilateral involvement of the muscles of upper arm, thorax, or abdomen with pain and weakness. Some improvement occurs following symptomatic treatment of diabetic radiculopathy but muscle weakness and atrophy persists. Peroneal, ulner, or median nerve mononeuropathy in extremities cause weakness, foot drop, and pain. Mononeuropathy of cranial nerves cause ptosis, diplopia, and facial palsy. The prognosis of mononeuropathy is good as most of the patients recover. Autonomic neuropathy of the gastrointestinal tract is troubling as some patients respond to the treatment but many are refractory to the treatment. This neuropathy manifests as gastroesophageal reflux disease., gastroparesis, diarrhea, steatorrhea, malabsorption syndrome, and fecal incontinence. In these diabetic patients, glycemic control becomes difficult due to erratic absorption of food. Metoclopramide and antiemetic drugs are used to treat gastroparesis whereas loperamide, codeine, and clonidine with fluids and electrolytes are used in the treatment of diarrhea. Toilet training, biofeedback, or anorectal sphincter surgery may require for fecal incontinence.

Orthostatic hypotension, loss of diurnal variation in blood pressure, resting tachycardia, exercise intolerance, silent myocardial ischemia, and infarction are manifestations of autonomic neuropathy involving cardiovascular system. Most patients are asymptomatic and many with symptoms of orthostatic hypotension respond to treatment. The autonomic neuropathy involving periphery manifests as trophic changes in skin and nail, noncardiac and nonrenal edema of feet, Charcot's joint, partial ptosis of upper eyelids, and disproportionate sweating with food ingestion. Early podiatric foot care is recommended to salvage foot from amputation. Genitourinary autonomic neuropathy causes mainly erectile dysfunction in male and dyspareunia in female patients. It causes urinary bladder dysfunction in both sexes. Phosphodiesterase inhibitors, vaginal estrogen cream, scheduled urination training, and bladder neck sphincter surgery are mainstay of the treatment of genitourinary autonomic neuropathy. Diabetic neuropathic cachexia, a rare complication of diabetes, has acute or subacute onset of symptoms of anorexia, marked weight loss, painful sensory peripheral neuropathy, and depression. Symptomatic and supportive treatment is effective with good prognosis as spontaneous recovery occurs within 24 months in most patients.

Metabolic and vascular factors play an important role in the pathophysiology of diabetic neuropathy. Some of the drugs used in the treatment of painful diabetic neuropathy are targeted to reverse the effects of these vascular and metabolic factors. A stepwise approach in the treatment of painful diabetic neuropathy is recommended.[27] Once nondiabetic or non-neuropathic causes of pain are treated, optimal glycemic control should be achieved. Next, tricyclic drugs, such as amitriptyline should be tried. Anticonvulsant drugs, pregabalin or valproic acid may be tried if tricyclic drugs are not effective. Use of topical agents, such as capsaicin cream may be used simultaneously with other agents. In the refractory cases, a trial with antioxidant drug alpha-lipoic acid therapy or transcutaneous electrical nerve stimulation may be useful. Because of recent controversies, use of gabapentin in the treatment of painful diabetic neuropathy is not recommended. Also, we prefer not to use opioids and other narcotic agents without referring the refractory diabetic patients with painful neuropathy to pain management experts.

REFERENCES

1. Callahan BC, Cheng HT, Stables CL, Smith AL, Feldman EL. Diabetic neuropathy: clinical manifestations and current treatments. *Lancet Neurol.* 2012;11(6):521-34.
2. Malik RA. The pathology of human diabetic neuropathy. *Diabetes.* 1997;46 Suppl 2:S50-3.
3. Dyck PJ, Karnes JL, O'Brien P, Okazaki H, Lais A, Engelstad J. The spatial distribution of fiber loss in diabetic polyneuropathy suggest ischemia. *Ann Neurol.* 1986;19(5):440-9.
4. Hanssen KF. Blood glucose control and microvascular and macrovascular complications in diabetes. *Diabetes.* 1997;46 Suppl 2:S101-3.
5. Genuth S. Insights form the diabetes control and complication trial/epidemiology of diabetes intervention and complications study on the use of intensive glycemic treatment to reduce the risk of complications of type 1 diabetes. *Endocr Pract.* 2006;12 Suppl 1:34-41.
6. Wiggin TD, Sullivan KA, Pop-Busui R, Amato A, Sima AA, Feldman EL. Elevated triglycerides correlate with progression of diabetic neuropathy. *Diabetes.* 2009;58(7):1634-40.
7. The Diabetes Control and Complication Trial Research Group. The effect of intensive treatment of diabetes on the development and progression of long-term complications in insulin-dependent diabetes mellitus. *New Engl J Med.* 1993;329(14):977-86.
8. Effect if intensive diabetes treatment on nerve conduction in the Diabetes Control and Complications Trial. *Ann Neurol.* 1995;38(6):869-80.
9. UK Prospective Diabetes Study (UKPDS) Group. Intensive blood-glucose control with sulphonylureas or insulin compared with conventional treatment and risk of complications in patients with type 2 diabetes (UKPDS 33). *Lancet.* 1998;352(9131): 837-53.
10. Tesfaye S, Chaturvedi N, Eaton SE, Ward JD, Manes C, Ionescu-Tirgoviste C, et al. Vascular risk factors and diabetic neuropathy. *N Engl J Med.* 2005;352(4):341-50.
11. Ahmed N, Thornalley PJ. Advanced glycation endproducts: what is their relevance to diabetic complications? *Diabetes Obes Metab.* 2007;9(3):233-45.
12. Thornalley PJ. Glycation in diabetic neuropathy: characteristics, consequences, causes and therapeutic options. *Int Rev Neurobiol.* 2002;50:37-57.
13. Sugimoto K, Yasujima M, Yagihashi S. Role of advanced glycation end products in diabetic neuropathy. *Curr Pharm Des.* 2008;14(10):953-61.
14. Singh R, Barden A, Mori T, Beilin L. Advanced glycation end-products: a review. *Diabetologia.* 2001;44(2):129-46.
15. Oates PJ. Aldose reductase, still a compelling target for diabetic neuropathy. *Curr Drug Targets.* 2008;9(1):14-36.
16. Das Evcimen N, King GL. The role of protein kinase C activation and the vascular complications of diabetes. *Pharmacol Res.* 2007;55(6):498-510.
17. Li F, Drel VR, Szabó C, Stevens MJ, Obrosova IG. Low dose poly (ADP-ribose) polymerase inhibitor-containing combination therapies reverses early peripheral diabetic neuropathy. *Diabetes.* 2005;54(5):1514-22.

18. Pracher P, Obrosova IG, Mabley JG, Szabó C. Role of nitrosative stress and peroxynitrite in the pathogenesis of diabetic complications. Emerging new therapeutical strategies. *Curr Med Chem.* 2005;12(3):267-75.

19. Brownlee M. Biochemistry and molecular cell biology of diabetic complications. *Nature.* 2001;414(6865):813-20.

20. Du X, Edelstein D, Brownlee M. Oral benfotiamine plus alpha-lipoic acid normalises complication causing pathway in type 1 diabetes. *Diabetologia.* 2008;51(10):1930-2.

21. Vincent AM, Russell JW, Low P, Feldman EL. Oxidative stress in the pathogenesis of diabetic neuropathy. *Endocr Rev.* 2004;25(4):612-28.

22. Edwards JL, Vincent AM, Cheng HT, Feldman EL. Diabetic neuropathy: mechanism to management. *Pharmacol Ther.* 2008;120(1):1-34.

23. Vracko R. A comparison of the microvascular lesions in diabetes mellitus with those in normal aging. *J Am Geriatr Soc.* 1982;30(3):201-5.

24. Newrick PG, Wilson AJ, Jakubowski J, Boulton AJ, Ward JD. Sural nerve oxygen tension in diabetes. *Br Med J (Clin Res Ed).* 1986;293(6554):1053-4.

25. Cameron NE, Cotter MA, Ferguson K, Robertson S, Radcliffe MA. Effect of chronic alpha-adrenergic receptor blockade on peripheral nerve conduction, hypoxic resistance, polyols, Na(+)-K(+)-ATPase activity, and vascular supply in STZ-D rats. *Diabetes.* 1991; 40(12):1652-8.

26. Kennedy JM, Zochodne DW. Impaired peripheral nerve regeneration in diabetes mellitus. *J Peripher Nerv Syst.* 2005;10(2):144-57.

27. Boulton AJ, Vinik AL, Arezzo JC, Bril V, Feldman EL, Freeman R, et al. Diabetic neuropathies: a statement by the American Diabetes Association. *Diabetes Care.* 2005;28(4):956-62.

28. Amthor KF, Dahl-Jørgensen K, Berg TJ, Heier MS, Sandvik L, Aagenaes O, et al. The effect of 8 year of strict glycemic control on peripheral nerve function in IDDM patients: the Oslo Study. *Diabetologia.* 1994;37(6):579-84.

29. Max MB, Culnane M, Schafer SC, Gracely RH, Walther DJ, Smoller B, et al. Amitriptyline relieves diabetic neuropathy pain in patients with normal or depressed mood. *Neurology.* 1987;37(4):589-96.

30. Kaur H, Hota D, Bhansali A, Dutta P, Bansal D, Chakrabarti A. A comparative evaluation of amitriptyline and duloxetine in painful diabetic neuropathy: a randomized, double-blind, cross-over clinical trial. *Diabetes Care.* 2011;34(4):818-22.

31. Freeman R, Durso-Decruz E, Emir B. Efficacy, safety and tolerability of Pregabalin treatment for painful diabetic peripheral neuropathy: findings from seven randomized, controlled trials across a range of doses. *Diabetes Care.* 2008;31(7):1448-54.

32. Kochar DK, Rawat N, Agrawal RP, Vyas A, Beniwal R, Kochar SK, et al. Sodium valproate for painful diabetic neuropathy: a randomized, double-blind, placebo-controlled study. *QJM.* 2004;97(1):33-8.

33. Vedula SS, Bero S, Sherer RW, Dickersin K. Outcome reporting in industry-sponsored trials of gabapentin for off-label use. *N Engl J Med.* 2009;361(20):1963-71.

34. Chou R, Ballantyne JC, Fanciullo GJ, Fine PG, Miaskowski C. Research gaps on use of opioids for chronic noncancer pain: findings from a review of the evidence for an American Pain Society and American Academy of Pain Medicine clinical practice guideline. *J Pain.* 2009;10(2):147-59.

35. Dunn KM, Saunders KW, Rutter CM, Banta-Green CJ, Merrill JO, Sullivan MD, et al. Opioid prescriptions for chronic pain and overdose: a cohort study. *Ann Intern Med.* 2010; 152(2):85-92.

36. The Capsaicin Study Group. Treatment of painful diabetic neuropathy with topical capsaicin. A multicenter, double-blind, vehicle-controlled study. *Arch Intern Med.* 1991; 151(11):2225-9.

37. Barbano RL, Herrmann DN, Hart-Gouleau S, Pennella-Vaughan J, Lodewick PA, Dworkin RH. Effectiveness, tolerability, and impact on quality of life of the 5% lidocaine patch in diabetic polyneuropathy. *Arch Neurol.* 2004;61(6):914-8.

38. Yuen KC, Baker NR, Rayman G. Treatment of chronic painful diabetic neuropathy with isosorbide dinitrate spray: a double-blind placebo-controlled cross-over study. *Diabetes Care.* 2002;25(10):1699-703.

39. Bril V, England J, Franklin GM, Backonja M, Cohen J, Del Toro D, et al. Evidence-based guideline: Treatment of painful diabetic neuropathy: report of the American Academy of Neurology, the American Association of Neuromuscular and Electrodiagnostic Medicine, and the American Academy of Physical Medicine and Rehabilitation. *Neurology.* 2011;76(20):1758-65.

40. Pascoe MK, Low PA, Windebank AJ, Litchy WJ. Subacute diabetic proximal neuropathy. *Mayo Clin Proc.* 1997;72(12):1123-32.

41. Kelkar P, Masood M, Parry GJ. Distinctive pathologic findings in proximal diabetic neuropathy (diabetic amyotrophy). *Neurology.* 2000;55(1):83-8.

42. Chan YC, Lo YL, Chan ES. Immunotherapy for diabetic amyotrophy. *Cochrane Database Syst Rev.* 2012;6:CD006521.

43. Brown MR, Dyck PJ, McClearn GE, Sima AA, Powell HC, Porte D. Central and peripheral nervous system complications. *Diabetes.* 1982;31(Suppl 1 Pt 2):65-70.

44. Adour K, Wingerd J, Doty HE. Prevalence of concurrent diabetes mellitus and idiopathic facial paralysis (Bell's palsy). *Diabetes.* 1975;24(5):449-51.

45. Bytzer P, Talley NJ, Hammer J, Young LJ, Jones MP, Horowitz M. GI symptoms in diabetes mellitus are associated with poor glycemic control and diabetic complications. *Am J Gastroenterol.* 2002;97(3):604-11.

46. Rayner CK, Samsom M, Jones K, Horowitz M. Relationship of upper gastrointestinal motor and sensory function with glycemic control. *Diabetes Care.* 2001;24(2):371-81.

47. Parkman HP, Hasler WL, Fisher RS, American Gastrointestinal Association. American Gastrointestinal Association technical review on the diagnosis and treatment of gastroparesis. *Gastroenterology.* 2004;127(5):1592-622.

48. Schvarcz E, Palmér M, Aman J, Horowitz M, Stridsberg M, Berne C. Physiological hyperglycemia slows gastric emptying in normal subjects and patients with insulin-dependent diabetes mellitus. *Gastroenterology.* 1997;113(1):60-6.

49. Russo A, Stevens JE, Chen R, Gentilcore D, Burnet R, Horowitz M, et al. Insulin-induced hypoglycemia accelerates gastric emptying of solids and liquids in long-standing type 1 diabetes. *J Clin Endocrinol Metab.* 2005;90(8):4489-95.

50. Wald A. Incontinence and anorectal dysfunction in patients with diabetes mellitus. *Eur J Gestroenterol Hepatol.* 1995;7(8):737-9.

51. Shanahan F, McKenna R, McCarthy CF, Drury MI. Coeliac disease and diabetes mellitus: a study of 24 patients with HLA typing. *Q J Med.* 1982;51(203):329-35.

52. Wald A, Tunuguntla AK. Anorectal sensorimotor dysfunction in fecal incontinence and diabetes mellitus. Modification with biofeedback therapy. *N Engl J Med.* 1984;310(20): 1282-7.

53. Vinik AI, Ziegler D. Diabetic cardiovascular autonomic neuropathy. *Circulation.* 2007; 115(3):387-97.

54. Wackers FJ, Young LH, Inzucchi SE, Chyun DA, Davey JA, Barrett EJ, et al. Detection of silent myocardial ischemia in asymptomatic diabetic subjects: the DIAD study. *Diabetes Care*. 2004;27(8):1954-61.

55. Pagkalos M, KoutlianosN, Koudi E, Pagkalos E, Mandroukas K, Deligiannis A. Heart rate variability modifications following exercise training in type 2 diabetic patients with definite cardiac autonomic neuropathy. *Br J Sports Med*. 2008;42(1):47-54.

56. Ten Harkel AD, van Lieshout JJ, Wieling W. Effects of leg muscle pumping and tensing on orthostatic arterial pressure: a study in normal subjects and patients with autonomic failure. *Clin Sci (Lond)*. 1994;87(5):553-8.

57. Grubb BP, Samoil D, Kosinski D, Wolfe D, Lorton M, Madu E. Fluoxetine hydrochloride for the treatment of severe refractory orthostatic hypotension. *Am J Med*. 1994;97(4):366-8.

58. Kaufmann H, Brannan T, Krakoff L, Yahr MD, Mandeli J. Treatment of orthostatic hypotension due to autonomic failure with peripheral alpha-adrenergic agonist (midodrine). *Neurology*. 1988;38(6):951-6.

59. Edmonds ME, Nicolaides K, Watkins PJ. The importance of autonomic neuropathy in the etiology of diabetic neuropathic foot ulceration. *Diabetologia*. 1981;21:506.

60. Shahani BT, Halperin JJ, Boulu P, Cohen J. Sympathetic skin responses–a method of assessing unmyelinated axon dysfunction in peripheral neuropathies. *J Neurol Neurosurg Psychiatry*. 1984;47(5):536-42.

61. Ziegler D, Papanas N, Roden M, GDC Study Group. Neuropad: evaluation of three cut-off points of sudomotor dysfunction for early detection of polyneuropathy in recently diagnosed diabetes. *Diabet Med*. 2011;28(11):1412-5.

62. Fealey RD, Low PA, Thomas JE. Thermoregulatory seating abnormalities in diabetes mellitus. *Mayo Clin Proc*. 1989;64(6):617-28.

63. Sarma AV, Kanaya A, Nyberg LM, Kusek JW, Vittinghoff E, Rutledge B, et al. Risk factor for urinary incontinence among women with type 1 diabetes: finding from the epidemiology of diabetes interventions and complications study. *Urology*. 2009;73(6):1203-9.

64. Van Den Eeden SK, Sarma AV, Rutledge BN, Cleary PA, Kusek JW, Nyberg LM, et al. Effect of intensive glycemic control and diabetes complication on lower urinary tract symptoms in men with type 1 diabetes: Diabetes Control and Complications Trial/Epidemiology of Diabetes Intervention and Complication (DCCT/EDIC) study. *Diabetes Care*. 2009;32(4):664-70.

65. Ellenberg M. Diabetic neuropathic cachexia. *Diabetes*. 1974;23(5):418-23.

66. Godil A, Berriman D, Knapik S, Norman M, Godil F, Firek AF. Diabetic neuropathic cachexia. *West J Med*. 1996;165(6):382-5.

67. Chandler PT, Singh RS, Schwetschenau RP. Diabetic neuropathic cachexia. *Acta Diabetol Lat*. 1978;15(3-4):212-6.

68. Wright DL, Shah JH. Diabetic neuropathic cachexia and hypothyroidism in a woman. *Mo Med*. 1987;84(3):143-5.

69. Blau RH. Diabetic neuropathic cachexia. Report of a woman with this syndrome and review of the literature. *Arch Intern Med*. 1983;143(10):2011-2.

70. D'Costa DF, Price DE, Burden AC. Diabetic neuropathic cachexia associated with malabsorption. *Diabet Med*. 1992;9(2):203-5.

Foot Care for Patients with Diabetes

14
Chapter

Joseph Fiorito, Brian Lekyum, Modassar Awan, David G Armstrong

ABSTRACT

With an ever-increasing population afflicted with diabetes, there is a need for all physicians treating these patients, to be able to identify and categorize those who are at increased risk for diabetic foot complications. This also includes understanding when to refer to a diabetic foot specialist, vascular surgeon, and what you can do to minimize the risk of those whom you treat who are at a lower risk. Simple screening by physicians and nurses, coupled with interdisciplinary care can lead to a reduced risk for amputation and a greater chance for a long, productive, ambulatory life for people with diabetes. The goal of this chapter is to aid the practitioner in understanding what constitutes an at risk diabetic foot, and to enable the practitioner to perform a clinical examination in order to stratify these patients based on an evidence based risk category.

INTRODUCTION

Diabetes mellitus is a disease with multisystem complications. Recent statistics by the American Diabetes Association (ADA) suggests that prevalence of diabetes in the United States is 26 million with the onset of type 2 diabetes mellitus preceding its diagnosis by a mean 7 years.[1] The diabetic foot is a major long-term complication of type 2 diabetes mellitus.

The development of diabetic foot ulceration with concomitant infection is the leading cause for diabetes-related hospital admission. The lifetime risk of a person with diabetes developing a foot ulcer may be as high as 25%, whereas the annual incidence of foot ulcer is approximately 2%.[2,3] With a majority of patients with type 2 diabetes, and of a more advanced age, 50% of these patients have one or more risk factors for foot ulceration.[2,4]

The goal of this chapter is to aid the practitioner in understanding what constitutes an at-risk diabetic foot, and to enable the practitioner to perform a clinical examination in order to stratify these patients on an evidence-based risk category.

WHAT MAKES UP AN AT-RISK DIABETIC FOOT?

Understanding the ultimate goal in treating the diabetic foot is to prevent foot ulceration, which in turn leads to infection with the possibility of eventual amputation. One must understand the initial casual pathway to this process in order to stop the progress.

The most common triad of causes that interact and ultimately result in ulceration has been identified as neuropathy, deformity, and trauma.[5] Being able to identify those patients who are at risk of foot problems is the first step in preventing such complications. This chapter will focus on the key components of foot examination primarily based on the task force report detailing a comprehensive diabetic foot examination (CDFE) and risk assessment.[6]

HISTORY

Obtaining a detailed history is an important component of risk assessment. Some of the essential features of the medical history are summarized in table 1. Of these questions, it is very important to help identify those items of the history that are specifically involved at increasing the risk a patient has for developing a foot ulcer

TABLE 1: Essential Features of History
Past history
• Ulceration
• Amputation
• Charcot joint
• Vascular surgery/intervention
• Cigarette smoking
Neuropathic symptoms
• Positive (e.g., burning or shooting pain, electrical or sharp sensations, etc.)
• Negative (e.g., numbness and feet feel dead)
Vascular symptoms
• Claudication
• Rest pain
• Nonhealing ulcer
Other diabetes complications
• Renal (dialysis and transplant)
• Retinal (visual impairment)

TABLE 2: Risk Factors for Foot Ulcers
• Previous amputation
• Past foot ulcer history
• Peripheral neuropathy
• Foot deformity
• Peripheral vascular disease
• Visual impairment
• Diabetic nephropathy (especially patients on dialysis)
• Poor glycemic control
• Cigarette smoking

(Table 2). Although the medical history is an important component of risk assessment, a careful foot examination remains the key component of this process.

DIABETIC FOOT EXAMINATION

General Inspection

Inspection of both feet with shoes and socks removed is paramount in assessing risk in the diabetic patient. The practitioner should look for signs of preulcerative lesions, such as erythema, callus, or blisters. These could be a direct result of musculoskeletal deformity, such as hammertoes, bunions, over or under subtalar joint pronation, as well as improper shoe gear. An inspection of the foot wear should include evaluation for proper width, length, depth, and wear pattern. Mostly, foot ulcerations develop as a direct result of mechanical irritation of the foot while wearing improper shoe gear. Specific features that should be assessed during the foot examination are outlined in table 3.

Vascular Assessment

Assessment of peripheral arterial disease (PAD) is very important in defining the overall extremity risk status. This is accomplished by palpation of the pedal arteries, which should be characterized as pulses being "present" or "absent".[7] Other elements of the vascular examination may include assessing the capillary refill time at the distal digits as well as noting the amount of lower extremity edema present, and the quality of the edema being "pitting" or "nonpitting" edema.

People with diabetes and signs or symptoms of vascular disease, or absent pedal pulses on screening examination, should undergo noninvasive vascular testing to include ankle brachial index (ABI), as well as toe pressures. Based on these results, the patient may be considered for referral to a vascular specialist. The ADA Consensus Panel on PAD recommended measurement of ABIs in patients with diabetes over 50 years of age, and consideration of ABI measurement in younger patients with

TABLE 3: Key Components of Diabetic Foot Examination

- Inspection
- Dermatologic
  - Skin status: color, thickness, dryness, and cracking
  - Sweating
  - Infection: check between toes for fungal infection
  - Ulceration
  - Calluses/blistering: hemorrhage into callus
- Musculoskeletal
  - Deformity, e.g., claw toes, prominent metatarsal heads, and Charcot joint
  - Muscle wasting (guttering between metatarsals)
- Neurological assessment
- 10 g monofilament and one of the following four:
  - Vibration using 128 Hz tuning fork
  - Pinprick sensation
  - Ankle reflexes
  - Vibration perception threshold
- Vascular assessment
  - Foot pulses
  - Ankle brachial index if indicated

multiple PAD risk factors, with repetition of normal tests every 5 years.[8] While evaluating ABI measurements in the diabetic patient, it is important to note that results may be misleading due to medial calcinosis of the blood vessels that can result in falsely elevated or suprasystolic ankle pressures.

Many studies have looked upon noninvasive vascular examinations as predictors of healing in patients with lower extremity wounds. Kalani and coworkers[9] found that toe pressures greater than 30 mm Hg demonstrated sensitivity, specificity, and positive predictive values of 15%, 97%, and 67%, respectively. In a study by Apelqvist and coworkers,[10] which evaluated 314 patients with diabetic foot wounds, primary healing was achieved in 85% of patients with a toe pressure greater than 45 mmHg. Only 36% of patients healed without amputation with a toe pressure less than 45 mmHg. While none of these examinations are completely accurate in predicting wound healing, they can assist the physician in deciding what the next best step is for a patient with a diabetic foot wound. If there is no limb threatening infection present, patients with low values for these examinations should be evaluated by vascular surgery for possible angiography and/or interventional surgery. Patients with ischemia and an overlying infection may need to undergo debridement to control this infection before immediate referral to a vascular surgeon to improve peripheral blood flow, which will aid in healing.

Neurologic Assessment

Testing for Neuropathy

Peripheral neuropathy in the diabetic foot is considered a polyneuropathy involving both axonal and demylenating nerve involvement. The usual presentation is a symmetrical "stocking and glove" distribution. There are five major functional classes of axons that may be assessed by neurophysiologic techniques. These classes include large myelinated motor axons (skeletal muscle control and reflexes), large myelinated sensory axons (vibration and proprioception), small myelinated sensory axons (cold and warmth sensation), unmyelinated sensory axons (pain), and autonomic axons (cardiac rate, blood pressure, and sweating).

In order to effectively diagnose neuropathy, one must ask subjective questions of patients as whether they are experiencing positive (pain, paraesthesia, and fasciculations) or negative symptoms (numbness, weakness, imbalance, and instability), and pursue an appropriate detailed neurologic examination of all the potentially affected nerve fibers. In regard to the neurologic examination, this would involve reliable testing procedures that are standardized, reproducible, simple, and noninvasive.

Large Fiber Neuropathy

Symptoms of large fiber neuropathy consist of tingling, numbness, and poor balance. Testing for large fiber neuropathy should include deep tendon reflex (DTR), vibration perception threshold (VPT), and proprioception testing.

Deep tendon reflexes can be helpful in identifying motor nerve involvement. One can test DTRs with a reflex hammer. The test provides information associated with the integrity of the central and peripheral nervous system. Generally, decreased reflexes indicate a peripheral problem.

Testing for VPT can be done by various methods. Perhaps the simplest method is the use of a 128 Hz tuning fork. Vibratory sensation is tested with the tuning fork placed over the tip of the great toe with an abnormal response being defined as the patient losing vibration sensation when the examiner still perceives it with the fork still in contact with the tip of the toe.[2,11]

One can test the VPT using a biothesiometer or vibration meter. The biothesiometer is tested over the pulp of the distal great toe. The stylus of the instrumentation is placed over the dorsal great toe and the amplitude is increased until the patient can detect the vibration; the resulting number is known as the VPT. This process should initially be done on the proximal site, and then the mean of three readings is taken over each hallux. If patients are unable to feel the device at greater than 25 volts, then they are at high risk for neuropathy. A measurement of 16–24 volts constitutes intermediate risk and less than 15 volts is considered low risk. A VPT greater then 25 volts has been shown to be strongly predictive of subsequent foot ulceration.[12,13]

Small Fiber Neuropathy

The Semmes Weinstein, 5.07–10 g monofilament (MF), is the most widely utilized tool for screening a patient for peripheral neuropathy in the world. The efficacy of this tool has been confirmed in a number of trials.[9,14-16] The MF test can assess whether a patient has lost the small fiber function of light, touch, and pain sensation. The examination is carried out having the patient close their eyes and asking for a response of "yes" or "no" when asked whether the MF is being applied to a particular site. This is typically on the plantar surface of the first, third, and fifth metatarsal heads and plantar surface of the distal hallux. It is important to avoid testing in areas of callus tissue as this may yield a false positive response. MFs are designed to buckle when a 10 g force is applied; loss of the ability to detect this pressure at one or more anatomic sites on the plantar surface of the foot is considered a positive result for loss of protective sensation (LOPS).

A recent study by Rayman et al. developed a simple touch test known as the Ipswich touch test (IpTT) that involves digital palpation of the distal toes to assess the protective sensation of the foot. Performing the IpTT involves lightly touching/resting the tip of the index finger for 1–2 s on the tips of the first, third, and fifth toes on both feet and defining neuropathy as greater than 2 insensate of the six sites. The IpTT was found to have a similar sensitivity, specificity, and operating characteristic as the MF when assessed against a VPT greater than or equal to 25. Furthermore, when compared directly with the MF, the IpTT was found to have excellent concordance.[17]

Jayaprakash et al. compared VPT (gold standard) with other previously mentioned modalities in the diagnosis of peripheral neuropathy in 1,044 patients with diabetes. When compared with VPT, ankle reflex was the most sensitive (90.7%) but least specific (37.3%). The tuning fork and MF tests, respectively, had lower sensitivity (62.5% and 62.8%) but better specificity (95.3% and 92.9%) and accuracy (78.9% and 77.9%). Significant correlations were observed between the VPT score and absent tuning fork sensation, MF sensation, and ankle reflex. This suggests that a simple bedside testing is useful in diagnosing peripheral neuropathy.[18]

It is important to remember that while testing small fiber neuropathy, a negative test does not rule out the presence of large fiber neuropathy. Therefore, one should only use it as an isolated test if the patient has a positive loss of protective threshold on examination. Perhaps the take home point in regard to testing small fiber neuropathy is not to use it as a single testing modality. A normal response to the 5.07 g Semmes Weinstein monofilament (SWM) does not rule out peripheral neuropathy. In 1998, Armstrong et al. found that combining VPT, SWM, and a subjective symptom score increases the specificity of predicting foot ulceration in comparison to using one of the above modalities alone.[19] The techniques are shown in figure 1.

Dermatological Assessment

There are many cutaneous signs and complications that occur on the lower extremity and foot in patient with diabetes. The initial foot inspection should focus on a global

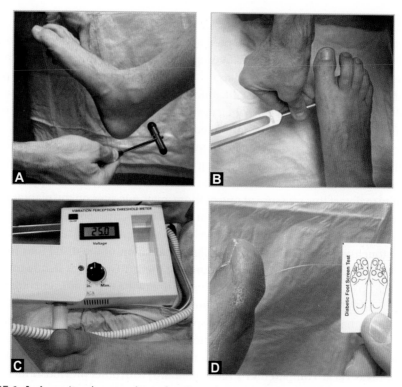

FIGURE 1 A, Assessing deep tendon reflex; **B,** Evaluating vibration perception threshold (VPT) with a tuning fork; **C,** Evaluating VPT with a biothesiometer; and **D,** testing small fiber function with a 10 g Semmes Weinstein monofilament.

evaluation of the lower limb and foot. Particular attention can be directed toward major weight-bearing areas of the foot to rule out ulceration or signs of preulceration, such as callus formation, increased temperature, erythema, induration, maceration, or bulla formation. Inspecting the interdigital spaces and the lower legs commonly reveal potential areas of skin breakdown. It is also important to look for signs of vascular cutaneous impairment, such as skin atrophy, coldness of the toes, loss of digital hair, dependent rubor of the foot, and dystrophy of the toe nails.

If there is an open wound upon inspection of the feet, it is recommended that the patient should see a foot specialist. However, understanding the severity of an open diabetic foot ulcer is important for physicians while determining the initial treatment at time of observation.

The University of Texas classification system is perhaps the most widely used diabetic foot ulcer (DFU) classification system (Table 4). This system categorizes diabetic foot ulcers based on the depth, infection, and vascular status of the wound as shown in figure 2. Along with classifying the DFU it is important to identify the severity of infection. This will help the practitioner to determine whether the patient

TABLE 4: University of Texas San Antonio Classification				
	Wound depth			
Class	**0**	**1**	**2**	**3**
A	Preulcerative lesion or healed ulcer site	Superficial wound; no tendon, capsule, or bone	Wound extends to tendon or capsule	Wound extends to bone or joint
B	+ Infection − PAD	+ Infection − PAD	+ Infection − PAD	+ Infection − PAD
C	− Infection + PAD	− Infection + PAD	− Infection + PAD	− Infection + PAD
D	+ Infection + PAD	+ Infection + PAD	+ Infection + PAD	+ Infection + PAD

PAD, peripheral arterial disease.
Source: Lavery LA, Armstrong DG, Harkless LB. Classification of diabetic foot wounds. *J Foot Ankle Surg.* 1996;35(6):528-31.

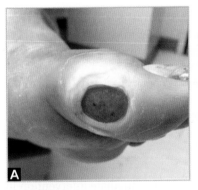

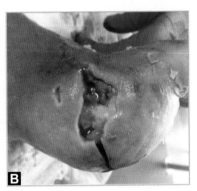

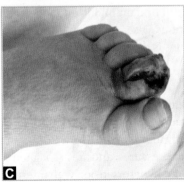

FIGURE 2 Wound classified by diabetes foot ulcers (DFU) as **A,** UT1A (superficial, noninfected and non-ischemic); **B,** UT2B (probes to closed joint capsule, infected, nonischemic); and **C,** UT3C (probes to bone, infected, ischemic).

TABLE 5: The Infectious Disease Society of America Classification System for Diabetic Foot Infections

Infection severity	Treatment recommendations
Uninfected ulcer	No antibiotics recommendations
Mild infection	
Involves skin and subcutaneous tissue, <2 cm of erythema surrounds ulcer Minimal necrosis	Gram-positive coverage with cephalexin, clindamycin, or trimethorpin-sulfamethoxazole; 7–14 days of antibiotic therapy
Moderate infection	
Penetrates to tendon, bone, or joint, >2 cm of erythema surrounds ulcer Deep abscess or local gangrene	• Broad-spectrum coverage • Hospital admission for incision and drainage or if oral therapies have failed • Amoxicillin-clavulanate, levofloxacin, piperacillin-tazobactam, ampicillin-sulbactam fluroquinolone with clindamycin MRSA; coverage if history of MRSA, risk factors, or positive culture: trimethoprim-sulfamethoxazole, ertapenem, linezolid, or vancomycin; 2–4 weeks of antibiotic therapy
Severe infection	
Systemic response to infection Fever, leukocytosis Metabolic complications	• Broad-spectrum antibiotics • Requires hospitalization • 2–4 weeks of antibiotic therapy for soft tissue infection • 4–6 weeks of antibiotic therapy for bone infection

MRSA, methicillin-resistant *Staphylococcus aureus*.
Source: Lipsky BA, Berendt AR, Cornia PB, Pile JC, Peters EJ, Armstrong DG, et al. 2012 Infectious Diseases Society of America clinical practice guideline for the diagnosis and treatment of diabetic foot infections. *Clin Infect Dis.* 2012;54(12):e132-73.

needs to be sent to the emergency department for immediate intervention involving intravenous antibiotics, or can be placed on an oral antibiotic and followed up with a foot specialist as an outpatient. The Infectious Disease Society of America (IDSA) classification system for diabetic foot infections is detailed in table 5.

Musculoskeletal Assessment

The musculoskeletal assessment should include evaluation for any gross deformity.[20] Rigid deformities are defined as any contractures that cannot easily be manually reduced. These deformities are most frequently found in the digits. Common forefoot deformities that are known to increase plantar pressures, and are associated with skin breakdown, include metatarsal phalangeal joint hyperextension with interphalangeal flexion (claw toe) or distal phalangeal extension (hammer toe).[12,21,22]

An important and often overlooked or misdiagnosed condition is Charcot arthropathy. This occurs in the neuropathic foot and most often affects the midfoot. This may present as a unilateral red, hot, swollen, and flat foot with profound deformity. A patient with suspected Charcot arthropathy should be immediately referred to a specialist for further assessment and care.

IDENTIFYING THE AT-RISK DIABETIC FOOT

While evaluating the diabetic foot, it is vital that there is a focused examination designed to classify patients into an evidence-based category in order to determine the risk for amputation.

International Working Group for the Diabetic Foot Classification

The most widely accepted risk classification for diabetic foot ulcers is based on consensus recommendations from the International Working Group for the Diabetic Foot (IWGDF) (Table 6). This system was adapted from the foot classification developed at the Carville Hansen Center. Foot complications and clinical outcomes change dramatically based on the risk profile of the population. In 2008, Lavery and colleagues[23] used the IWGDF's risk classification to demonstrate that the frequency of foot complications increases as the risk criteria increases. This was demonstrated by a significant increase in the incidence of foot ulceration, reulceration, infection, amputation, and hospitalization compared with patients with neuropathy and foot deformity but without previous foot pathology and PAD.

TABLE 6: Diabetic Foot Risk Classification

| Classification | Risk group | | | | |
	0	1	2	3	4
International Working Group on Diabetic Foot	• No neuropathy • No PAD	• Peripheral neuropathy • No deformity or PAD	Peripheral neuropathy and deformity or PAD	History of ulcer or amputation	–
Modified International Working Group on the Diabetic Foot	• No neuropathy • No PAD	• Peripheral neuropathy • No deformity or PAD	• 2A: Peripheral neuropathy and deformity • 2B: PAD	• 3A: History of ulcer • 3B: History of amputation	–
Modified IWGDF system	–	• No neuropathy • No PAD	• Neuropathy ± deformity • No PAD	PAD ± neuropathy	History of ulcer or amputation

PAD, peripheral arterial disease, IWGDF, International Working Group for the Diabetic Foot.

COMPLICATIONS AND RISKS OF DIABETIC FOOT

Diabetic Foot Ulcer

Foot ulcers can be classified as neuropathic, neuroischemic, and ischemic. It is suggested that on an average, the rate of occurrence for neuropathic ulcers is 40%, whereas the rate of occurrence for ischemic ulcers is just 10%.[24]

Ulcers invariably occur as a consequence of interaction between environmental hazards and specific changes in the lower limbs of certain patients. Factors, such as microangiopathy and autonomic neuropathy, together with loss of sensation, high foot pressures, local deformity, trauma, and susceptibility to infection lead to a propensity for foot ulcers.

Diabetic Foot Ulcer with Infection

The challenging task is to diagnose soft tissue and bone infection in persons with diabetes. The diagnosis of infection is based on the presence of two or more local signs of inflammation (erythema, swelling, local warmth, local pain, and purulent drainage). Due to the presence of neuropathy, lack of pain, vascular disease, and impaired cellular immunity in patients with diabetes, these symptoms are not clearly noticed. Thus, diagnosis of infection is based on subtle signs and high index of suspicion. Even in the presence of abscess and extensive tissue necrosis, patients with diabetes have a lack of normal systemic or local inflammation response. They often do not feel ill or appear to be unwell. They are often afebrile, with only minimal or mild local signs of redness and swelling. There may be a subtle history of malaise or flu-like symptoms. In the diagnosis of infection, superficial swabs of the wound bed are unreliable because wounds are colonized by a variety of microorganisms that fail to reflect the true bacterial pathogen when a clinical infection is present. The widespread use of antibiotics has demonstrated the increase in prevalence of antibiotic-resistant infection.

Osteomyelitis

As discussed above, diagnosis of infection including osteomyelitis in patients with diabetes is also challenging and difficult task to clinically assess it alone. Data reported sensitivity of clinical examination to diagnose bone infection ranges from 0 to 54. Ancillary resting is needed to improve diagnostic accuracy. The "gold standard" is bone biopsy. However, the use of extensive methods of diagnosis in clinic and hospital settings, bone scans, and magnetic resonance imaging (MRI) are often ordered before plain radiographs. Percutaneous bone biopsy is inexpensive and more accurate in both establishing a definitive diagnosis and identifying bacterial pathogens.

Probe to Bone

The "probe-to-bone" test has been widely adopted to diagnose bone infections in the foot. Palpation with a sterile metallic probe can increase the accuracy of diagnosing osteomyelitis. The technique is simple and inexpensive. However, the positive and negative predictive values and sensitivity and specificity of this test are controversial and are dependent on the clinical setting. A landmark study by Grayson and coworkers used this technique in a group of 76 patients admitted to the hospital for limb-threatening infections. As might be expected, there was a high prevalence of bone infection (66%) that was proved by bone biopsy, surgical exploration, or radiologic studies. The authors reported a very high positive predictive value (89%) and low negative predictive value (56%), with a sensitivity of 66% and a specificity of 85% if the bone was palpable with a sterile probe.[25] "Lavery and associates" and "Shone and colleagues" reported data on two groups treated as outpatients with a much lower prevalence of osteomyelitis (20%).[26] A positive probe-to-bone test improves the pretest probability only slightly, but a negative test most likely rules out a bone infection.

Imaging Studies

Changes in plain film radiographs may lag several weeks behind the clinical course. In the setting of acute osteomyelitis, typical findings include soft tissue swelling, periosteal reaction, irregularity of the bony cortex, and demineralization. Chronic osteomyelitis is characterized radiographically by thick sclerotic bone and interspersed radiolucencies, periosteal elevation, and sinuses. Positive plain radiographs, radionuclide tests, technetium 99m leukocyte labeling techniques and MRI are highly used for diagnosing bone infection, with a high values of sensitivity and specificity, but the reliability of both radiographs and bone scans is diminished in the presence of arterial disease or Charcot arthropathy or after recent surgery or trauma.

Bacteriology

Host immunity, mechanism of injury, wound depth, and severity of infection is strongly associated with the type and variety of bacterial pathogens in diabetic foot infections. *Staphylococcus aureus* and *Streptococcus* species are often found in mild to moderate infections. Puncture wounds that result from penetrating injuries through footwear are usually associated with a high prevalence of *Pseudomonas* infection in patients without diabetes. However, most puncture-related infections in persons with diabetes are due to *Staphylococcus* and *Streptococcus* species. Mixed and polybacterial growth of Gram-positive and Gram-negative aerobic and anaerobic pathogens are found in limb-threatening infections.

Wound Cultures

The IDSA has produced a useful classification system for diabetic foot infections that addresses obtaining cultures as well as guidelines for treatment. Ulcers that are not infected should not be cultured or treated with antibiotics. Superficial wound swabs should not be used for culture and sensitivity because these often provide cultures representative of superficial colonization. Mild to moderate community-acquired infections usually require empirical therapy so the cultures are not done. If the infection is not responding to empirical therapy, the wound is deep, or there is extensive tissue necrosis, a fetid odor or crepitus, then deep tissue aerobic and anaerobic cultures are required. The ideal tissues for cultures are obtained from debrided base of wounds.

Charcot Arthropathy

Sensory and autonomic neuropathy in patients with diabetes can lead to the neuroarthorpathy, fracture, and dislocation process of foot and ankle known as Charcot arthropathy. Patients with Charcot arthropathy classically present with a painless, hot, and swollen foot. It may present as unilateral foot deformity, with the arch of foot "suddenly" collapsing. Patients may have excellent arterial pulses with severe sensory neuropathy.

Diagnosis

Charcot arthropathy is often misdiagnosed as infection unless the treating physician has a high index of suspicion. The differential diagnosis includes infection, osteomyelitis, deep venous thrombosis, posterior tibialis tendon dysfunction, and even bone tumor. Imaging studies can be misleading, especially early. Plain film radiographs often show periosteal elevation, multiple fractures and, in some cases, osteopenia that can be misinterpreted as osteomyelitis by an inexperienced radiologist or surgeon. Many patients are treated for osteomyelitis even though they have never had a wound (injury). Bone scans and MRI are usually not reliable to differentiate bone infection, trauma, fracture, and postsurgical inflammation. The surgeon should have a clear diagnosis of bone infection versus Charcot fracture before planning an amputation, especially in the absence of a wound. A bone biopsy is the "gold standard" to diagnose bone infection. A Jamshidi bone marrow aspirate needle used under fluoroscopy permits the surgeon to obtain a bone specimen for a definitive diagnosis; it also often helps reduce the ambiguity associated with imaging techniques, which may be expensive. It is important to note, however, that no diagnostic tool, even a bone biopsy, is entirely infallible at identifying either Charcot or osteomyelitis.[27]

Radiographically, Charcot fracture is most common at midfoot. The result is often a convex arch, with the head of the talus and navicular bones or the cuboid projecting from the bottom of the foot. In advanced cases, these midfoot bones may be destroyed, with the weight of the extremity borne by the malleoli. Ulcers often occur at these sites because of the abnormal pressure and shear forces created by the collapse of the arch. Failure of these wounds to heal is usually due to the combination of neuropathy, bony abnormality, pressure, shear, and repetitive local trauma.

Treatment

The treatment for Charcot arthropathy is cast immobilization with a total-contact cast. This therapy allows patients to continue to ambulate while preventing progressive deformity. Charcot fractures in people with diabetes may take (on average) two to three times longer to heal than fractures at the same site in persons without diabetes. Casts must be checked and changed weekly to evaluate the fit, assess the ulcer, and perform debridement when required. Serial plain radiographs should be obtained during the acute phase. A total-contact cast is generally required for 3–6 months to reach a state of quiescence for acute Charcot arthropathy. Metal braces and ankle-foot orthosis have also been used but are less effective than casts.

Management after cast removal is focused on life-long protection of the involved extremity. Patient education and specialized regular foot care are integral. Following cast removal, a protective foot brace or accommodative footwear should be prescribed, such as a modified ankle-foot orthosis, a Charcot restraint orthotic walker, or a double metal upright ankle-foot orthosis. Custom footwear includes extra-deep shoes with rigid soles and a plastic or metal shank. If ulcers are present, a rocker-bottom sole can be used, with the addition of Plastazote inserts for those with insensate feet. Continued use of custom footwear in the postacute phase is essential for foot protection and support. Surgical procedures are uncommonly performed, but are based on the location of the disease and on the surgeon's preferences and experience with Charcot arthropathy. They include osteotomy, exostectomy of a bony prominence, arthrodesis, screw and plate fixation, open reduction and internal fixation, major arch reconstructive surgery, Achilles tendon lengthening with fusion, autologous bone grafting, and rarely, major amputation. Healing times are frequently prolonged after surgery. Total-contact casts and pressure reduction remain the cornerstones of therapy.[28-30]

PREVENTION OF DIABETIC FOOT COMPLICATIONS

Neuropathy

Good glycemic control is fundamental in the prevention of diabetic foot ulcers. While there is no evidence that any treatment can reverse diabetic neuropathy, efforts to keep a patient euglycemic may promote other habits surrounding prevention. It is proposed that it can be reversed by means of peripheral nerve decompression, but the American Academy of Neurology published position statement cautioning against the use of invasive procedures that lack any supportive evidence and are based entirely on misconceptions regarding the pathophysiology of diabetic neuropathy.[31] There have been ongoing trials in investigating the role of vitamin B and E, magnesium, and zinc in restoring the sensory loss in diabetic neuropathy. Perhaps even more importantly, hypertriglyceridemia may predict risk for development of neuropathy.[32] It is possible that early treatment may alter the natural history of the disease and neuropathic complications.[33]

Pressure Reduction

The reduction of high plantar pressure in the presence of sensory neuropathy can reduce the risk for a diabetic foot ulcer. Pressure reduction can be internal (surgical) or external (bracing and shoes). The surgical approach has already been discussed earlier in this chapter.

Use of custom and noncustom shoes or braces composes the external offloading. Custom insoles and footwear reduce plantar pressure in diabetic with neuropathy with or without foot deformity.

PATIENT EDUCATION

Educating patients with diabetes is important in the prevention of the lower extremity ulceration or trauma. Patients with diabetes should be instructed to look at their feet everyday to check for cuts, scrapes, redness, or blisters. If they have trouble seeing their feet, they should ask a family member to look for them, or use a mirror. Many patients with diabetes suffer from dry skin as a result of autonomic neuropathy. This dryness can lead to cracks or fissures with eventual ulceration or infection. Patients should be instructed to keep skin moisturized daily. In severe cases, prescription strength cream or lotions may be necessary.

The diabetic patient should be instructed to wear shoes and socks at all times. This will reduce the risk of trauma to the patient's foot, especially in those with neuropathy. If a patient has been prescribed custom molded shoes or a brace, compliance with these devices needs to be reinforced. These patients should also be instructed to test the temperature of bath water before stepping inside in order to reduce the risk of burns.

Based on the diabetic foot risk classification previously discussed, patients with diabetes should visit a foot specialist at least yearly. These patients need to understand their risk level, and the importance of keeping the appointments with their foot specialist. Carls and coworkers, in a study of patients at risk for developing a diabetic foot ulcer visited a podiatrist once before complications set in, and the United States health care system saved $3.5 billion in 1 year.[34] Similarly, Sloan and colleagues,[35] in a nationwide United States Medicare sample reported large, long-term (6 years) risk reductions ranging from 19% to 64% in patients who saw a podiatrist along with another diabetes specialist in the year preceding assessment.

In patients with a previous history of Charcot arthropathy, home measurement of skin temperature is an important strategy in prevention of future foot complications. An increase in temperature of about 2°C, or 4°F can indicate the presence of inflammation, and possibly the early stages of Charcot arthropathy. This measurement of skin temperatures by the doctor and patient seems to reduce risk for other people with neuropathy and diabetes as well.[36-41]

CONCLUSION

With an ever-increasing population afflicted with diabetes, there is a need for all physicians treating these patients to be able to identify and categorize those who are at increased risk for diabetic foot complications. This also includes understanding when to refer to a diabetic foot specialist, vascular surgeon and what you can do to minimize the risk of those whom you treat and who are at a lower risk. Simple screening by physicians and nurses, coupled with interdisciplinary care can lead to a reduced risk for amputation and a greater chance for a long, productive, and ambulatory life for people with diabetes.

REFERENCES

1. O'Brien JA, Patrick AR, Caro J. Estimates of direct medical costs for microvascular and macrovascular complications resulting from type 2 diabetes mellitus in the United States in 2000. *Clin Ther.* 2003;25(3):1017-38.
2. Singh N, Armstrong DG, Lipsky BA. Preventing foot ulcers in patients with diabetes. *JAMA.* 2005;293(2):217-28.
3. Reiber GE. Epidemiology of foot ulcers and amputations in the diabetic foot. In: Bowker JH, Pfeifer MA, editors. The Diabetic Foot. St. Louis: Mosby; 2001. p. 13-32.
4. Boulton AJ, Kirsner RS, Vileikyte L. Clinical practice. Neuropathic diabetic foot ulcers. *N Engl J Med.* 2004;351(1):48-55.
5. Reiber GE, Vileikyte L, Boyko EJ, del Aguila M, Smith DG, Lavery LA, et al. Causal pathways for incident lower-extremity ulcers in patients with diabetes from two settings. *Diabetes Care.* 1999;22(1):157-62.
6. Boulton AJ, Armstrong DG, Albert SF, Frykberg RG, Hellman R, Kirkman MS, et al. Comprehensive foot examination and risk assessment: a report of the task force of the foot care interest group of the American Diabetes Association, with endorsement by the American Association of Clinical Endocrinologists. *Diabetes Care.* 2008;31(8):1679-85.
7. Khan NA, Rahim SA, Anand SS, Simel DL, Panju A. Does the clinical examination predict lower extremity peripheral arterial disease? *JAMA.* 2006;295(5):536-46.
8. Uccioli L, Mancini L, Giordano A, Solini A, Magnani P, Manto A, et al. Lower limb arterio-venous shunts, autonomic neuropathy and diabetic foot. *Diabetes Res Clin Pract.* 1992;16(2):123-30.
9. Kalani M, Brismar K, Fagrell B, Ostergren J, Jörneskog G. Transcutaneous oxygen tension and toe blood pressure as predictors for outcome of diabetic foot ulcers. *Diabetes Care.* 1999;22(1):147-51.
10. Apelqvist J, Castenfors J, Larsson J, Stenström A, Agardh CD. Prognostic value of systolic ankle and toe blood pressure levels in outcome of diabetic foot ulcer. *Diabetes Care.* 1989;12(6):373-8.
11. Abbott CA, Carrington AL, Ashe H, Bath S, Every LC, Griffiths J, et al. The North-West Diabetes Foot Care Study: incidence of, and risk factors for, new diabetic foot ulceration in a community-based patient cohort. *Diabet Med.* 2002;19(5):377-84.

12. Young MJ, Breddy JL, Veves A, Boulton AJ. The prediction of diabetic neuropathic foot ulceration using vibration perception thresholds. A prospective study. *Diabetes Care.* 1994;17(6):557-60.

13. Armstrong DG, Lavery LA, Vela SA, Quebedeaux TL, Fleischli JG. Choosing a practical screening instrument to identify patients at risk for diabetic foot ulceration. *Arch Intern Med.* 1998;158(3):289-92.

14. Mayfield JA, Sugarman JR. The use of the Semmes-Weinstein monofilament and other threshold tests for preventing foot ulceration and amputation in persons with diabetes. *J Fam Pract.* 2000;49(11 Suppl):S17-29.

15. Booth J. Assessment of peripheral neuropathy in the diabetic foot. *J Tissue Viability.* 2000; 10(1):21-5.

16. Boyko EJ, Ahroni JH, Cohen V, Nelson KM, Heagerty PJ. Prediction of diabetic foot ulcer occurrence using commonly available clinical information: the Seattle Diabetic Foot Study. *Diabetes Care.* 2006;29(6):1202-7.

17. Rayman G, Vas PR, Baker N, Taylor CG Jr, Gooday C, Alder AI, et al. The Ipswich Touch Test: a simple and novel method to identify inpatients with diabetes at risk of foot ulceration. *Diabetes Care.* 2011;34(7):1517-8.

18. Jayaprakash P, Bhansali A, Bhansali S, Dutta P, Anantharaman R, Shanmugasundar G, et al. Validation of bedside methods in evaluation of diabetic peripheral neuropathy. *Indian J Med Res.* 2011;133645-9.

19. Armstrong DG, Hussain SK, Middleton J, Peters EJ, Wunderlich RP, Lavery LA. Vibration perception threshold: are multiple sites of testing superior to single site testing on diabetic foot examination? Ostomy Wound Manage. 1998;44(5):70-4, 76.

20. Frykberg RG, Zgonis T, Armstrong DG, Driver VR, Giurini JM, Kravitz SR, et al. Diabetic foot disorders. A clinical practice guideline (2006 revision). *J Foot Ankle Surg.* 2006; 45(5 Suppl):S1-66.

21. Mueller MJ, Hastings M, Commean PK, Smith KE, Pilgram TK, Robertson D, et al. Forefoot structural predictors of plantar pressures during walking in people with diabetes and peripheral neuropathy. *J Biomech.* 2003;36(7):1009-17.

22. Lavery LA, Armstrong DG, Vela SA, Quebedeaux TL, Fleischli JG, et al. Practical criteria for screening patients at high risk for diabetic foot ulceration. *Arch Intern Med.* 1998;158(2):157-62.

23. Lavery LA, Peters EJ, Williams JR, Murdoch DP, Hudson A, Lavery DC; International Working Group on the Diabetic Foot. Reevaluating the way we classify the diabetic foot: restructuring the diabetic foot risk classification system of the International Working Group on the Diabetic Foot. *Diabetes Care.* 2008;31(1):154-6.

24. Grunfield C. Diabetic foot ulcers: etiology, treatment, and prevention. *Adv Int Med.* 1992; 37:103-32.

25. Grayson ML, Gibbons GW, Balogh K, Levin E, Karchmer AW. Probing to bone in infected pedal ulcers. A clinical sign of underlying osteomyelitis in diabetic patients. *JAMA.* 1995; 273(9):721-3.

26. Lavery LA, Armstrong DG, Peters EJ, Lipsky BA. Probe-to-bone test for diagnosing diabetic foot osteomyelitis: reliable or relic? *Diabetes Care.* 2007;30(2):270-4.

27. Meyr AJ, Singh S, Zhang X, Khilko N, Mukherjee A, Sheridan MJ, et al. Statistical reliability of bone biopsy for the diagnosis of diabetic foot osteomyelitis. *J Foot Ankle Surg.* 2011; 50(6):663-7.

28. Rogers LC, Frykberg RG, Armstrong DG, Boulton AJ, Edmonds M, Van GH, et al. The charcot foot in diabetes. *Diabetes Care.* 2011;34(9):2123-9.

29. Nielsen D, Armstrong DG. The Natural History of Charcot Arthropathy. *Clin Podiatr Med Surg*. 2008;25(1):53-62.

30. Armstrong DG, Todd WF, Lavery LA, Harkless LB, Bushman TR. The Natural History of Acute Charcot's Arthropathy in a Diabetic Foot Specialty Clinic. *Diabet Med*. 1997;14(5): 357-63.

31. Chaudhry V, Stevens JC, Kincaid J, So YT. Practice Advisory: utility of surgical decompression for treatment of diabetic neuropathy: report of the Therapeutics and Technology Assessment Subcommittee of the American Academy of Neurology. *Neurology*. 2006; 66(12):1805-8.

32. Wiggin TD, Sullivan KA, Pop-Busui R, Amato A, Sima AA, Feldman EL. Elevated triglycerides correlate with progression of diabetic neuropathy. *Diabetes*. 2009;58(7):1634-40.

33. Rajamani K, Colman PG, Li LP, Best JD, Voysey M, D'Emden MC. Effect of fenofibrate on amputation events in people with type 2 diabetes mellitus (FIELD study): a prespecified analysis of a randomised controlled trial. *Lancet*. 2009;373(9677):1780-8.

34. Carls GS, Gibson TB, Driver VR, Wrobel JS, Garoufalis MG, Defrancis RR. The economic value of specialized lower-extremity medical care by podiatric physicians in the treatment of diabetic foot ulcers. *J Am Podiatr Med Assoc*. 2011;101(2):93-115.

35. Sloan FA, Feinglos MN, Grossman DS. Receipt of care and reduction of lower extremity amputations in a nationally representative sample of U.S. *Elderly Health Serv Res*. 2010; 45(6 Pt 1):1740-62.

36. Armstrong DG, Lavery LA, Liswood PJ, Todd WF, Tredwell JA. Infrared dermal thermometry of the high risk diabetic foot. *Phys Ther*. 1997;77(2):169-77.

37. Armstrong DG, Lavery LA. Monitoring healing of acute Charcot's arthropathy with infrared dermal thermometry. *J Rehabil Res Dev*. 1997;34(3):317-21.

38. Armstrong DG, Lipsky BA, Polis AB, Abramson MA. Does dermal thermometry predict clinical outcome in diabetic foot infection? Analysis of data from the SIDESTEP* trial. *Int Wound J*. 2006;3(4):302-7.

39. Bharara M, Cobb JE, Claremont DJ. Thermography and thermometry in the assessment of diabetic neuropathic foot: a case for furthering the role of thermal techniques. *Int J Low Extrem Wounds*. 2006;5(4):250-60.

40. Armstrong DG, Holtz-Neiderer K, Wendel C, Mohler MJ, Kimbriel HR, Lavery LA. Skin temperature monitoring reduces the risk for diabetic foot ulceration in high-risk patients. *Am J Med*. 2007;120(12):1042-6.

41. Arad Y, Fonseca V, Peters A, Vinik A. Beyond the monofilament for the insensate diabetic foot: a systematic review of randomized trials to prevent the occurrence of plantar foot ulcers in patients with diabetes. *Diabetes Care*. 2011;34(4):1041-6.

Management of Eye Disorders in Diabetic Patients

15
Chapter

Alexander A Izad

ABSTRACT

Diabetes mellitus is the leading cause of blindness between ages of 20 and 64 years in developed countries. Visual loss has a major health, psychological, and financial impact on the life of affected patients and their families. Significant visual loss makes the delivery of the health care much more challenging for the diabetic patients and health care team involved. Diabetes can affect the ocular system in various ways. In this chapter, the most common and serious ophthalmic conditions directly related to diabetes mellitus are reviewed, with more emphasis given to its most dangerous and common ocular complication, i.e., diabetic retinopathy. Since the optimal management of diabetic patients is team oriented, some additional knowledge of these ocular conditions might lead to timely referral and treatment of these conditions.

INTRODUCTION

Diabetes mellitus is the leading cause of blindness between ages of 20 and 64 years in developed countries. Visual loss has a major health, psychological, and financial impact on the life of affected patients and their families. Significant visual loss makes the delivery of the health care much more challenging for the diabetic patients and health care team involved. Diabetes can affect the ocular system in various ways. In this chapter, the most common and serious ophthalmic conditions directly related to diabetes mellitus are reviewed, with more emphasis given to its most dangerous and common ocular complication, i.e., diabetic retinopathy. Since the optimal management of diabetic patients is team oriented, some additional knowledge of these ocular conditions might lead to timely referral and treatment of these conditions.

DIABETIC RETINOPATHY

Diabetic retinopathy is by far the most common and serious ocular complication, even though diabetes mellitus (DM) affects the eyes in many ways, e.g., it increases the risk of cataract development.[1] Diabetic retinopathy is one of the leading causes of visual loss in many developed countries.[2,3] Almost one-third of the 366 million people with diabetes worldwide have signs of diabetic retinopathy.[4] A third of these patients could potentially have severe retinopathy and/or macular edema that could be vision threatening.[5] Economic and human cost on the society will increase substantially as the number of the visually impaired rises.

Disease Definition

Diabetic retinopathy is a disease that develops in nearly all diabetic patients to some degree. Microaneurysms and retinal hemorrhages are the earliest visible clinical signs. Vascular irregularities progress to capillary nonperfusion, venous anomalies, and intraretinal microvascular abnormalities. As the disease progresses, the arterioles and venules close and new vessels proliferate on the optic nerve, retina, iris, and filtration angle. During the course of the disorder retinal thickening (edema) can occur due to increased permeability of the vessels. Loss of vision can result due to several reasons, such as vitreous hemorrhage, distortion of the retina, tractional retinal detachment, macular edema, and ischemia.

Epidemiology

Diabetes is the leading cause of preventable blindness in many countries among working-aged adults (20–64 years).[6] An estimated 86% of patients with type 1 diabetes have diabetic retinopathy (42% of type 1 patients have vision-threatening retinopathy). The corresponding numbers for type 2 diabetes are 40% and 8%, respectively, in the United States.[7,8] The estimated prevalence is similarly high in Asian countries.[9] In some developing countries, such as India,[10,11] lower prevalence rates have been reported. This most likely changes with shifting socioeconomic circumstances, increasing obesity rate, and growing lifespan of the diabetic patients (i.e., longer duration of diabetes) in those countries. African, Mexican, and native Americans have a higher prevalence of DM compared to Caucasians in the United States. The National Health and Nutrition Examination Survey III of type 2 diabetes found that the rate of diabetic retinopathy was higher among non-hispanic Blacks and Mexican Americans than non-hispanic Caucasians.[12]

It is estimated that 90–95% of diabetic patients overall have type 2 diabetes. Due to this large disparity between the two groups, type 2 diabetic patients comprise the considerably larger proportion of visually impaired patients secondary to diabetic retinopathy, despite the fact that type 1 diabetes causes more severe and numerous ocular complications.[13,14]

Risk Factors

The key risk factors for development of diabetic retinopathy are the duration of diabetes and the degree of hyperglycemia.[15-24] Hyperglycemia becomes a more important factor for the progression of the disease rather than the duration, once the retinopathy has developed.[25] Additionally, thorough management of hypertension and intensive control of serum lipids have been shown to slow the progression of retinopathy.[26-30] In recent trials, Evaluating How the Treatment in the Action to Control Cardiovascular Risk in Diabetes (ACCORD) Study Affect Diabetic Retinopathy (The ACCORD Eye Study) and Finofibrate Intervention and Event Lowering Diabetes (FIELD) study, a lower proportion of diabetic patients showed progression of retinopathy while treated with fenofibrate. This protective effect was independent of blood glucose, blood pressure, and lipid values.[31,32] Fenofibrate decreased the triglyceride levels compared with placebo. The FIELD study result was limited by several factors, such as incomplete reporting of degree of retinopathy and indications for laser treatment. Further research would be needed to substantiate these findings.

Pregnancy is an independent risk factor as well. There is less consensus among studies regarding the importance of other factors, such as type of diabetes, clotting factors, renal disease, physical inactivity, age, and use of specific type of blood pressure medication (i.e., angiotensin-converting enzyme inhibitors).[33-36] However, since these factors affect the cardiovascular morbidity and mortality along with other aspects of the diabetic patients' health, it would be sensible to recommend them to address all medical treatment aspects of their condition.

The long-term benefit of tight glycemic control has been confirmed by many studies; however, it has been observed that during the first year of intensive treatment with insulin, there is often a temporary worsening of the retinopathy.[37,38]

Pathogenesis

The exact cause of diabetic retinopathy is still not known. Our understanding of the pathophysiological mechanisms is continuously evolving with new research.[39,40] It is understood that the process is multifactorial. The chronic exposure to hyperglycemia over time causes multiple biochemical and physiological changes that will lead not only to primarily vascular damage but also to neurosensory retinal injury.[41] It is well known that these insults over time will result in specific retinal capillary changes, such as selective loss of pericytes and thickening of the basement membrane. This will in turn not only lead to capillary nonperfusion and occlusion but also to breakdown of the endothelial barrier function. The result will be serum leakage and retinal edema. The vascular occlusion leads to ischemia and neovascularization might develop over time.

Hyperglycemia can damage the retina in many possible ways. Cellular metabolism and signaling and growth factors are all affected. Possible pathways include accumulation of sorbitol within the retinal cells and advanced glycosylation end products in the extracellular fluid, impaired autoregulation of retinal blood flow, oxidative stress, inflammation, microthrombosis, altered regulation of various growth factors [e.g., vascular endothelial growth factor (VEGF), erythropoietin, insulin-like growth factor-1 (IGF-1)] along with genetic influence.[42-50] In the Diabetes Control and Complications Trial (DCCT), severe retinopathy was three times more frequent among the relatives of the patients with documented diabetic retinopathy than diabetic patients without retinopathy.

One medication has been implicated in developing diabetic macular edema (DME). Rosiglitazone has been reported in several case reports.[51,52] Its incidence is unknown. Patients with heart or renal insufficiency (i.e., that are at risk for fluid retention) appear to have the highest risk of developing macular edema. It is advised to discontinue thiazolidinediones in individuals who develop DME.

Diabetes can negatively affect the entire neurosensory retina. In experimental models, it has been shown that it can induce apoptosis or alter the metabolism of neuroretinal supporting cells. The neuroretinal decline could occur early in the course of the disease even before the onset of microvascular abnormalities.[38]

Clinical Assessment

Most diabetic patients who develop retinopathy are asymptomatic until the very late stage. Sometimes at that stage, an effective treatment is limited. To regain lost vision is often more challenging and sometimes impossible, even with maximal systemic and ocular treatment. By the time the patient notices loss or change of vision, the individual could be already at the late stage of the disease. It is important to screen diabetic patients regularly since diabetic retinopathy can progress rapidly and the therapy could both decrease the symptoms and reduce the rate of progression.

Diabetic retinopathy can be divided into two major groups: (1) nonproliferative and (2) proliferative (Table 1). It refers to absence or presence of new abnormal blood vessels in retina or anterior segment of the eye. Nonproliferative diabetic retinopathy (NPDR) (Figure 1) can display with various signs, such as microaneurysms, intraretinal hemorrhages, dilated or tortuous vessels, nerve-fiber layer infarcts (cotton-wool spots), and hard exudates (lipid deposits). Loss of vision in NPDR occurs by macular edema or ischemia.

In proliferative diabetic retinopathy (PDR), new blood vessels grow at the optic nerve or elsewhere in the retina. These vessels can bleed easily and cause preretinal and vitreous hemorrhage. They also can lead to tractional retinal detachment as they undergo fibrosis. Neovascularization sometimes occurs on the iris and anterior chamber angle structures and leads to neovascular glaucoma.

Diabetic macular edema is retinal thickening with or without hard exudates that specifically involves the macula. It is diagnosed primarily by a particular fundus examination with stereoscopic viewing. The diagnosis can be furthermore investigated by fluorescein angiography and optical coherence tomography (OCT). Fluorescein

TABLE 1: Diabetic Retinopathy Classification by Severity[53]	
Degree of severity of diabetic retinopathy	**Clinical findings**
No visible retinopathy	No lesions
Mild nonproliferative diabetic retinopathy (NPDR)	Only microaneurysms
Moderate NPDR	Microaneurysms along other microvascular lesions, but not severe NPDR
Severe NPDR	• Many intraretinal hemorrhages and microaneurysms in all four quadrants of retina, or • Venous beading in two or more quadrants, or • Intraretinal microvascular abnormalities in one or more quadrants
Proliferative diabetic retinopathy	Neovascularization and/or vitreous/preretinal hemorrhage

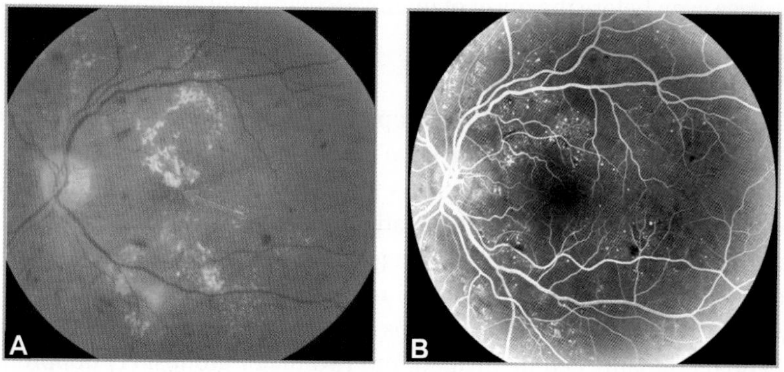

FIGURE 1 Nonproliferative diabetic retinopathy with corresponding fluorescein angiography. Severe diabetic macular edema with intraretinal hemorrhages and hard exudates extending into the fovea (arrow).

dye is injected intravenously and its transit is recorded with a special camera. OCT is a noninvasive low energy laser imaging modality that offers a precise and reproducible optical biopsy of the retina (Figure 2). It allows exact measurement of the retinal thickness. DME can be present at any level of retinopathy. The patient could be asymptomatic initially with preserved vision despite having a significant DME.

The symptoms vary depending on the nature of the pathology. With DME, patients might see distortion of images, such as wavy lines or experience reduced vision. With vitreous hemorrhage, a curtain in the visual field or floaters could be seen. Massive hemorrhage could result in sudden loss of vision.

Regular eye examinations are essential for early detection and treatment of asymptomatic vision-threatening diabetic retinopathy. The gold standard is a

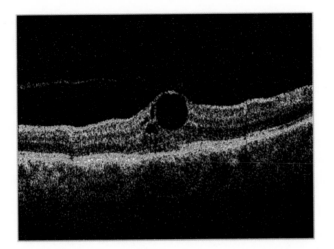

FIGURE 2 Foveal cyst with vitreomacular traction on an image by optical coherence tomography.

TABLE 2: Ophthalmic Examination Schedule for Diabetic Patients		
Patient class	**Recommend first eye examination**	**Advised routine follow-up***
Type 1	Within 5 years after diagnosis[15]	Annually[15]
Type 2	Upon diagnosis of diabetes mellitus[16]	Annually[16]
Pregnancy (type 1 or 2)	Before conception and early in the first trimester[59-61]	1–12 months depending on the degree of retinopathy at initial examination[59-61]

*Upon abnormal findings many more examinations are necessary.
Source: Modified from American Academy of Ophthalmology Retina Panel. Preferred Practice Pattern Guidelines. Diabetic Retinopathy. San Francisco, CA: American Academy of Ophthalmology. 2008.

complete dilated ophthalmic evaluation by a trained ophthalmologist. Seven-field stereoscopic fundus photography or digital imaging with stereoscopic capabilities also have good sensitivity and specifity for detecting diabetic retinopathy.[54-58] These screening methods can serve very well to identify the patients who would need referral for ophthlamic evaluation and management. The screening methods are very valuable when access to ophthalmic care is limited.

The examination schedule in table 2 shows the suggested intervals endorsed by the American Academy of Ophthalmology and the American Diabetes Association. However, more frequent examinations are necessary depending on the severity of diabetic retinopathy and threat to the visual function. Many factors play a role in determining the follow-up interval. Both systemic factors, such as control of hyperglycemia, hypertension, and ocular findings are important in the decision making process by the ophthalmologist. The ocular findings include severity of diabetic retinopathy and presence or absence of DME.

Pregnancy has been shown in several studies to accelerate the advancement of diabetic retinopathy. Diabetic patients who are planning pregnancy should be informed about the risk of developing diabetic retinopathy or its accelerated progression due to pregnancy. The above guideline does not apply to women who develop gestational diabetes, since they do not have the same risk profile.

Treatment of Diabetic Retinopathy

Treatment of diabetic retinopathy should encompass both the systemic causes and the resulting ocular complications. All the modifiable risk factors need to be addressed. There is a consensus that tight control of hyperglycemia and blood pressure prevent and slow down the progression of diabetic retinopathy. Many studies also indicate that lipid lowering therapy is another important factor.[6,15-30] However, strict control of these factors does not preclude development of diabetic retinopathy, and regular eye examination is still necessary.

In the DCCT, the progression of mild and moderate diabetic retinopathy was slowed down by strict glycemic control, which was defined a mean of glycosylated hemoglobin (HbA1c) of 7%.[36] In the Epidemiology of Diabetes Interventions and Complications (EDIC) study, a continuing follow-up of the DCCT cohort, it was seen that the beneficial effects of strict glycemic control persisted as long as 10 years after the study, despite the fact that the HbA1c difference between the treatment and control group had dissipated. This is referred to as "metabolic memory".[62]

When it comes to control of hypertension, there is insufficient data to recommend any one specific antihypertensive agent. Good blood pressure control is the main goal. Many studies have been performed, specifically regarding angiotensin inhibition versus other agents.[63-66]

Aspirin has not been shown to alter the progression of diabetic retinopathy, nor does it increase the risk of vitreous hemorrhage.[67,68] Aspirin is certainly an important medication to reduce the cardiovascular morbidity and mortality risk.

As mentioned previously, glitazones should be avoided in patients with DME. Ultimately, a multifactorial risk reduction is the optimal way to treat the patient both from the ocular standpoint and the overall health status. The results from the Steno 2 diabetes study suggest that aggressive treatment of hyperglycemia, hypertension, hyperlipidemia, and nephropathy also prevent the long-term development and progression of diabetic retinopathy. This study also confirmed that the metabolic memory is present as the DCCT trial did.[69]

Ocular Therapy

Laser Photocoagulation

Laser photocoagulation is the most established treatment for vision-threatening diabetic retinopathy. Treatment aims to induce regression of new blood vessels and promote closure of leaking capillaries. It also reduces retinal thickening. Thus, it can help to prevent visual loss from PDR and DME. Although its efficacy is remarkable, the visual loss still occurs. It also has some visual side-effects due to its destructive nature.

The two main types of laser treatment are panretinal photocoagulation (PRP) and focal/grid laser treatment. In the Diabetic Retinopathy Study, the risk of severe visual loss decreased by 50% over 6 years by applying PRP in patients with advanced diabetic retinopathy.[70] The Early Treatment of Diabetic Retinopathy Study showed significant reduction of visual loss when focal laser photocoagulation was used for patients with significant DME.[71] Unfortunately, focal laser treatment is not effective for improvement of visual acuity. Despite the great benefits of laser treatment, side-effects can occur. Side-effects for PRP treatment are difficulty with light-dark adaption, decrease of central visual acuity, loss of peripheral vision with subsequent decreased night vision, and difficulty driving. Paracentral scotomas, subfoveal fibrosis, and accidental foveal photocoagulation (with resulting immediate reduction of vision) are among the side-effects for focal laser treatment.

Pharmacologic Therapy

Intravitreal anti-VEGF drugs have emerged as a great additional treatment tool that can work on their own and in conjunction with laser treatment and surgery for treatment of diabetic retinopathy. Anti-VEGF agents include pegaptanib (Macugen), bevacizumab (Avastin), and ranibizumab (Lucentis). VEGF is a potent mediator for vascular leakage and neovascularization. Intraocular VEGF levels are elevated when retinal ischemia is present and its levels decrease after PRP treatment is applied.[72] Multiple studies have documented regression of active intraocular neovascularization with or without subsequent standard PRP treatment.[73-75] Some benefit has also been documented upon intraocular application of anti-VEGF drugs for DME.[76-83] Studies performed by the Diabetic Retinopathy Clinical Research Network (DRCR.net) indicate that combination treatment of laser plus intravitreal anti-VEGF could increase the chance of visual gain and decrease the number of the injections needed to achieve this. Most of the larger studies have so far not shown any systemic side-effects; nevertheless, the long-term safety is not known.[84] Ocular adverse events include infection, vitreous hemorrhage, and retinal detachment. However, the overall rate of the ocular complications is very low. A portion of the intravitreally injected anti-VEGF drug gets into the systemic circulation. Many times, repeated injections are needed. Partial inhibition of systemic angiogenesis is a potential risk with these injections, especially in diabetic patients. Systemic vascular complications include stroke, myocardial infarction, or renal hemorrhage.[84-86] So far, the safety profile of these injections has been comparable to the control groups in all major studies.

Inflammation is a major component of diabetic retinopathy.[38] The practice of intraocular administration of glucocorticoids for treatment of DME is very common. In a large multicenter study done by the DRCR.net, it was found that focal laser was superior to intravitreal triamcinolone acetonide (IVTA) alone over-long term (2 years). The eyes treated with intravitreal triamcinolone initially (i.e., first 4 months) had a better response.[38,87,88] However, this study did not look at the combination treatment of both macular focal/grid photocoagulation and intravitreal triamcinolone. So far, there is no consensus on the combination treatment. Some studies show sustained visual improvement with the combination treatment[89,90] than IVTA alone while others do not.[91,92] Intravitreal glucocorticoids lead to higher rates of accelerated cataract formation and glaucoma.

Surgery

Pars plana vitrectomy is the primary treatment for vision-threatening tractional retinal detachment and nonclearing vitreous hemorrhage (Figure 3). It has substantial benefits with some negative effects. It restores vision in many ways but it does accelerate the formation of cataract and rarely it also increases the risk of iris neovascularization.[93] In the largest randomized clinical trial that assessed the timing and the indications for surgical intervention, it was clear that early surgical intervention (less than 6 months) was beneficial for patients with severe persistent vitreous hemorrhage.[94,95] It also showed that patients with very severe neovascularization would benefit from early vitrectomy. The benefits of this relatively old study were obtained at the time when the technology did not allowed application

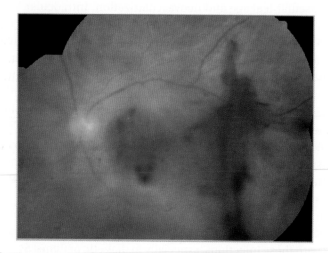

FIGURE 3 Vitreous hemorrhage in a diabetic patient. *Courtesy:* RetinaGallery.com – Steven Cohen, MD.

of endolaser during surgery and advanced vitrectomy machines with small gauge instruments were not available.

Vitrectomy seems to be beneficial for some types of DME as well, especially if there is evidence of vitreomacular traction or presence of epiretinal membrane.[6,96]

OTHER OCULAR CONDITIONS ASSOCIATED WITH DIABETES

Cataract

The development of cataract can be another important cause of visual impairment in diabetic patients. There are many studies documenting association between diabetes and cataract. There is association between posterior subcapsular and to some degree cortical cataract, but not with nuclear cataract.[97-103] The evidence also exists that the prolonged duration and severity of diabetes increase the progression of cataract.[104,105] Cataract becomes visually significant at a younger age for diabetic patients and it progresses more rapidly.[106,107]

Once the cataract becomes visually significant, surgery is recommended. Overall cataract surgery has excellent results. However, some diabetic patients might have suboptimal visual recovery due to worsening of the preexisting DME or active PDR. Therefore, any clinically significant diabetic retinopathy needs to be addressed before any planned cataract extraction.[118,109] Diabetic patients also need to be monitored more carefully postoperatively.

Diabetic patients have an increased risk to develop endophthalmitis (severe intraocular infection), which is one of the most devastating postoperative complication after cataract surgery.[110,111]

Glaucoma

Glaucoma is a progressive optic neuropathy with characteristic optic disc changes and associated visual field defects. PDR is one of the leading causes of neovascular glaucoma, which is an uncommon secondary glaucoma.[112,113] Neovascular glaucoma is a devastating disease and normally would require glaucoma surgery alongside topical glaucoma medication. PDR needs to be addressed as well. Therefore, any neovascularization of the iris and/or anterior chamber angle, which is a precursor of neovascular glaucoma, is aggressively treated.

Whether DM is an independent risk factor for development of primary open angle glaucoma, which is by far the most common type of glaucoma, is still controversial. There are population-based studies from various parts of the world that confirm an association[114,115] while others do not.[116-118]

Diabetic Papillopathy

Diabetic papillopathy is a rare optic neuropathy that presents with sudden optic disc edema and possibly some mild painless visual disturbance (Figure 4).[119] It can

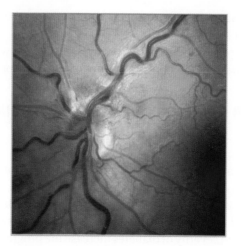

FIGURE 4   Diabetic papillopathy. Optic nerve with superior hyperemic, irregular border.

be bilateral. An afferent pupillary defect might be absent. Mild visual field defect, such as an enlarged blind spot, might be present. This should not be mistaken for papilledema or neovascularization of the optic disc. It usually improves over a period of 2–10 months and can leave minor optic disc atrophy. The visual prognosis is usually good, but ultimately depends on the associated diabetic retinopathy.[120] Case reports have been published with intraocular steroid or anti-VEGF injections as treatment method.[121,122]

Ocular Motor Cranial Nerve Disorders

Diabetes can be a contributing cause of extraocular muscle palsies, i.e., pupil-sparing third, fourth, or sixth nerve palsy in 25–30% of patients aged 45 years and older.[123] Ischemic neuropathy secondary to microvascular disease is then the underlying mechanism.[124,125] Patients present with binocular diplopia. Recovery usually occurs in 3 months in diabetic cranial nerve palsies.[126] Reasons to pursue further work-up and obtain neurology or neuro-ophthalmology consultation are involvement of the pupil in the third nerve palsy, presence of other neurological signs, multiple cranial nerve palsies, or palsy in a young patient (<45 years).

CONCLUSION

Diabetes mellitus can affect the visual system in numerous manners. An effective team approach of its management can prevent, resolve, delay, and/or ameliorate the visual symptoms and decline due to this chronic disease. Regular ophthalmic examinations and screening are essential for early detection and management of its ocular complications. The ophthalmic complications of diabetes mellitus could progress silently for many years. The reversal of that process is usually impossible. Early detection and treatment is crucial. With proper systemic and ophthalmic management of this condition, many of these disorders can be kept in control for many years.

REFERENCES

1. Jeganathan VS, Wang JJ, Wong TY. Ocular associations of diabetes other than diabetic retinopathy. *Diabetes Care.* 2008;31(9):1905-12.

2. Congdon NG, Friedman DS, Lietman T. Important causes of visual impairment in the world today. *JAMA.* 2003;290(15):2057-60.

3. Fong DS, Aiello LP, Ferris FL 3rd, Klein R. Diabetic retinopathy. *Diabetes Care* 2004; 27(10):2540-53.

4. International Diabetes Federation. Diabetes Atlas 2007. [online] Available from www. eatlas.idf.org. (Accessed June, 2013).

5. Saaddine JB, Honeycutt AA, Narayan KM, Zhang X, Klein R, Boyle JP. Projection of diabetic retinopathy and other major eye diseases among people with diabetes mellitus: United States, 2005-2050. *Arch Ophthalmol.* 2008;126(12):1740-7.

6. Mohamed Q, Gillies MC, Wong TY. Management of diabetic retinopathy: a systemic review. *JAMA.* 2007;298(8):902-16.

7. Kempen JH, O'Colmain BJ, Leske MC, Haffner SM, Klein R, Moss SE, et al. The prevalence of diabetic retinopathy among adults in the United States. *Arch Ophthalmol.* 2004;122(4):552-63.

8. Roy MS, Klein R, O'Colmain BJ, Klein BE, Moss SE, Kempen JH. The prevalence of diabetic retinopathy among adult type 1 diabetic persons in the United States. *Arch Ophthalmol.* 2004;122(4):546-51.

9. Raymond NT, Varadhan L, Reynold DR, Bush K, Sankaranarayanan S, Bellary S, et al. Higher prevalence of retinopathy in diabetic patients of South Asian ethnicity compared with white Europeans in the community: a cross-sectional study. *Diabetes Care.* 2009; 32(3):410-5.

10. Rema M, Premkumar S, Anitha B, Deepa R, Pradeepa R, Mohan V. Prevalence of diabetic retinopathy in urban India: the Chennai Urban Rural Epidemiology Study (CURES) eye study, I. *Invest Ophthalmol Vis Sci.* 2005;46(7):2328-33.

11. Raman R, Rani PK, Reddi Rachepalle S, Gnanamoorthy P, Uthra S, Kumaramanickavel G, et al. Prevalence of diabetic retinopathy in India: Sankara Nethralaya Diabetic Retinopathy Epidemiology and Molecular Genetics Study report 2. *Ophthalmology.* 2009;116(2):311-8.

12. Harris MI, Klein R, Cowie CC, Rowland M, Byrd-Holt DD. Is the risk of diabetic retinopathy greater in non-Hispanic blacks and Mexican Americans than in non-Hispanic whites with type 2 diabetes? A U.S. population study. *Diabetes Care.* 1998;21(8):1230-5.

13. Klein R, Klein BE, Moss SE. Visual impairment in diabetes. *Ophthalmology.* 1984;91(1):1-9.

14. Eppens MC, Craig ME, Cusumano J, Hing S, Chan AK, Howard NJ, et al. Prevalence of diabetes complications in adolescents with type 2 compared with type 1 diabetes. *Diabetes Care.* 2006;29(6):1300-6.

15. Klein R, Klein BE, Moss SE, Davis MD, DeMets DL. The Wisconsin epidemiologic study of diabetic retinopathy. II. Prevalence and risk of diabetic retinopathy when age at diagnosis is less than 30 years. *Arch Ophthalmol.* 1984;102(4):520-6.

16. Klein R, Klein BE, Moss SE, Davis MD, DeMets DL. The Wisconsin epidemiologic study of diabetic retinopathy. III. Prevalence and risk of diabetic retinopathy when age at diagnosis is 30 or more years. *Arch Ophthalmol.* 1984;102(4):527-32.

17. Diabetes Control and Complications Trial Research Group. Progression of retinopathy with intensive versus conventional treatment in the Diabetes Control and Complication Trial. *Ophthalmology.* 1995;102(4):647-61.

18. Diabetes Control and Complications Trial/Epidemiology of Diabetes Interventions and Complications Research Group. Retinopathy and nephropathy in patients with type 1 diabetes four years after a trial of intensive therapy. *N Engl J Med.* 2000;342:381-9.

19. The relationship of glycemic exposure (HbA1c) to the risk of development and progression of retinopathy in the diabetes control and complications trial. *Diabetes.* 1995;44(8):968-83.

20. Writing team for the Diabetes Control and Complications Trial/Epidemiology of Diabetes Interventions and Complications Research Group. Effect of intensive therapy on the microvascular complications of type 1 diabetes mellitus. *JAMA.* 2002;287(19):2563-9.

21. UK Prospective Diabetes Study (UKPDS) Group. Intensive blood-glucose control with sulphonylureas or insulin compared with conventional treatment and risk of complications in patients with type 2 diabetes (UKPDS 33). *Lancet.* 1998;352(9131):837-53.

22. Varma R, Torres M, Peña F, Klein R, Azen SP; Los Angeles Latino Eye Study Group. Prevalence of diabetic retinopathy in adults Latinos: the Los Angeles Latino eye study. *Ophthalmology.* 2004;111(17):1298-306.

23. Kohner EM, Stratton IM, Aldington SJ, Holman RR, Matthews DR; UK Prospective Diabetes Study (IKPDS) Group. Relationship between the severity of retinopathy and progression to photocoagulation in patients with Type 2 diabetes mellitus in the UKPDS (UKPDS 52). *Diabet Med.* 2001;18(3):178-84.

24. Wong TY, Liew G, Tapp RJ, Schmidt MI, Wang JJ, Mitchell P, et al. Relation between fasting glucose and retinopathy for diagnosis of diabetes: three population-based cross-sectional studies. *Lancet.* 2008;371(9614):736-43.

25. Davis MD, Fisher MR, Gangnon RE, Barton F, Aiello LM, Chew EY, et al. Risk factors for high-risk proliferative diabetic retinopathy and severe visual loss: Early Treatment Diabetic Retinopathy Study Report # 18. *Invest Ophthalmol Vis Sci.* 1998;39(2):233-52.

26. UK Prospective Diabetes Study Group. Tight blood pressure control and risk of macrovascular and microvascular complications in type 2 diabetes: UKPDS 38. *BMJ.* 1998;317(7160):703-13.

27. Snow V, Weiss KB, Mottur-Pilson C. The evidence base for tight blood pressure control in the management of type 2 diabetes mellitus. *Ann Intern Med.* 2003;138(7):587-92.

28. van Leiden HA, Dekker JM, Moll AC, Nijpels G, Heine RJ, Bouter LM, et al. Blood pressure, lipids, and obesity are associated with retinopathy: the Hoorn Study. *Diabetes Care.* 2002;25(8):1320-5.

29. Lyons TJ, Jenkins AJ, Zheng D, Lackland DT, McGee D, Garvey WT, et al. Diabetic retinopathy and serum lipoprotein subclasses in the DCCT/EDIC cohort. *Invest Ophthalmol Vis Sci.* 2004;45(3):910-8.

30. Chew EY, Klein ML, Ferris FL 3rd, Remaley NA, Murphy RP, Chantry K, et al. Association of elevated serum lipid levels with retinal hard exudate in diabetic retinopathy. Early Treatment Diabetic Retinopathy Study (ETDRS) Report 22. *Arch Ophthalmol.* 1996;114(9): 1079-84.

31. Keech AC, Mitchell P, Summanen PA, O'Day J, Davis TM, Moffitt MS, et al. Effect of fenofibrate on the need for laser treatment for diabetic retinopathy (FIELD study): a randomised control trial. *Lancet.* 2007;370(9600):1687-97.

32. ACCORD Study Group, ACCORD Eye Study Group, Chew EY, Ambrosius WT, Davis MD, Danis RP, et al. Effects of medical therapies on retinopathy progression in type 2 diabetes. *N Engl J Med*. 2010;363(3):233-44.

33. Klein R, Sharrett AR, Klein BE, Moss SE, Folsom AR, Wong TY, et al. The association of atherosclerosis, vascular risk factors, and retinopathy in adults with diabetes: the atherosclerosis risk in communities study. *Ophthalmology*. 2002;109(7):1225-34.

34. Klein R, Klein BE, Moss SE, Davis MD, DeMets DL. The Wisconsin Epidemiologic Study of Diabetic retinopathy. IX. Four-year incidence and progression of diabetic retinopathy when age at diagnosis is less than 30 years. *Arch Ophthalmol*. 1989;107(2):237-43.

35. Klein R, Klein BE, Moss SE, Davis MD, DeMets DL. The Wisconsin Epidemiologic Study of Diabetic retinopathy. X. Four-year incidence and progression of diabetic retinopathy when age at diagnosis is 30 years or more. *Arch Ophthalmol*. 1989;107(2):244-9.

36. Kriska AM, LaPorte RE, Patrick SL, Kuller LH, Orchard TJ. The association of physical activity and diabetic complications in individuals with insulin-dependent diabetes mellitus: the Epidemiology of Diabetes Complications Study—VII. *J Clin Epidemiol*. 1991; 44(11):1207-14.

37. The effect of intensive treatment of diabetes on the development and progression of long-term complications in insulin-dependent diabetes mellitus. The Diabetes Control and Complications Trial Research Group. *N Engl J Med*. 1993;329(14):977-86.

38. Early worsening of diabetic retinopathy in the Diabetes Control and Complication Trial. *Arch Ophthalmol*. 1998;116(7):874-86.

39. Antonetti DA, Barber AJ, Bronson SK, Freeman WM, Gardner TW, Jefferson LS, et al. Diabetic retinopathy: seeing beyond glucose-induced microvascular disease. *Diabetes*. 2006;55(9):2401-11.

40. Ciulla TA, Amador AG, Zinman B. Diabetic retinopathy and diabetic macular edema: pathophysiology, screening, and novel therapies. *Diabetes Care*. 2003;26(9):2653-64.

41. Frank RN. Diabetic retinopathy. *N Engl Med*. 2004;350(1):48-58.

42. Kohner EM, Patel V, Rassam SM. Role of blood flow and impaired autoregulation in the pathogenesis of diabetic retinopathy. *Diabetes*. 1995;44(6):603-7.

43. Ko BC, Lam KS, Wat NM, Chung SS. An (A-C)n dinucleotide repeat polymorphic maker at the 5′ end of the aldose reductase gene is associated with early-onset diabetic retinopathy in NIDDM patients. *Diabetes*. 1995;44(7):727-32.

44. Brownlee M. Lilly Lecture 1993. Glycation and diabetic complications. *Diabetes*. 1994; 43(6):836-41.

45. Boeri D, Maiello M, Lorenzi M. Increased prevalence of microthromboses in retinal capillaries of diabetic individuals. *Diabetes*. 2001;50(6):1432-9.

46. Smith LE, Shen W, Perruzzi C, Soker S, Kinose F, Xu X, et al. Regulation of vascular endothelial growth factor-dependent retinal neovascularization by insulin-like growth factor-1 receptor. *Nat Med*. 1999;5(12):1390-5.

47. Aiello LP. Angiogenic pathways in diabetic retinopathy. *N Engl J Med*. 2005;353(8):839-41.

48. Hernández C, Fonollosa A, García-Ramírez M, Higuera M, Catalán R, Miralles A, et al. Erythropoietin is expressed in the human retina and it is highly elevated in the vitreous fluid of patients with diabetic macular edema. *Diabetes Care*. 2006;29(9):2028-33.

49. Matsubara Y, Murata M, Maruyama T, Handa M, Yamagata N, Watanabe G, et al. Association between diabetic retinopathy and genetic variations in alpha2beta1 integrin, a platelet receptor for collagen. *Blood*. 2000;95(5):1560-4.

50. Clustering of long-term complications in families with diabetes in the diabetes control and complication trial. The Diabetes Control and Complication Trial Research Group. *Diabetes*. 1997;46(11):1829-39.

51. Kendall C, Wooltorton E. Rosiglitazone (Avandia) and macular edema. *CMAJ*. 2006; 174(5):623.

52. Colucciello M. Vision loss due to macular edema induced by rosiglitazone treatment of diabetes mellitus. *Arch Ophthalmo*. 2005;123(9):1273-5.

53. Wilkinson CP, Ferris FL 3rd, Klein RD, Lee PP, Agardh CD, Davis M, et al. Proposed international clinical diabetic retinopathy and diabetic macular edema disease severity scales. *Ophthalmology*. 2003;110(9):1677-82.

54. Moss SE, Klein R, Kessler SD, Richie KA. Comparison between ophthalmoscopy and fundus photography in determining severity of diabetic retinopathy. *Ophthalmology*. 1985;92(1):62-7.

55. Ahmed J, Ward TP, Bursell SE, Aiello LM, Cavallerano JD, Vigersky RA. The sensitivity and specificity of nonmydriatic digital stereoscopic retinal imaging in detecting diabetic retinopathy. *Diabetes Care*. 2006;29(10):2205-9.

56. Vujosevic S, Benetti E, Massignan F, Pilotto E, Varano M, Cavarzeran F, et al. Screening for diabetic retinopathy: 1 and 3 nonmydritic 45-degree digital fundus photographs vs 7 standard early treatment diabetic retinopathy study fields. *Am J Ophthalmol*. 2009; 148(1):111-8.

57. Bragge P, Gruen RL, Chau M, Forbes A, Taylor HR. Screening for presence or absence of diabetic retinopathy: a meta-analysis. *Arch Ophthalmol*. 2011;129(4):435-44.

58. Taylor CR, Merin LM, Salunga AM, Hepworth JT, Crutcher TD, O'Day DM, et al. Improving diabetic retinopathy screening ratios using telemedicine-based digital retinal imaging technology: the Vine Hill study. *Diabetes Care*. 2007;30(3):574-8.

59. Klein BE, Moss SE, Klein R. Effect of pregnancy on progression of diabetic retinopathy. *Diabetes Care*. 1990;13(1):34-40.

60. Chew EY, Mills JL, Metzger BE, Remaley NA, Jovanovic-Peterson L, Knopp RH, et al. Metabolic control and progression of retinopathy. The Diabetes in Early Pregnancy Study. National Institute of Child Health and Human Development Diabetes in Early Pregnancy Study. *Diabetes Care*. 1995;18(5):631-7.

61. Diabetes Control and Complications Trial Research Group. Effect of pregnancy on microvascular complications in the diabetes control and complications trial. *Diabetes Care*. 2000;23(8):1084-91.

62. White NH, Sun W, Cleary PA, Danis RP, Davis MD, Hainsworth DP, et al. Prolonged effect of intensive therapy on the risk of retinopathy complications in patients with type 1 diabetes mellitus: 10 years after the Diabetes Control and Complications Trial. *Arch Ophthalmol*. 2008;126(12):1707-15.

63. Mathews DR, Stratton IM, Aldington SJ, Holman RR, Kohner EM. Risks of progression of retinopathy and vision loss related to tight blood pressure control in type 2 diabetes mellitus: UKPDS 69. *Arch Ophthalmol*. 2004;122(11):1631-40.

64. Estacio RO, Jeffers BW, Gifford N, Schrier RW. Effect of blood pressure control on diabetic microvascular complications in patients with hypertension and type 2 diabetes. *Diabetes Care*. 2000;23 Suppl 2:B54-64.

65. Chaturvedi N, Porta M, Klein R, Orchard T, Fuller J, Parving HH, et al. Effect of candesartan on prevention (DIRECT-Prevent 1) and progression (DIRECT-Protect 1) of retinopathy in type 1 diabetes: randomised, placebo-controlled trials. *Lancet*. 2008;372(9647):1394-402.

66. Sjølie AK, Klein R, Porta M, Orchard T, Fuller J, Parving HH, et al. Effect of candesartan on progression and regression of retinopathy in type 2 diabetes (DIRECT-Protect 2): a randomised placebo-controlled trial. *Lancet*. 2008;372(9647):1385-93.

67. Early Treatment Diabetic Retinopathy Study Research Group. Effects of aspirin treatment on diabetic retinopathy. ETDRS report number 8. *Ophthalmology*. 1991;98(5 Suppl): 757-65.

68. Bergerhoff K, Clar C, Richter B. Aspirin in diabetic retinopathy. A systemic review. *Endocrinol Metab Clin North Am*. 2002;31(3):779-93.

69. Gaede P, Lund-Andersen H, Parving HH, Pedersen O. Effect of a multifactorial intervention on mortality in type 2 diabetes. *N Engl J Med*. 2008;358(6):580-91.

70. Photocoagulation treatment of proliferative diabetic retinopathy. Clinical application of Diabetic Retinopathy Study (DRS) findings, DRS report number 8. The Diabetic Retinopathy Study Research Group. *Ophthalmology*. 1981;88(7):583-600.

71. Photocoagulation for diabetic macular edema. Early Treatment Diabetic Retinopathy Study report number 1. Early Treatment Diabetic Retinopathy Study research group. *Arch Ophthalmol*. 1985;103(12):1796-806.

72. Aiello LP, Avery RL, Arrigg PG, Keyt BA, Jampel HD, Shah ST, et al. Vascular endothelial growth factor in ocular fluid of patients with diabetic retinopathy and other retinal disorders. *N Engl J Med*. 1994;331(22):1480-7.

73. Avery RL, Pearlman J, Pieramici DJ, Rabena MD, Castellarin AA, Nasir MA, et al. Intravitreal bevacizumab (Avastin) in the treatment of proliferative diabetic retinopathy. *Ophthalmology*. 2006;113(10):1695.e1-15.

74. Mason JO 3rd, Nixon PA, White MF. Intravitreal injection of bevacizumab (Avastin) as adjunctive treatment of proliferative diabetic retinopathy. *Am J Ophthalmol*. 2006; 142(4):685-8.

75. Mirshahi A, Roohipoor R, Lashay A, Mohammadi SF, Abdoallahi A, Faghihi H. Bevacizumab-augmented retinal laser photocoagulation in proliferative diabetic retino-pathy: a randomized double-masked clinical trial. *Eur J Ophthalmol*. 2008;18(2):263-9.

76. Salam A, DaCosta J, Sivaprasad S. Anti-vascular endothelial growth factor agents for diabetic maculopathy. *Br J Ophthalmol*. 2010;94(7):821-6.

77. Arevalo JF, Fromow-Guerra J, Quiroz-Mercado H, Sanchez JG, Wu L, Maia M, et al. Primary intravitreal bevacizumab (Avastin) for diabetic macular edema: results from the Pan-American Collaborative Retina Study Group at 6-month follow-up. *Ophthalmology*. 2007;114(4):743-50.

78. Cunningham ET, Adamis AP, Altaweel M, Aiello LP, Bressler NM, D'Amico DJ, et al. A phase II randomized double-masked trial of pegaptanib, an anti-vascular endothelial growth factor aptamer, for diabetic macular edema. *Ophthalmology*. 2005;112(110): 1747-57.

79. Diabetic Retinopathy Clinical Research Network, Scott IU, Edwards AR, Beck RW, Bressler NM, Chan CK, Elman MJ, et al. A phase II randomized clinical trial of intravitreal bevacizumab for diabetic macular edema. *Ophthalmology*. 2007;114(10):1860-7.

80. Michaelides M, Kaines A, Hamilton RD, Fraser-Bell S, Rajendram R, Quhill F, et al. A prospective randomized trial of intravitreal bevacizumab or laser therapy in the manage-ment of diabetic macular edema (BOLT study) 12-month data: report 2. *Ophthalmology*. 2010;117(6):1078-86.

81. Massin P, Bandello F, Garweg JG, Hansen LL, Harding SP, Larsen M, et al. Safety and efficacy of ranibizumab in diabetic macular edema (RESOLVE Study): a 12-month,

randomized, controlled, double-masked, multicenter phase II study. *Diabetes Care*. 2010; 33(11):2399-405.

82. Nguyen QD, Shah SM, Khwaja AA, Channa R, Hatef E, Do DV, et al. Two-year outcomes of the ranibizumab for edema of the mAcula in diabetes (READ-2) study. *Ophthalmology*. 2010;117(11):2146-51.

83. Diabetic Retinopathy Clinical Research Network, Elman MJ, Aiello LP, Beck RW, Bressler NM, Bressler SB, et al. Randomized trial evaluating ranibizumab plus prompt or deferred laser or triamcinolone plus prompt laser for diabetic macular edema. *Ophthalmology*. 2010;117(6):1064-77.

84. Wong TY, Liew G, Mitchell P. Clinical update: new treatments for age-related macular degeneration. *Lancet*. 2007;370(9583):204-06.

85. Gillies MC, Wong TY. Ranibizumab for neovascular age-related macular degeneration. *N Engl J Med*. 2007;356(7):748-50.

86. Wirostko B, Wong TY, Simo R. Vascular endothelial growth factor and diabetic complications. *Prog Retin Eye Res*. 2008;27(6):608-21.

87. Diabetic Retinopathy Clinical Research Network. A randomized trial comparing intravitreal triamcinolone acetonide and focal/grid photocoagulation for diabetic macular edema. *Ophthalmology*. 2008;115(9):1447-49.

88. Diabetic Retinopathy Clinical Research Network (DRCR.net), Beck RW, Edwards AR, Aiello LP, Bressler NM, Ferris F, et al. Three-year follow-up of a randomized trial comparing focal/grid photocoagulation and intravitreal triamcinolone for diabetic macular edema. *Arch Ophthalmol*. 2009;127(3):245-51.

89. Kang SW, Sa HS, Cho HY, Kim JI. Macular grid photocoagulation after intravitreal triamcinolone acetonide for diffue macular edema. *Arch Ophthalmol*. 2006;124(5):653-8.

90. Maia OO, Takahashi BS, Costa RA, Scott IU, Takahashi WY. Combined laser and intravitreal triamcinolone for proliferative diabetic retinopathy and macular edema: one-year results of a randomized clinical trial. *Am J Ophthalmol*. 2009;147(2):291-7.

91. Lam DS, Chan CK, Mohamed S, Lai TY, Lee VY, Liu DT, et al. Intravitreal triamcinolone plus sequential grid laser versus triamcinolone or laser alone for treating diabetic macular edema: six-month outcomes. *Ophthalmology*. 2007;114(12):2162-7.

92. Avitabile T, Longo A, Reibaldi A. Intravitreal triamcinolone compared with macular grid laser photocoagulation for the treatment of cystoid macular edema. *Am J Ophthalmol*. 2005;140(4):695-702.

93. Stefansson E. Physiology of vitreous surgery. *Graefes Arch Clin Exp Ophthalmol*. 2009; 247(2):147-63.

94. Early vitrectomy for severe vitreous hemorrhage in diabetic retinopathy. Two-year results of a randomized trial. Diabetic Retinopathy Vitrectomy Study report 2. The Diabetic Retinopathy Vitrectomy Study Research Group. *Arch Ophthalmol*. 1985;103(11):1644-52.

95. Early vitrectomy for severe proliferative diabetic retinopathy in eyes with useful vision. Results of a randomized trial—Diabetic Retinopathy Vitrectomy Report 3. The Diabetic Retinopathy Vitrectomy Study Research Group. *Ophthalmology*. 1988;95(10):1307-20.

96. Diabetic Retinopathy Clinical Research Network Writing Committee, Haller JA, Qin H, Apte RS, Beck RR, Bressler NM, et al. Vitrectomy outcomes in eyes with diabetic macular edema and vitreomacular traction. *Ophthalmology*. 2010;117(6):1087-93.

97. Rowe NG, Mitchell PG, Cumming RG, Wans JJ. Diabetes, fasting blood glucose and age-related cataract: the Blue Mountains Eye Study. *Ophthalmic Epidemiol*. 2000;7(2): 103-14.

98. Hiller R, Sperduto RD, Ederer F. Epidemiologic associations with nuclear, cortical and posterior subcapsular cataracts. *Am J Epidemiol*. 1986;124(6):916-25.

99. Klein BE, Klein R, Wang Q, Moss SE. Older-onset diabetes and lens opacities. The Beaver Dam Eye Study. Ophthalmic Epidemiol. 1995;2(1):49-55.

100. Mukesh BN, Le A, Dimitrov PN, Ahmed S, Taylor HR, McCarty CA. Development of cataract and associated risk factors: the Visual Impairment Project. *Arch Ophthalmol.* 2006;124(1):79-85.

101. Foster PJ, Wong TY, Machin D, Johnson GJ, Seah SK. Risk factors for nuclear, cortical and posterior subcapsular cataracts in Chinese population of Singapore: the Tanjong Pagar Survey. *Br J Ophthalmol.* 2003;87(9):1112-20.

102. Nirmalan PK, Robin AL, Katz J, Tielsch JM, Thulasiraj RD, Krishnadas R, et al. Risk factors for age related cataract in a rural population of southern India: the Aravind Comprehensive Eye Study. *Br J Ophthalmol.* 2004;88(8):989-94.

103. Leske MC, Wu SY, Hennis A, Connell AM, Hyman L, Schachat A. Diabetes, hypertension, and central obesity as cataract risk factors in a black population. The Barbados Eye Study. *Ophthalmology.* 1999;106(1):35-41.

104. Negahban K, Chern K. Cataracts associated with systemic disorders and syndromes. *Curr Opin Ophthalmol.* 2002;13(6):419-22.

105. Kato S, Shiokawa A, Fukushima H, Numaga J, Kitano S, Hori S, et al. Glycemic control and lens transparency in patients with type 1 diabetes mellitus. *Am J Ophthalmol.* 2001; 131(3):301-4.

106. Klein BE, Klein R, Moss SE. Incidence of cataract surgery in the Wisconsin Epidemiologic Study of Diabetic Retinopathy. *Am J Ophthalmol.* 1995;119(3):295-300.

107. Murtha T, Cavallerano J. The management of diabetic eye disease in the setting of cataract surgery. *Curr Opin Ophthalmol.* 2007;18(1):13-8.

108. Hykin PG, Gregson RM, Stevens JD, Hamilton PA. Extracapsular cataract extraction in proliferative diabetic retinopathy. *Ophthalmology.* 1993;100(3):394-9.

109. Chew EY, Benson WE, Remaley NA, Lindley AA, Burton TC, Csaky K, et al. Results after lens extraction in patients with diabetic retinopathy: early treatment diabetic retinopathy study report number 25. *Arch Ophthalmol.* 1999;117(12):1600-6.

110. Kattan HM, Flynn HW, Pflugfelder SC, Robertson C, Forster RK. Nosocomial endophthalmitis survey. Current incidence of infection after intraocular surgery. *Ophthalmology.* 1991;98(2):227-38.

111. Montan PG, Koranyi G, Setterquist HE, Stridh A, Philipson BT, Wiklund K. Endophthalmitis after cataract surgery: risk factors relating to technique and events of the operation and patient history: a retrospective case-control study. *Ophthalmology.* 1998;105(12):2171-7.

112. Schertzer RM, Wang D, Bartholomew LR. Diabetes mellitus and glaucoma. *Int Ophthalmol Clin.* 1998;38(2):69-87.

113. Brown GC, Magargal LE, Schachat A, Shah H. Neovascular glaucoma. Etiologic considerations. *Ophthalmology.* 1984;91(4):315-20.

114. Dielemans l, de Jong PT, Stolk R, Vingerling JR, Grobbee DE, Hofman A. Primary openangle glaucoma, intraocular pressure, and diabetes mellitus in the general elderly population. The Rotterdam Study. *Ophthalmology.* 1996;103(8):1271-5.

115. Mitchell P, Smith W, Chey T, Healey PR. Open-angle glaucoma and diabetes: the Blue Mountains eye study, Australia. *Ophthalmology.* 1997;104(4):712-8.

116. Tielsch JM, Katz J, Quigley HA, Javitt JC, Sommer A. Diabetes, intraocular pressure, and primary open-angle glaucoma in the Baltimore Eye Survey. *Ophthalmology.* 1995; 102(1):48-53.

117. Vijaya L, George R, Paul PG, Baskaran M, Arvind H, Raju P, et al. Prevalence of open-angle glaucoma in a rural south Indian population. *Invest Ophthalmol Vis Sci.* 2005;46(12): 4461-7.

118. Armaly MF, Krueger DE, Maunder L, Becker B, Hetherington J, Kolker AE, et al. Biostatistical analysis of the collaborative glaucoma study. I. Summary report of the risk factors for glaucomatous visual-field defects. *Arch Ophthalmol.* 1980;98(12):2163-71.

119. Regillo CD, Brown GC, Savino PJ, Byrnes GA, Benson WE, Tasman WS, et al. Diabetic papillopathy. Patient characteristics and fundus findings. *Arch Ophthalmol.* 1995;113(7): 889-95.

120. Pavan PR, Aiello LM, Wafai MZ, Briones JC, Sebestyen JG, Bradbury MJ. Optic disc edema in juvenile-onset diabetes. *Arch Ophthalmol.* 1980;98(12):2193-5.

121. Al-Haddad CE, Jurdi FA, Bashshur ZF. Intravitreal triamcinolone acetonide for the management of diabetic papillopathy. *Am J Ophthalmol.* 2004;137(6):1151-3.

122. Ornek K, Oðurel T. Intravitreal bevacizumab for diabetic papillopathy. *J Ocul Pharmacol Ther.* 2010;26(2):217-8.

123. Rush JA. Extraocular muscle palsies in diabetes mellitus. *Int Ophthalmol Clin.* 1984;24(4): 155-9.

124. Watanabe K, Hagura R, Akanuma Y, Takasu T, Kajinuma H, Kuzuya N, et al. Characteristics of cranial nerve palsies in diabetic patients. *Diabetes Res Clin Pract.* 1990;10(1):19-27.

125. Patel SV, Holmes JM, Hodge DO, Burke JP. Diabetes and hypertension in isolated sixth nerve palsy: a population-based study. *Ophthalmology.* 2005;112(5):760-3.

126. Burde RM. Neuro-ophthalmic associations and complications of diabetes mellitus. *Am J Ophthalmol.* 1992;114(4):498-501.

Management of Diabetic Nephropathy

16
Chapter

Mordecai M Popovtzer

ABSTRACT

Diabetes is the leading cause of chronic kidney disease and end stage renal disease (ESRD). Diabetic kidney disease has been listed as the major etiology of ESRD, even though the vast majority of diabetic patients with ESRD lack tissue diagnosis of classic diabetic nephropathy. This assumption, however, is warranted as almost all diabetic patients with ESRD manifest marked proteinuria, which is a salient feature of diabetic glomerulopathy. Persistent proteinuria is the hallmark of diabetic nephropathy and the degree of proteinuria is closely related with the deterioration of kidney function. Increased urinary protein excretion is not only an indication of glomerular damage but has been proposed as a factor in the progression of diabetic renal disease. Since the beginning of 1990s, the number of patients beginning chronic dialysis has increased more rapidly due to type 2 diabetes more than any other condition. Clinically, diabetic nephropathy is characterized by persistent proteinuria (>300 mg/24 h), hypertension and progressive loss of kidney function. More recently, the definition of diabetic nephropathy for both type 1 and 2 has been modified. Accordingly, making of the clinical diagnosis of diabetic nephropathy has to meet the following criteria: presence of proteinuria, presence of diabetic retinopathy, and absence of other kidney diseases. Interestingly, the requirement for hypertension has been replaced with the presence of diabetic retinopathy. Accordingly, the presence of diabetic retinopathy is an absolute requirement for the diagnosis of diabetic nephropathy. This criterion will be discussed further in more detail. Diabetic nephropathy seldom is diagnosed before 10 years after emergence of diabetes in type 1 diabetes and is diagnosed in nearly 3% in newly diagnosed patients with type 2 diabetes.

INTRODUCTION

Diabetes is a major public health challenge. Over the last 25 years, the prevalence of type 2 diabetes has doubled in the United States and has increased almost fourfold in India and Far East.[1] Diabetes is the leading cause of chronic kidney disease (CKD) and end-stage renal disease (ESRD). Diabetic kidney disease has been listed as the major etiology of ESRD, even though the vast majority of diabetic patients with ESRD lack tissue diagnosis of classic diabetic nephropathy. This assumption, however, is warranted as almost all diabetic patients with ESRD manifest marked proteinuria, which is a salient feature of diabetic glomerulopathy. Persistent proteinuria is the hallmark of diabetic nephropathy and the degree of proteinuria is closely related with the deterioration of kidney function. Increased urinary protein excretion is not only an indication of glomerular damage but has been proposed as a factor in the progression of diabetic renal disease. Since the beginning of 1990s, the number of patients on chronic dialysis has increased more rapidly due to type 2 diabetes more than any other condition. Clinically, diabetic nephropathy is characterized by persistent proteinuria (>300 mg/24 h), hypertension, and progressive loss of kidney function. More recently, the definition of diabetic nephropathy for both type 1 and 2 has been modified. Accordingly, making of the clinical diagnosis of diabetic nephropathy has to meet the following criteria: presence of proteinuria, presence of diabetic retinopathy, and absence of other kidney diseases. Interestingly, the requirement for hypertension has been replaced with the presence of diabetic retinopathy. Accordingly, the presence of diabetic retinopathy is an absolute requirement for the diagnosis of diabetic nephropathy. This criterion will be discussed further in more detail. Diabetic nephropathy is seldom diagnosed 10 years after emergence of type 1 diabetes and is diagnosed in nearly 3% in newly diagnosed patients with type 2 diabetes.[2-5]

PATHOGENESIS OF DIABETIC NEPHROPATHY

Functional Changes

Hyperfiltration is an early abnormality in diabetes, and is believed to be a risk factor leading to diabetic kidney disease. It is observed in patients with type 1 and type 2 diabetes.[6-15] Likewise, it is observed in animal models featuring both type 1 and type 2 diabetes.[16-20] Hyperfiltration is mainly observed in patients with type 1 diabetes. The magnitude of increase in glomerular filtration may amount up to 50% of normal rate. Hyperfiltration is usually associated with glomerular hypertrophy and enlarged kidney size. Treatment with insulin and normalization of blood glucose restores the excessive filtration rate to normal in men. It has been postulated that glomerular hyperfiltration may adversely affect the structural integrity of the kidney and lead to progressive renal damage. The mechanism of hyperfiltration remains enigmatic. Both in clinical and experimental diabetes with hyperglycemia and increased filtered load of glucose, tubular reabsorption of glucose is markedly increased. In diabetic patients, very often substantial hyperglycemia is not associated with glycosuria because of altered threshold and tubular maximum for glucose absorption (TmG).

There is an intimate relationship between glucose and sodium reabsorption in the proximal nephron. Augmented glucose reabsorption enhances sodium reabsorption via a luminal sodium-glucose cotransporter which is driven by transcellular sodium gradient. This avid proximal sodium reabsorption sets in motion a sequence of alterations along the nephron that lead to sustained hyperfiltration state. Experimental data provide evidence supporting reduced sodium delivery to macula densa as a trigger for vasodilation of afferent arteriole. Vasodilation of afferent arteriole augments glomerular filtration rate (GFR) leading to increased filtered load of sodium. However, the increased filtered load of sodium is reabsorbed at Henle's loop, thus perpetuating reduced delivery of sodium to macula densa leading to sustained hyperfiltration. Maintenance of increased intraglomerular pressure due to vasodilation of the afferent arteriole results in hyperfiltration. Hyperfiltration is associated with microalbuminuria possibly due to increased mechanical stress altering the structural integrity of the glomerular filtering elements. Subsequently, glomerular filtration drops, presumably due to mechanical damage in glomerular capillaries, and albuminuria (>300 mg/24 h) appears. At this stage, kidney function deteriorates progressively leading to ESRD.[21-24] In this regard, it is of interest to refer to the reported autopsy findings in diabetic patients in whom unilateral renal artery stenosis prevented development of diabetic nephropathy in the underperfused kidney, while diabetic nephropathy was evident in the contralateral kidney with patent renal artery.[25] Similarly, using experimental model of rats with streptozotocin-induced diabetes, unilateral clipping of renal artery protected the underperfused kidney from developing diabetic nephropathy while the contralateral kidney with patent renal artery developed severe diabetic nephropathy.[26]

Recent long-term study evaluated the clinical course of type 2 diabetic patients with glomerular hyperfiltration and biopsy proven diabetic nephropathy. Glomerular hyperfiltration was associated with increased glomerular filtration surface. This longitudinal study of normo- and microalbuminuric type 2 diabetics demonstrated that hyperfiltration was associated with subsequent linear decline in GFR. This is one of the few studies in type 2 diabetics presenting with hyperfiltration. Furthermore, it showed that hyperfiltration predicts subsequent deterioration in kidney function independent of changes in urinary albumin excretion.[27] Above observations have served as rationale for conducting clinical trials employing either angiotensin converting enzyme (ACE) inhibitors or angiotensin receptor blockers (ARBs) not only as antihypertensive agents but also as potential vasodilators of the efferent arterioles. Vasodilation of the efferent arterioles caused by blocking angiotensin-induced efferent vasoconstriction is believed to reduce intraglomerular hypertension rendering protection to the glomerular capillary loops against hydraulic mechanical damage.

Impaired renal autoregulation of GFR and renal plasma flow has been demonstrated in type 1 and type 2 diabetic patients.[28] Blunted autoregulation may allow more aortic pressure to be transmitted to the glomeruli and exert a mechanical stress on glomerular capillary network leading to structural trauma of the filtering elements.

Hyperfiltration is more common in patients with type 1 diabetes and is less frequent in type 2 diabetes. Hyperfiltration appears to be an important factor involved in the pathogenesis of diabetic nephropathy.

Hypertension

In diabetic patients, hypertension is a risk factor for large vessel disease, leading to atherosclerotic lesions in coronary, cerebral, renal, and other peripheral arteries. Hypertension plays a major role in the progression of microvascular complications, including diabetic retinopathy, diabetic nephropathy, and diabetic neuropathy. The pathogenesis of hypertension in the setting of diabetic nephropathy can be construed in the framework of Guyton's hypothesis.[29] This hypothesis suggests that CKD is associated with decreased natriuretic capacity. This leads to renal sodium retention which results in extracellular volume expansion. The latter causes a rise in cardiac output. Increased cardiac output enhances arterial perfusion which triggers arterial autoregulation. The latter results in arterial vasoconstriction and systemic hypertension. Hypertension is detrimental to kidney function as it increases glomerular capillary pressure and hydraulic stress which accelerate glomerular damage.

The magnitude of hypertension is inversely related to the kidney function. As CKD develops, the prevalence of hypertension in type 1 diabetics exceeds 90%. Similar to other glomerular diseases, the pathophysiology of hypertension is related to sodium retention. As alluded to above, renal sodium retention is at least partly triggered by enhanced activity of sodium-glucose cotrasporters in the proximal nephron as well as enhanced sodium reabsorption in the loop of Henle. In type 2 diabetics, essential hypertension may precede the onset of diabetes. High levels of insulin in type 2 diabetes enhance renal tubular sodium reabsorption, partly by activating tubular Na^+-K^+-ATPase. This leads to sodium retention and extracellular volume expansion. Consonant with Guyton's hypothesis, in type 2 diabetes, hypertension is also sodium sensitive and an impaired natriuresis accounts for the development of hypertension; hence, the importance of dietary sodium restriction in the management of hypertension in type 1 and type 2 diabetics.[30-32]

Hyperglycemia

Hyperglycemia alters lipids and proteins via nonenzymatic covalent binding of sugar elements resulting in the synthesis of advanced glycation end products (AGEs).[33] Elevated levels of AGEs are present in diabetic patients and in experimental animals with diabetes. Evidence has accumulated suggesting that AGEs cause injury to glomerular mesangial cells and podocyte by upregulating gene expression of collagen and transforming growth factor beta one (TGF beta-1).[34] AGEs exert their effects by receptor-dependent or independent actions. The receptors for AGEs are expressed on podocytes and blocking their activity diminishes the expression of TGF beta-1, reduces mesangial expansion, and thickening of glomerular basement membrane.[35] Therefore, interference with AGE formation may be a potential therapeutic option to slow progression of diabetic nephropathy. Interestingly, ACE inhibitors and ARBs reduce tissue levels of AGEs in addition to their hemodynamic effects. In addition to the actions mediated by TGF beta-1, AGEs by binding to their receptor [receptor for advanced glycation end products (RAGE)] have been shown to set off a signaling pathway leading to increased expression of connective tissue growth factor (CTGF) independent of TGF beta-1. CTGF is the downstream mediator of cellular effect of TGF beta-1; it plays a key role in cellular processes leading to diabetic nephropathy. Additional effects of high levels AGEs include stimulation of oxygen-free radicals, cytokines, chemokines, and adhesion molecules.[36]

Renin-Angiotensin-Aldosterone in Diabetes

Systemic renin-angiotensin levels are downregulated in diabetes while intrarenal angiotensinogen is upregulated in diabetes. This increase in intrarenal renin-angiotensin system can contribute to the progression of diabetic nephropathy by hemodynamic, tubular, and growth-promoting actions. Angiotensin II induces insulin resistance. Angiotensin II type 1 and type 2 receptors are downregulated in chronic diabetes. Decreased type 2 receptor expression might contribute to early diabetic nephropathy by reducing type 2 receptor-mediated beneficial actions that are counter-regulatory to those of type 1 receptor. Type 2 receptor stimulation may explain partially the renal protection observed with type 1 receptor blockade. Experimental data indicate that renin-angiotensin blockade prevents intrarenal renin-angiotensin activation, hypertension, and progression of diabetic nephropathy.[37-39] High glucose has been shown to induce renin and angiotensin II production in mesangial and podocyte cultures.[40-42] Accumulation of angiotensin II in diabetic kidneys induces renal injury by promoting glomerular oxidative and inflammatory stress leading to fibrosis and loss of glomeruli. Inhibitors of the renin-angiotensin system by interfering with negative feedback loop lead to increased renin which can activate the renin receptor and induce renal damage independent of angiotensin II.[43-45] Active derivatives of vitamin D have been shown to suppress renin gene transcription as well as to block glucose-stimulated angiotensinogen production.[46,47] In this regard, the combined use of inhibitors of renin-angiotensin system with active vitamin derivatives in experimental model of type 2 diabetes have been shown to preempt the compensatory rise in renin following angiotensin receptor blockade.[48]

Mounting evidence suggests that aldosterone causes oxidative stress, inflammation, and fibrosis resulting in renal injury.[49] Mineralocorticoid receptor blockers when added to ACE inhibitors or ARBs induce further decrease in proteinuria in patients with CKD.[50] The enzyme responsible for synthesis of aldosterone, cytochrome P450 11 beta-2 (CYP11beta2) has been reported to be present in rat kidney glomerulus, mainly in podocytes.[51] Upregulation of renal CYP11beta2 was reported to occur in rat model of type 1 diabetes.[52] Aldosterone has been shown to activate signaling pathway of mammalian target of rapamycin (mTOR) which promotes cell proliferation, interstitial inflammation, and fibrosis.[53]

Genetic Predisposition

Only a portion of diabetic patients develop diabetic nephropathy in their lifetime. Diabetic nephropathy clusters in families. Furthermore, the familial aggregation of diabetic nephropathy has suggested an important role for hereditary factors in developing this trait. The likelihood of developing diabetic nephropathy is increased when parents or siblings are affected by diabetic nephropathy. The familial predisposition cannot be explained by the duration of diabetes, hypertension, or glucose control; however, genetic abnormalities in renal sodium handling and hypertension may be important. Most of the early studies were based on searching for candidate genes. The polymorphism of the gene which codes ACE has been the subject of many studies. The DD polymorphism of the ACE alleles has been associated with increased risk for development of diabetic nephropathy in patients with type 2 diabetes.[54,55] Subsequent studies, however, failed to confirm this association.[56] Another candidate gene, the angiotensin II type 2 receptor gene, on chromosome X was evaluated. Male type 1 diabetics with AA haplotype of that gene had lower kidney function than those with GT haplotype. This association was not found in female diabetics.[57] Additional candidate gene that has been implicated is inheritance of one allele of the aldose reductases gene. Homozygosity for the Z-2 allele was associated with diabetic nephropathy.[58] As opposed to picking candidate genes approach as referred to above, a genome-wide scan has been used as an alternative approach. A genome scan has become a standard unbiased method for searching for linkage between genetic regions and phenotypes of interest. The results of a genome-wide scan based on diabetic type 1 siblings discordant for nephropathy trait suggest that 3q locus most likely contains a susceptibility gene for diabetic nephropathy.[59]

PATHOLOGY OF DIABETIC NEPHROPATHY

There are several histological glomerular changes in diabetic nephropathy; glomerular basement membrane thickening is the earliest abnormality, it is followed by mesangial matrix expansion which leads to glomerular sclerosis. Additional observed changes, the so called exudative lesions, caused insinuation of plasma components (fibrin, immunoglobulins, proteins, and complement) into vascular wall. These include subendothelial hyaline caps, capsular drops along parietal surface of Bowman's capsule (hence capsular), and afferent and efferent arteriolar hyalinosis. Occasionally, glomerular capillary aneurysms (similar to retinal microaneurysms) are observed. These lesions are most likely caused by mesangiolysis leading to detachment of glomerular capillary wall from mesangial anchoring attachment.

Recent studies based on high power electron microscopy have emphasized the role of podocytopathy in the pathogenesis of proteinuria in diabetic kidneys.[60-63] Podocyte detachment from the glomerular basement membrane has been demonstrated in kidney biopsies from type 2 diabetics. This detachment may be responsible for podocyte loss. Podocyte number and podocyte numerical density are reduced both in type 1 and type 2 diabetes. Above abnormalities may lead to secondary focal segmental glomerulosclerosis with worsening proteinuria in diabetic nephropathy. The latter may also account for the presence of atubular glomeruli, possibly due to focal adhesions (tip type lesions) that block tubular take-off from glomeruli, resulting in perfused but nonfiltering glomeruli.

Abnormalities in podocyte-specific insulin signaling may play a role in diabetic nephropathy. Animal models with deleted insulin receptor-specific fashion were studied. Affected animals developed proteinuria, effacement of foot processes, apoptosis, glomerular basement membrane thickening, accumulation of mesangial matrix, and glomerulosclerosis. Intact insulin receptor is crucial for remodeling of the actin cytoskeleton and preservation of glomerular structural integrity.[64] Likewise, decreases in renal nephrin expression have been reported in diabetic nephropathy.[65] The accumulating data emphasize abnormalities in podocyte structure and function in diabetic nephropathy.

The following is modified sequential numeric histological classification of glomerular lesions that reflects the pathological progression of diabetic nephropathy as established by Renal Pathology Society.[66]

- Class I: Isolated glomerular basement thickening. There is no evidence of mesangial expansion, increased mesangial matrix, or global glomerulosclerosis (involving more than 50% of glomeruli)
- Class II: Mild (Class IIa) or severe (Class IIb) mesangial expansion. A lesion is considered severe if areas of expansion larger than the mean area of capillary lumen are present in greater than 25% of the total mesangium
- Class III: At least one Kimmelstiel-Wilson lesion (nodular intercapillary glomerulosclerosis) is observed on biopsy and there is less than 50% global glomerulosclerosis (Figures 1 and 2)
- Class IV: Advanced diabetic glomerulosclerosis. There is more than 50% global glomerulosclerosis.

The severities of vascular and interstitial abnormalities are also rated.

Scores 0, 1, or 2 were assigned if no arteriolar hyalinosis, one arteriole, or more than one arteriole with hyalinosis was present.

Scores 0, 1, 2, or 3 were assigned if interstitium had no areas of fibrosis, less than 25%, 25–50%, or more than 50%, respectively.

Scores 0, 1, or 2 were assigned if no lymphocytes or macrophage infiltrate was present, if infiltrate was limited to areas surrounding atrophic tubules, or if infiltrate was not limited, respectively.

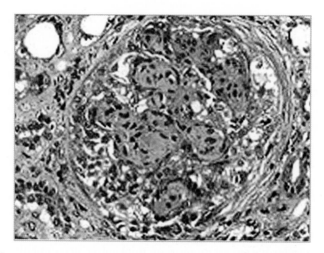

FIGURE 1 Glomerular lesion characteristic of class III diabetic glomerulosclerosis.

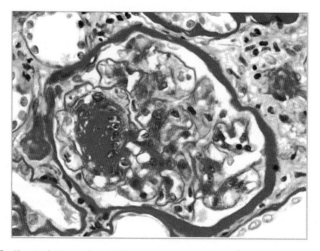

FIGURE 2 Classical Kimmelstiel-Wilson glomerular diabetic sclerotic nodule class III diabetic nephropathy.

It has been suggested that glomerular disease in type 2 diabetes is more heterogeneous than that in type 1 diabetes. Likewise, it has been estimated that close to 40% of patients with type 2 diabetes manifest a wide variety of glomerular pathologies, including immunoglobulin A nephropathy, minimal change disease, membranous nephropathy, and focal segmental glomerulosclerosis.

Data has accumulated indicating that in glomerular diseases, including diabetic nephropathy, the decline in kidney function correlates closely with degree of interstitial disease. The interaction between glomerular disease and interstitial disease has been attributed to the effect of proteinuria on tubular epithelial cells.

Endocytosis of protein components activates proinflammatory cytokines, such as increased expression of TGF-beta and chemokines. This leads to interstitial inflammation, fibrogenesis, and interstitial scarring. It may be speculated that tight control of blood pressure and use of ACE inhibitors which put tab on proteinuria may slow the progression of renal disease by minimizing the expression of TGF-beta.

REVERSIBILITY OF DIABETIC NEPHROPATHY

Steffes et al. reported amelioration of diabetic glomerular lesions in diabetic rats following islet transplantation.[67] Lee et al. removed kidneys with diabetic lesions from rats with streptozotocin-induced diabetes and transplanted them into normal nondiabetic syngeneic animals. Two months later, the histological lesion had regressed.[68] Abouna et al. reported reversal of diabetic nephropathy in two cadaveric kidneys after transplantation into nondiabetic recipients. Two kidneys were removed from a deceased donor with 17-year history of type 1 diabetes. At the time of death, the donor had proteinuria but normal serum creatinine. Histological examination of the kidneys showed typical lesions of diffuse intercapillary glomerulosclerosis. Seven months after transplantation, the kidneys showed almost complete resolution of the diabetic intercapillary glomerulosclerosis in both recipients.[69] These observations underscore the importance of normal metabolic environment not only in preventing glomerular diabetic lesions but even in reversing those lesions once they have occurred. The mechanism of reversal sclerotic lesions in glomeruli is not well understood. Taken together, these observations strongly support the importance of metabolic control of diabetes in minimizing the microvascular complications.

CLINICAL DIAGNOSIS OF DIABETIC NEPHROPATHY

Microalbuminuria (urinary albumin excretion of 30–300 mg/day) precedes the appearance of macroalbuminuria (>300 mg/day).[70] Checking for microalbuminuria may be considered as a screening test but not as a diagnostic test for diabetic nephropathy. Epidemiologic studies suggest that negative test for microalbuminuria has 99% probability of not having the target condition, whereas positive test for microalbuminuria has only 27% probability of having the target condition.[71] Recently, the pattern of the sequential steps of progression of diabetic nephropathy starting with microalbuminuria, followed by proteinuria with subsequent decline in kidney function terminating in ESRD, has been re-evaluated.[72] In a long-term study of 79 patients with type 1 diabetes and new-onset microalbuminuria after 12 years, 23 cases (viz., 29%) progressed to CKD stage 3–5 [estimated glomerular filtration rate (eGFR) 60 to less than 15 mL/min]. This outcome matches very closely the findings of the epidemiologic study cited above indicating that the presence of microalbuminuria portends 27% probability of having the target condition, which refers in this case to diabetic nephropathy. Accordingly, 71% of patients with type 1 diabetes and microalbuminuria do not progress to CKD. Interestingly, 11 patients in above study who developed CKD, microalbuminuria regressed to normal protein excretion. In absence of kidney biopsies, it is questionable whether CKD in these patients was due to diabetic nephropathy. Similarlar to type 1 diabetes, some patients with microalbuminuria and type 2 diabetes return to normal albumin excretion. In a study involving 216 patients with type 2 diabetes and microalbuminuria, after 6 years, return to normal urinary albumin excretion was observed in 51% while progression to macroalbuminuria occurred in 28%.[73] This observation bears striking resemblance to the rate of progression of microalbuminuria to CKD in type 1 diabetes. One cannot ignore, however, the progress in treatment of diabetes in recent years, which may also influence the progression of microalbuminuria to CKD. In most cases, albuminuria is the earliest sign of diabetic renal disease; however, there are reports of functional renal impairment in the absence of albuminuria. In the UK Prospective Diabetes Study, 51% of those who developed CKD stage 3 did not have preceding albuminuria.[74] Vice versa, classical nodular glomerusclerosis has been reported in type 2 diabetics with normoalbuminuria and impaired kidney function.[75] In fact, many type 2 diabetics with early CKD (eGFR 60–45 mL/min) during follow-up period may reverse to normal kidney function.[76] In absence of tissue diagnosis, it is uncertain whether in these patients the kidneys are affected by diabetic lesions. As painful peripheral diabetic neuropathy affects many diabetics, the use nonsteroidal anti-inflammatory drugs (NSAIDs) is widespread in this patient population. Likewise, obesity which is present in many type 2 diabetics is very often associated with lower back changes causing pain and disability prompting use of NSAIDs. The combined use of NSAIDs with blood pressure lowering diuretics appears to be predisposing to renal ischemia leading to analgesic nephropathy. Thus, the occurrence of analgesic nephropathy should not be underestimated in these patients. Often cessation of NSAIDs leads to improved kidney function.

Diabetic Nephropathy and Retinopathy

It is obvious that microvascular pathology is involved in the pathogenesis of diabetic retinopathy, diabetic neuropathy, and diabetic nephropathy. Parving et al. have suggested that the presence of retinopathy is a prerequisite for the diagnosis of diabetic nephropathy. They have argued that proteinuric patients without retinopathy may have high incidence of atypical renal biopsy features or other renal diseases. In this regard, proteinuric patients with type 1 diabetes of less than 10 years and type 2 diabetics without retinopathy should be thoroughly investigated for other diseases, and renal biopsy for diagnosis, prognosis, and amenability to targeted therapy should be strongly contemplated. In view of this strong recommendation, we have performed kidney biopsies in six patients with type 2 diabetes and persistent proteinuria but lacking diabetic retinopathy on serial retinal ophthalmologic examinations. In all six patients, renal biopsies were interpreted as typical diabetic nodular glomerulosclerosis (unpublished observation). It appears that there may be certain inconsistency in the proposed dependence of the clinical diagnosis of diabetic nephropathy on the presence of diabetic retinopathy; further studies may shed light on that uncertainty. In above cohort study, high glycosylated hemoglobin and proteinuria were strongly associated with the risk of advanced CKD. Thus, it appears that less than one-third of patients with type 1 diabetes and microalbuminuria progress to CKD. Most frequently, microalbuminuria regresses to normoalbuminuria.[2]

CLINICAL CHARACTERISTICS OF PATIENTS WITH DIABETIC NEPHROPATHY

Diabetic nephropathy occurs in 30–40% of type 1 diabetic patients, 20–25 years after the onset of diabetes, and in about 20–25% of type 2 diabetic patients within 20 years.[77] Approximately, 20–30% of patients with diabetic nephropathy progress to ESRD while the rest may die from coronary artery disease or other cardiovascular causes before the onset of ESRD.[78,79] The prognosis of diabetic patients with ESRD is very poor. About 30% of diabetic patients undergoing dialysis die within 2 years, while 15% of diabetic patients receiving their first deceased donor transplant die within 2 years.[79]

Previous studies suggested that minority of patients with type 2 diabetic nephropathy progress to ESRD requiring renal replacement therapy (RRT). This has been explained by high incidence of cardiovascular mortality preceding the development of ESRD.[80,81] Recently published information from the Diabetes Mellitus Treatment for Renal Insufficiency Consortium (DIAMETRIC) database provides more precise analysis regarding progression of type 2 diabetic nephropathy to ESRD. ESRD occurred in only 6% of patients with initial urinary albumin excretion of 1 or less than 1 g/24 h, as compared with initial urinary albumin of more than 2 g/24 h. Likewise, if initial eGFR was more than 45 mL/min, only 5% developed ESRD, whereas with eGFR equal or less than 30 mL/min 48%, developed ESRD. These findings suggest that only patients with nephrotic range proteinuria and CKD stage 4 are more likely to develop ESRD. Thus, the degree of proteinuria and the severity of renal insufficiency predict the risk of ESRD.[82]

MANAGEMENT OF PATIENTS WITH CHRONIC KIDNEY DISEASE AND DIABETIC NEPHROPATHY

Control of Hypertension

Intensive control of hypertension plays a major role in slowing the progression of diabetic nephropathy. Thirty six years ago, Mogensen[83] demonstrated a marked decrease in proteinuria in type 1 diabetic patients following lowering hypertension with propanolol and hydralazine. Subsequently, in a landmark study, he demonstrated slowing of decline in GFR from 1.24 mL/min/month before antihypertensive treatment to 0.45 mL/min/month during treatment, using the same antihypertensive agents.[84,85] Parving et al. confirmed these observations later.[86] Thus control of hypertension remains the cornerstone therapy that slows the progression of diabetic nephropathy but fails to stop it (Figures 3 and 4).

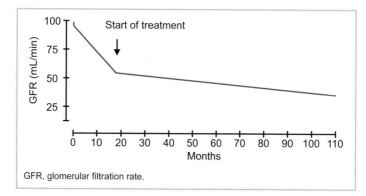

GFR, glomerular filtration rate.

FIGURE 3 Antihypertensive treatment reduces the rate of decline in the glomerular filtration rate in diabetic nephropathy. The figure depicts the course of changes over 110 months . *Modified from* Mogensen GE. Long-term antihypertensive treatment inhibiting progression of diabetic nephropathy. *Br Med J (Clin Res Ed).* 1982;285(6343):685-8.

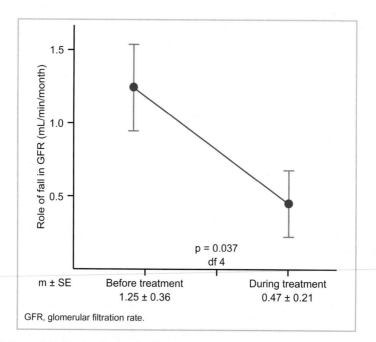

GFR, glomerular filtration rate.

FIGURE 4 Rate of decline in glomerular filtration before and during antihypertensive treatment. Before treatment, the mean rate of decline was 1.24 mL/min/month; during treatment it decreased to 0.49 mL/min/month. *Modified from* Mogensen CE. Long-term antihypertensive treatment inhibiting progression of diabetic nephropathy. *Br Med J (Clin Res Ed).* 1982;285(6343):685-8.

Data from clinical trials suggest that ACE inhibitors may be beneficial in the treatment of diabetic nephropathy through a mechanism that is not limited to their effect on systemic hypertension.

The Collaborative Study Group[87] evaluated the response to ACE inhibitor in type 1 diabetics with diabetic nephropathy (proteinuria of 500 mg/day or more) and serum creatinine of 2.5 mg/dL or less. Four hundred and nine patients were randomized to therapy with either captopril or placebo. Further antihypertensive drugs were added as required. Captopril was given at the dose of 25 mg three times daily. The blood pressure goal was less than 140/90 mmHg. The blood pressure in the captopril group was by less than 4 mmHg lower than that in the placebo group over a period of 4 years. The primary end-point of the trial was a doubling of the serum creatinine which was recorded in 25 patients in the captopril treated group and in 43 patients in the placebo group (p < 0.01). Captopril treatment was associated with 48% reduced relative risk of doubling of serum creatinine, and 50% reduction in relative risk of ESRD or death.

In the Irbesartan in Diabetic Nephropathy Trial, 1,715 patients with nephropathy associated with type 2 diabetes (mean serum creatinine 1.7 mg/dL) were randomized to treatment with ARB irbesartan (300 mg daily), to calcium channel blocker (CCB) amlodipine (10 mg daily), or placebo. Blood pressure was controlled at the target of 135/85 mmHg with the addition of antihypertensive drugs of classes other than ARBs/ACE inhibitor or CCBs if required. Treatment with irbesartan was associated with 20% (compared with placebo) or 23% (compared with amlodipine) reduction in unadjusted risk of reaching the composite end-point of doubling of baseline serum creatinine level, development of ESRD, or death from any cause (p < 0.05). The risk of doubling serum creatinine was 33% lower in the irbesartan group than in the placebo group and 37% lower than in the amlodipine group. The relative risk of ESRD was 23% lower in the irbesartan than with either amlodipine or placebo. The irbesartan group had a 33% decrease in daily protein excretion compared with 6% in the amlodipine group and 10% in the placebo group. These differences were not explained by the levels of blood that were recorded between the respective groups.[88]

In the Reduction of End points in NIDDM with Angiotensin II Antagonist Losartan Trial (RENAAL) 1,513 patients with type 2 diabetes and nephropathy (mean serum creatinine 1.9 mg/dL) were randomized to losartan (50 mg titrating up to 100 mg daily) or placebo, in addition to conventional antihypertensive therapy excluding ACE inhibitors. Losartan reduced the incidence of doubling serum creatinine by 25% and ESRD by 28%.[89]

Unlike above two large-scale randomized studies which evaluated head-on the effect of two angiotensin receptor blocking agents on progression of diabetic nephropathy as a primary outcome, no similar trials addressing the effect ACE inhibitors on progression of diabetic nephropathy in type 2 diabetes have been reported. In this regard, most of the information on the renoprotective effect of ACE inhibitors in type 2 diabetes stems from subgroup analysis and as a secondary outcome.

The renal outcomes with telmisartan, ramipril, or both in people at high vascular risk [the Ongoing Telmisartan Alone or in Combination with Ramipril Global Endpoint Trial (ONTARGET)] randomized 25,019 subjects with established atherosclerotic vascular disease or with diabetes with end-organ damage into three corresponding groups. The patients were followed for 56 months. The definition of the outcomes in this large mixed group was rather vague. The primary composite outcome was the first occurrence of any dialysis, the doubling of serum creatinine, or death. The secondary renal outcomes included the composite of any dialysis and doubling of serum creatinine, components of the composite outcomes, changes in GFR and progression of proteinuria (defined as new development of microalbuminuria or macroalbuminuria). Renal impairment was not defined but was based on reports from clinical investigators. The secondary renal outcome, dialysis, or doubling of serum creatinine was similar with telmisartan and ramipril, and more frequent with combination therapy (p = 0.038). Estimated GFR declined least with ramipril compared with telmisartan (p < 0.0001). The increase in urinary albumin excretion was less with telmisartan (p = 0.004) or with combination therapy (p = 0.001) than with ramipril. The interpretation of these results by the ONTARGET investigators suggested that in people at high vascular risk, telmisartan's effects on major renal outcomes are similar to ramipril. Combination therapy diminishes proteinuria more than monotherapy; however, it worsens major renal outcomes. Thus, the major concerns raised by above findings refer to the combination therapy. The combination therapy is associated with worse renal outcomes and increased risk of death. In view of the above, the use of combination therapy should be discouraged.[90]

Of interest is the dissociation between effects on proteinuria and kidney function. While ramipril monotherapy was associated with better preservation of kidney function as compared with telmisartan; by contrast, telmisartan therapy showed advantage over ramipril with respect to reduction of proteinuria. Thus, proteinuria and kidney function do not always follow a similar course. In this regard, it is noteworthy that proteinuria in diabetic nephropathy has been considered as surrogate for kidney function.

In the MICRO-HOPE substudy of the Heart Outcomes Prevention Evaluation (HOPE), 3,577 peoples were included. The subjects were randomly assigned to ramipril or placebo. The combined primary outcome was myocardial infarction, stroke, or cardiovascular death. Overt nephropathy was main outcome in a substudy. Overt nephropathy was diagnosed if the 24-hour urine albumin was 300 mg or more or if 24-hour urine total protein excretion was 500 mg or more. eGFR was not included. Ramipril reduced the risk of combined microvascular outcome of overt nephropathy, dialysis or laser therapy by 16% (p = 0.036); 117 (7%) on ramipril, and 149 (8%) on the placebo developed overt nephropathy (p = 0.027). Blood pressure in the ramipril group, however, was lower than that in the placebo group.[91]

In the Action in Diabetes and Vascular Disease: preterAx and diamicron-MR Controlled Evaluation (ADVANCE) study, type 2 diabetic patients were randomized to combination of perindopril-indapamide (ACEI + thiazide) or placebo regardless of their blood pressure at entry.[92] Lower systolic blood pressure, even less than 110 mmHg was associated with progressively lower rates of renal events. A total of 1,243 (22.3%) patients in the active treatment group and 1,500 (26.9%) in the placebo group developed the composite renal outcome of new-onset microalbuminuria, new-onset nephropathy (defined by macroalbuminuria), doubling of serum creatinine, and ESRD. The mean blood pressure during the follow-up was 134/74 mmHg in the active treatment group and 140/77 mmHg in the placebo group (p < 0.0001).

Tight control of hypertension targeting levels equal to or lower than 130/80 mmHg is beyond doubt the mainstay therapeutic modality proven to slow the progression of diabetic nephropathy.[93-96] The reported lower blood pressure levels achieved with ACE inhibitors or angiotensin receptor blocking agents compared with placebo control questioned their specific therapeutic efficacy beyond blood pressure control.[97] This question has not been resolved entirely despite the myriad of randomized controlled studies. Despite about uncertainties, there is a strong theoretical and experimental evidence to support the renoprotective therapeutic advantage of inhibitors of renin-angiotensin system over other antihypertensive agents.[98,99]

The effect of renin-angiotensin blockers has been primarily tested in type 1 and 2 diabetics with clinical diagnosis of diabetic nephropathy featuring proteinuria and impaired kidney function. Recent study addressed the question regarding the effect of renin-angiotensin blockers in primary prevention of diabetic nephropathy in type 1 diabetics without hypertension, normal kidney function, and without microalbuminuria. The Renin-Angiotensin System Study (RASS) addressed the question whether blockade of renin-angiotensin system in type 1 diabetes could slow progression of early histopathological changes of diabetic nephropathy.[100] RASS was based on the assumption that slowing the pathological abnormalities responsible for renal impairment would modify the progression of renal dysfunction. This is one of the very few studies of diabetic kidney that included two-spaced kidney biopsies which indeed are the real "hard evidence" regarding the presence and progression of diabetic glomerular abnormalities. Two hundred eighty five normotensive patients with type 1 diabetes and normoalbuminuria were randomized to losartan 100 mg daily, enalapril 20 mg daily, or placebo with a 5-year follow-up. The primary end-point was change in the fraction of glomerular volume occupied by mesangium in kidney biopsy specimens. Over the 5-year period the changes in mesangial fractional volume in placebo group was not significantly different from that with either enalapril or losartan. The microalbuminuria incidence was higher with losartan than with placebo, but was not higher with enalapril. As opposed to lack of effect on progression of glomerular disease, blockade of renin-angiotensin system slowed significantly the progression of diabetic retinopathy. However, the achieved blood pressure levels with enalapril and with losartan were significantly lower than in the placebo group. The RASS study questions the utility of renin-angiotensin blockade in the primary prevention of diabetic kidney disease in type 1 diabetic patients. Similarly, in normotensive type 2 diabetics blockade of angiotensin II receptors for 4.7 years failed to prevent microalbuminuria.[101]

The role of renin-angiotensin blockade as the first line for treatment of hypertension in diabetic patients is widely acknowledged. In clinical practice, however, the occurrence of hyperkalemia is of concern. Recent study addressed the adverse effect of hyperkalemia. Treatment with losartan increased the serum potassium concentration. Furthermore, the appearance of hyperkalemia not only increased its cardiotoxicity but also increased the risk of adverse renal outcomes and counteracted the beneficial renoprotective action of losartan.[102-104] Some diabetic patients with hyporeninemic-hypoaldosteronism are likely to be more prone to manifest this complication. Monitoring of serum potassium levels, especially when initiating the treatment with renin-angiotensin blockers is mandatory. In this regard, multidisciplinary treatment plan involving counseling by renal dieticians is indispensable. Like in other areas of renal medicine enforcement of dietary guidelines is of paramount importance. Furthermore, dietary sodium restriction plays a key role in the control of hypertension in diabetic patients. Endothelial dysfunction with capillary leak predisposes to edema formation in diabetic patients. Adding a diuretic to the therapeutic regimen may be of some help as well.

The addition of spironolactone to ACE inhibitors or ARBs decreased proteinuria. This antiproteinuric effect was not related to further decrease blood pressure. Aldosterone in addition to its effects on electrolyte transport has been shown to activate profibrotic cytokines leading to tissue scarring. What remains to be shown is whether mineralocorticoid receptor blockers slow progression of diabetic nephropathy. In view of the risk of hyperkalemia in diabetics treated with renin-angiotensin system inhibitors, addition of spironolactone may potentiate even more this adverse side effect.[105,106]

Glucose Control

The Diabetes Control and Complications Trial (DCCT) evaluated the effect of intensive treatment of diabetes on the development and progression of long-term complications in 1,441 persons with type 1 diabetes over 6.5 years. The intensive therapy reduced the incidence of microalbuminuria by 39% and the occurrence of overt nephropathy by 54%. Mean glycated hemoglobin in the intensive therapy group was 7.3 while in the conventional therapy group, it was 9.1%. Intensive therapy slowed the progression of nephropathy, retinopathy, and neuropathy.[107] The extension of DCCT, the observational Epidemiology of Diabetes Interventions and Complications (EDIC) study followed these patients for a total period of 22 years. The EDIC study focused on the cumulative incidence of impaired GFR in the intensive and conventional therapy group. At year 16 of EDIC, the mean glycated hemoglobin in the intensive therapy group was 7.9 and in the conventional therapy 8.0%. Despite the parity in glucose control during the EDIC observational follow-up study, the beneficial effect of intensive therapy during the six years of DCCT persisted and even improved. Over a median follow-up of 22 years in the DCCT combined with EDIC studies, impairment of GFR was evident in 24 patients of the intensive therapy group and in 46 of the conventional therapy group (p = 0.006). ESRD developed in eight patients of the intensive therapy and in 16 of the conventional therapy group (p < 0.001). This long-term study lends support to the role of early glucose control in slowing progression of diabetic nephropathy and reducing by 50% the occurrence of ESRD.[108]

The UK Prospective Diabetes Study (UKPDS) involving 3,867 type 2 diabetics evaluated intensive treatment of diabetes with sulfonylureas or insulin. Intensive therapy was associated with a decrease in microvascular complications but not in macrovascular complications. There was a decrease in doubling of serum creatinine in the intensive glucose group after 12 years of follow-up.[109]

In the ADVANCE Collaborative study, 11,140 patients with type 2 diabetes were randomized to standard glucose control or to intensive glucose control, defined as targeting glycated hemoglobin of 6.5%. After a median of five years, the achieved level glycated hemoglobin in the intensive control was 6.5% and in the standard control 7.3%. The regimen of intensive glucose control decreased the incidence of combined major macrovascular and microvascular events; 18.1% against 20% with standard control (p = 0.01), as well as of major microvascular events (p = 0.01), primarily because of a drop in the incidence of nephropathy (p = 0.006). The relative reduction in the incidence of nephropathy amounted to 21%.[110]

The Veterans Affairs Diabetes Trial (VADT) randomized 1,791 patients with long-standing poorly controlled type 2 diabetes to receive either standard or intensive glucose control therapy.[111] Following 5.6 years of trial the median glycated hemoglobin in the standard control group was 8.4% while in the intensive control it was 6.9%. The intensive glucose control failed to change the rates of major cardiovascular events; however, it reduced the progression of albuminuria (p = 0.01).

Effects of Multifactorial Intervention (The Steno-2 Study)

In the Steno-2 study, 160 patients with type 2 diabetes and persistent micro-albuminuria were randomized to receive either intensive therapy or conventional therapy.[112] The mean treatment duration was 7.8 years with an observational extension for another 5.5 years. The intensive therapy included well-defined goals like glycated hemoglobin of less than 6.6%, fasting serum cholesterol of 175 mg/dL, serum triglycerides of less than 150 mg/dL, systolic blood pressure of less than 130 mmHg and diastolic blood pressure of less than 80 mmHg. Patients were treated with inhibitors renin-angiotensin system regardless of blood pressure and received low-dose aspirin. The tertiary end-points were incident diabetic nephropathy or development of diabetic retinopathy or neuropathy. Diabetic nephropathy was defined as urinary albumin excretion rate of more than 300 mg/24 h. Nine patients in the intensive therapy group, while 19 patients in the conventional-therapy group died from cardiovascular causes (p = 0.03). During the entire study period, diabetic nephropathy occurred in 20 patients in intensive therapy group, and in 37 patients in the conventional therapy group (p = 0.04). One patient in the intensive therapy group as opposed to six patients in the conventional therapy group developed ESRD requiring dialysis (p = 0.04). Thus, early multifactorial therapy holds a promise for better outcomes including microvascular complications. The decrease in microvascular complications included an absolute risk reduction of 6.3% in the need for dialysis. In comparison with trials involving treatment of single risk factor, the results of multifactorial intervention reached more impressive risk reduction. Whether initiation of intensive therapy at more advanced stages of diabetes with associated CKD could improve renal outcomes is of great clinical interest.

The Action to Control Cardiovascular Risk in Diabetes (ACCORD) study randomized 10,251 high-risk type 2 diabetics with mean age of 62.2 years and median glycated hemoglobin 8.1% to intensive therapy and/or standard therapy group. The intensive therapy targeted glycated hemoglobin below 6%, systolic blood pressure below 120 mmHg, and tight lipid control by adding fenofibrate to statin therapy. The intensive therapy motivated to achieve normal glycated hemoglobin, increased all-cause mortality by 22%, and did not reduce major cardiovascular events. High incidence of hypoglycemia was observed in the intensive therapy group. The finding of higher mortality in the intensive therapy group led to discontinuation of intensive therapy after a mean of 3.5-year follow-up. At the end of five-year follow-up, intensive treatment had no effect on outcomes of advanced microvascular disease, including renal failure (serum creatinine more than 3.3 mg/dL), dialysis, or renal transplantation. The intensive treatment reduced the incidence of microalbuminuria and macroalbuminuria. Neither microalbuminuria nor macroalbuminuria predicted subsequent development of renal failure. Approximately half of all patients who developed renal failure had neither microalbuminuria nor macroalbuminuria at baseline. Thus, these results do not lend support to the presence of macroalbuminuria as an absolute surrogate marker of diabetic nephropathy. The findings of ACCORD study have identified a previously unrecognized harm of intensive glucose lowering in elderly high-risk patients with type 2 diabetes. It is noteworthy, however, that severe hypoglycemic episodes were a risk factor for mortality and occurred three times as often in the intensive glycemic treatment group as compared with the standard care group. Thus, the potential benefits of adequate glucose control might have been overshadowed by excessive lowering of blood glucose to life-threatening levels. Likewise, excessive lowering of blood pressure in elderly diabetics with advanced cardiovascular disease and poor arterial autoregulation may have precarious side effects as opposed to the beneficial effect of moderate blood pressure reduction. Additional comments regarding the findings of ACCORD trial underscore the importance to a balanced approach, avoidance of overzealous overdoing in the control of blood glucose, and hypertension in the management of high-risk elderly diabetics.[113-117]

Nutritional Intervention

Studies in experimental diabetes show that increase in total body sodium and activation of renal renin-angiotensin system induced by high sodium intake blunt the antihypertensive and the antiproteinuric effects of renin-angiotensin inhibitors. Observational studies in patients with CKD have demonstrated that increased dietary sodium intake increases proteinuria and enhances progression of CKD. Sodium overload increases ACE activity in renal and vascular tissues which augments vascular conversion of angiotensin I to angiotensin II. High sodium intake blunts the effects of ACE inhibitors in rats and in humans.[118-120]

Recent analysis of data obtained from the ramipril efficacy in nephropathy (REIN) and REIN-2 showed that in patients with CKD treated with ACE inhibitor, high salt intake led to accelerated progression to ESRD. The incidence of ESRD per 100 patient years was three times higher in the high sodium diet (more than 200 mEq) than in the low sodium (less than 100 mEq) group. The increased risk of rapid progression to ESRD appeared to be mediated by blunted antiproteinuric actions of ACE inhibitor.[121] Avoiding excess sodium intake may be important to slow CKD progression to ESRD. Sodium restriction to 70 mEq per day has been reported to enhance the antiproteinuric effect of angiotensin receptor inhibitors.[122] Compliance with restricted sodium diet can be verified by measurements of 24-hour urinary sodium excretion. In general, sodium restriction is strongly recommended in patients with diabetic nephropathy who fail to respond to the antiproteinuric effects of renin-angiotensin inhibitors.

Vitamin D Analogs

Paricalcitol (19-nor-1,25-dihydroxyvitamin D2) (Zemplar), an active analog of vitamin D has been reported to exert an antiproteinuric effect in patients with CKD. This beneficial effect was observed in patients who were already on ACE inhibitors or ARBs. In fact, this effect was additive to those of renin-angiotensin inhibitors in decreasing proteinuria. The antiproteinuric effect of paricalcitol subsequently was also demonstrated in double-blinded trial in patients with CKD stage 2 and 3. This antiproteinuric effect of vitamin D was associated with significant fall in urinary TGF-beta-1, a known profibrotic cytokine, which plays a role in the progression of diabetic nephropathy.[123,124] As alluded to above, the presumed mechanism underlying the renoprotective effect of vitamin D analogs is its renin-blocking effect. Thus, evidence is supporting a possible therapeutic effect of active vitamin D metabolites as antiproteinuric agents in addition to their widespread use for improvement of mineral and bone metabolism in CKD. Untoward adverse side-effects of vitamin D include hypercalcemia, hyperphosphatemia, and soft tissue calcifications. As vitamin D analogs are recommended by Kidney Disease Outcomes Quality Initiative (K/DOQI) for treatment of secondary hyperparathyroidism, they are frequently prescribed for CKD patients. Very often, this recommendation is overlooked by providers. In view of the potential renoprotective effect of vitamin D, it might be beneficial to use vitamin D as recommended.

Peroxisome Proliferator-Activated Receptors Gamma Agonists

Diabetes is associated with insulin resistance. Insulin signaling in the visceral glomerular epithelial cells, the podocytes, is crucial for preserving the function and structural integrity of glomeruli. Impaired insulin signaling leads to glomerular abnormalities characteristic of diabetic nephropathy. Peroxisome proliferator-activated receptors (PPAR), which are ligand activated transcription factors, enhance the sensitivity to insulin, and are used in the treatment of diabetes. PPAR-gamma agonists reduce urinary albumin excretion and lower blood pressure in different stages of diabetic nephropathy.[125-129] Whether this effect translates to slowing progression of diabetic nephropathy remains to be determined by clinical trials in the future.

Obesity

Obesity has been associated with increased risk of diabetic kidney disease. Furthermore, weight loss may decrease the diabetic metabolic burden. In addition, diet and weight loss may diminish proteinuria and improve kidney function in patients with diabetes.[129-131] The effect of weight loss on progression of diabetic nephropathy is unknown.

MANAGEMENT OF PATIENTS WITH DIABETIC NEPHROPATHY UNDERGOING CHRONIC DIALYSIS

About 45% of all new patients with ESRD in United States initiating RRT are diabetics. Survival of diabetic patients on chronic dialysis is lower than in nondiabetics with ESRD. Only 30% of patients with diabetic nephropathy survive five years after starting dialysis.[132-134] Comorbidities related to diabetes contribute to the relatively high mortality. Cardiovascular complications are the most common cause of mortality accounting for more than 50% of all cases of death. Nondifference was found between hemodialysis and peritoneal dialysis in death rate. Compared with dialysis, kidney transplantation is accompanied by better survival and better quality of life.[135]

Starting Renal Replacement Therapy

Patients with ESRD and their families face a difficult decision of becoming dependent on RRT, which limits their freedom and independence. Multidisciplinary support is required to help the patient to cope with this far-reaching change in their life. First, education is a key element in preparing the patient to adjust to the new situation which may be a challenging and demanding experience. Second, a support team including a social worker, nephrology nurse, dietician, nephrologist, dialysis technician, or a clergy-person if required should dedicate time and effort to help the patient in these stressful circumstances.

The K/DOQI clinical practice guidelines actions of National Kidney Foundation recommend preparing for RRT at eGFR levels of 15–29 mL/min (CKD stage 4) and starting RRT at eGFR levels when eGFR falls below 15 mL/min[136] Diabetics with ESRD are usually started earlier on RRT than nondiabetics with ESRD. Earlier start allows better control of hypertension, fluid overload, and congestive heart failure which are common in diabetics with ESRD. Better control of hypertension reduces the progression of diabetic retinopathy leading to blindness. Likewise, RRT corrects the uremic bleeding diathesis which leads to rapid progression of retinopathy. Control of volume-dependent hypertension by RRT reduces cardiovascular complications related to hypertension, such as myocardial infarction, congestive heart failure, and stroke. Poor appetite and poor nutrition due to the uremic state contribute to high mortality. Evidence based on randomized controlled studies indicating survival advantage with earlier RRT is lacking. Likewise, the use of heparin during hemodialysis may pose a risk for retinal bleeding. In this regard peritoneal dialysis has been reported to provide a better protection with respect to progression of diabetic retinopathy. Taken together, the optimal timing of initiating RRT has to be determined, case by case, on individual basis. Refractory congestive heart failure with recurrent pulmonary edema which occurs often in diabetics with ischemic heart disease is obviously an indication for earlier dialysis. If a patient opts for peritoneal dialysis as long-term RRT, peritoneal catheter should be inserted 2–4 weeks before starting therapy.

Arterial-Venous Fistula "First"

Surgery to construct vascular access for hemodialysis is the most important step in preparing for maintenance hemodialysis. This has to be planned several months ahead of starting hemodialysis as maturation of arterial-venous fistula (AVF) may require several months. The rate of primary failures of AVFs is high, which requires corrective surgery or surgery attempting to create a new AVF. Peripheral vascular disease, which is common in diabetics, may be a serious impediment to successful surgical creation of AVF. Even patients who are hesitant or refuse the option dialysis should be encouraged to have AVF. Having an AVF is not tantamount to commitment to acceptance of RRT; however, it leaves the patient with the option to accept the treatment on temporary or permanent manner when the need arises. The alternative to AVF is cannulation of central veins with catheters. This is associated with frequent life-threatening infections and substandard quality of dialysis due to poor blood flow through the filtering dialyzers. AVF remains the optimal vascular access to dialysis. Line infections are the second most common causes of mortality in dialysis patients. When creation of AVF fistula is hindered by poor venous network, arterial-venous graft (AVG) would be the best second choice. However, three-year survival of an AVF is 80% whereas for AVG it is 47%.[137] Likewise, thrombosis is more frequent in venous catheters and AVGs than in AVFs.

Hemodialysis-Related Complications

Hypotension

Diabetic patients have a 20% higher frequency of hypotension during hemodialysis treatment than nondiabetics. Hypotension may be associated with muscle cramps, abdominal and back pain, anginal pain, dizziness, nausea, and vomiting.[138] Hypotension may trigger arrhythmia and acute myocardial infarction. Hemodialysis-induced hypotension is an independent risk factor for 2-year mortality in patients with ESRD.[139] Contrary to normal individuals who respond to hypotension with accelerated heart beat rate, diabetics with ESRD fail to respond to drop in blood pressure with reflex tachycardia. This contributes to hypotension during hemodialysis with ultrafiltration. Diabetic autonomous dysfunction may at least partly account for this hemodynamic abnormality. Likewise, poor myocardial contractility due to systolic or diastolic dysfunction in diabetics with ESRD may compromise the reflex physiological response to hypotension.[140] Furthermore, the reduced oncotic pressure due to hypoalbuminemia may prevent the refill of intravascular compartment that is contracting during ultrafiltration. Failure to refill the intravascular compartment to match the fluid volume removed with ultrafiltration leads to hypovolemia with resulting hypotension. Monitoring changes in hematocrit during hemodialysis may assist in assessment of intravascular volume. Furthermore, rapid increase in hematocrit may signal fast decrease in intravascular volume requiring reducing the rate of ultrafiltration. On the other hand, unchanging hematocrit during ultrafiltration suggests that the rate of refill matches the rate of ultrafiltration with possible excessive accumulation of fluid in interstitial compartment. Acute hypotensive episodes are usually treated by placing the patient in Trendelenburg position; a bolus of 0.9% saline is rapidly administered through the venous line and ultrafiltration is reduced to zero. Once the vital signs have stabilized ultrafiltration can be resumed at a lower rate.

Some of the following therapeutic measures have been employed to improve the hemodynamic balance and avoid hypotension during hemodialysis sessions. Slow rate of ultrafiltration minimizes the fluid shifts and improves hemodynamic balance. The patients hold the morning or predialysis antihypertensive medications. The patients are encouraged not to consume food during dialysis as it leads to pooling blood in the gastrointestinal blood vessels lowering systemic blood pressure, determining the accurate "dry weight" and avoiding ultrafiltration below patient's "dry weight". Educating patients to reduce sodium and associated water intake would decrease interdialytic weight gains and thus minimize the need for aggressive ultrafiltration that causes hypertension. In refractory cases, alpha-adrenergic agonists (e.g., midodrine) administered before dialysis may be helpful.

Hypertension

Hypertension is more common in diabetic than in nondiabetic patients undergoing hemodialysis. While 50% of diabetics on hemodialysis require antihypertensive medication, only 27% of nondiabetic patients require antihypertensive treatment.[141] Hypertension is volume dependent in vast majority diabetics undergoing hemodialysis. Persistent gradual removal of excess sodium and water with slow ultrafiltration may, on the long run, normalize the blood pressure and stop or reduce the need for antihypertensive medications. Few diabetics undergoing hemodialysis may paradoxically experience a rise in blood pressure during hemodialysis treatment.[142] This phenomenon is poorly understood. Endothelial dysfunction, which is common in diabetics, expressed with failure to respond properly to vascular changes by releasing vasodilator nitric oxide, and paradoxically releasing vasoconstrictor endothelin instead could contribute to this abnormality. Sublingual nitrates have been helpful in some patients with this phenomenon.[142,143] Caution, however, has to be exercised to avoid precipitous drops in blood pressure. Excessive response of renin-angiotensin system to hypovolemia induced by ultrafiltration may be an alternative explanation for this rise in blood pressure. Pretreatment with blockers of renin-angiotensin activity may be useful in this situation.

Excessive Interdialytic Weight Gain

High interdialytic weight gain is very common in diabetics undergoing hemodialysis. Close relation between the level of hyperglycemia and amount of weight gain has been observed.[143,144] High intracellular sodium due to failure of sodium pump or increased cellular membrane back leak causes increased thirst in diabetics. Increased interdialytic weight gain is independently associated with decreased survival in diabetic patients undergoing hemodialysis.[145] Noncompliance with dietary sodium and water restrictions are the leading causes for interdialytic weight gain. Excessive weight gain contributes to resistant hypertension, cardiovascular morbidity, and mortality. Peritoneal dialysis offers an advantage with regard to the risk of excessive weight gain, as gradual rather than rapid ultrafiltration avoids salt and water accumulation.

Hypoglycemia

Many diabetic patients undergoing dialysis manifest reduction in insulin requirements due to decreased urinary excretion and reduced degradation of endogenous and exogenous insulin by the kidneys. This leads to decreased dosing of oral hypoglycemic agents and insulin to avoid hypoglycemia. Reduced appetite, diabetic gastroparesis, enteropathy leading to malnutrition may further increase the risk of hypoglycemia. In diabetic patients, hemodialysis solution should always contain 200 mg/dL glucose. If glucose is not added, then severe hypoglycemia during or soon after the hemodialysis session can result. With control of uremia and improved appetite, this trend may be partially reversed.

Hyperglycemia

The presentation of hyperglycemia is altered when renal function is absent as in dialysis patients. The absence of the modifying effect of glycosuria may lead to severe hyperglycemia. Hyperosmolarity with altered mental status is unusual because of the absence of water loss induced by osmotic diuresis. However, manifestations may include weight and pulmonary edema due to expansion of extracellular fluid volume. Hyperglycemia is very often accompanied by life-threatening hyperkalemia due to lack of insulin effect on sodium pump, and shifts of intracellular fluids rich in potassium to extracellular compartment as a result of extracellular hyperosmolarity. Sustained hyperglycemia leads to the progression of all diabetic complications. Nonenzymatic glycolysation of proteins forms advanced glycosylation end-products which increase synthesis of growth factors and cytokines which impair the structure and function of vascular basement membranes and intracellular proteins resulting in widespread diabetic complication. Hence, metabolic control of diabetes is important in diabetics undergoing dialysis.

Peripheral Vascular Disease

Poor blood glucose control, peripheral vascular disease and peripheral neuropathy, and nonhealing infected ischemic ulcers are the main risk factors for multiple amputations in diabetics undergoing dialysis. Life-threatening bacteremias may result from dissemination of local infections.[146,147] In these circumstances, and in the presence of central venous catheter used as vascular access for hemodialysis, uncertainty regarding the origin of the infection results in a therapeutic dilemma. Eventually, the central venous vascular access may be lost, even though the systemic infection originates from the diabetic foot and not from the venous line. Secondary hyperparathyroidism on one hand, and adynamic bone, which is common in diabetics on the other, contribute to hyperphosphatemia and to elevated calcium x phosphate product.[148] This abnormality may be aggravated by poor compliance with dietary phosphate restrictions and failure to take the prescribed phosphate binders. Above derangements in mineral balance predispose to vascular complication in diabetics with ESRD. Calcific urenic arteriolopathy consists of small arterial vessel calcifications with secondary occlusive thrombosis leading to widespread soft tissue and fat necrosis with secondary life-threatening infections.[149]

CONCLUSION

Diabetic nephropathy is the leading etiology of CKD and ESRD worldwide and the major single cause of ESRD in the US. In the US, it accounts for almost half of patients initiating dialysis each year. The current therapies address the metabolic abnormalities associated with diabetes including hyperglycemia, hyperlipidemia, obesity, vitamin D deficiency, and obesity. Control of hypertension and inhibition of renin-angiotensin-aldosterone system have proven to be highly effective to slow the progression of diabetic nephropathy. The latter remain currently the mainstay therapies for diabetic kidney disease. These therapies, however, have been largely unsuccessful in preventing, arresting, or reversing diabetic nephropathy. This shortcoming is not entirely unexpected as diabetic nephropathy appears to be a complex disorder stemming from a broad spectrum of intertwined pathological factors. An ever growing number of these derangements are a subject of ongoing research. Recent animal studies[150] and past sporadic reports[67-69] on reversal of diabetic nephropathy focus on complete restoration of metabolic environment as key factor for reversal of structural and functional damage of diabetic nephropathy. Even though this therapeutic approach shows some promise, many questions remain unanswered. One of these questions is why a large portion of diabetic patients with identical metabolic abnormalities do not develop diabetic nephropathy during many years of follow up. Evaluation of these diabetic patients who are not susceptible to the similar diabetic environment and comparison with patients who develop diabetic nephropathy perhaps may help define better factors involved in the pathogenesis of diabetic nephropathy.

REFERENCES

1. Atkins RC, Zimmet P. World Kidney Day 2010: diabetic kidney disease-act now or pay later. *Am J Kidney Dis.* 2010;55(2):205-8.
2. Parving HH, Gall MA, Scøtt P, Jørgensen HE, Løkkegaard H, Jørgensen F, et al. Prevalence and causes of albuminuria in non-insulin-dependent diabetic patients. *Kidney Int.* 1992; 41(4):758-62.
3. Rossing P. The changing epidemiology of diabetic microangiopathy in type 1 diabetes. *Diabetologia.* 2005;48(8):1439-44.
4. Rossing P. Prediction, progression and prevention of diabetic nephropathy. The Minkowski Lecture 2005. *Diabetologia.* 2006;49(1):11-9.
5. Coresh J, Selvin E, Stevens LA, Manzi J, Kusek JW, Eggers P, et al. Prevalence of chronic kidney disease in the United States. *JAMA.* 2007;298(17):2038-47.
6. Mogensen CE, Andersen MJ. Increased kidney size and glomerular filtration rate in untreated juvenile diabetes: normalization by insulin-treatment. *Diabetologia.* 1975; 11(3):221-4.
7. Mogensen CE. Early glomerular hyperfiltration in insulin-dependent diabetics and late nephropathy. *Scand J Clin Lab Invest.* 1986;46(3):201-6.
8. Mogensen CE, Christensen CK. Predicting diabetic nephropathy in insulin-dependent patients. *N Engl J Med.* 1984;311(2):89-93.
9. Rudberg S, Persson B, Dahlquist G. Increase glomerular filtration rate as a predictor of diabetic nephropathy—an 8-year prospective study. *Kidney Int.* 1992;41(4):822-8.
10. Mauer M, Drummond K. The early natural history of nephropathy in type 1 diabetes: I. Study design and baseline characteristics of the study participants. *Diabetes.* 2002; 51(5):1572-9.
11. Magee GM, Bilous RW, Cardwell CR, Hunter SJ, Kee F, Fogarty DG. Is hyperfiltration associated with the future risk of developing diabetic nephropathy? A meta-analysis. *Diabetologia.* 2009;52(4):691-7.

12. Gragnoli S, Signorini AM, Tanganelli I, Fondelli C, Borgogni P, Borgogni L, et al. Prevalence of glomerular hyperfiltration and nephromegaly in normo- and microalbuminuric type 2 diabetic patients. *Nephron*. 1993;65(2):206-11.

13. Bruce R, Rutland M, Cundy T. Glomerular hyperfiltration in young Polynesians with type 2 diabetes. *Diabetes Res Clin Pract*. 1994;25(3):155-60.

14. Playle R, Ollerton RL, Dunstan FD, Evans WD, Burch A, Luzio SD, et al. Determining true glomerular filtration status in newly presenting type 2 diabetic subjects using age and sex adjustments. *Diabetes Care*. 1998;21(11):1893-6.

15. Lee KU, Park JY, Hwang IR, Hong SK, Kim GS, Moon DH, et al. Glomerular hyperfiltration in Koreans with non-insulin-dependent diabetes mellitus. *Am J Kidney Dis*. 1995;26(5): 722-6.

16. Wald H, Popovtzer MM. The effect of streptozotocin-induced diabetes mellitus on urinary excretion of sodium and renal Na^+-K^+-ATPase activity. *Pflugers Arch*. 1984;401(1):97-100.

17. Wald H, Scherzer P, Popovtzer MM. Enhanced renal tubular ouabain-sensitive APTase in streptozotocin diabetes mellitus. *Am J Physiol*. 1986;251(1 Pt 2):F164-70.

18. Popovtzer MM, Wald H, Scherzer P. The diabetic kidney–A lesson from the resetting of tubuloglomerular feedback. In: Jinhong Z, Xuehai D, Zhihong L, Leishi L (Eds). Nephrology. Proceedings of the 4th Asian-Pacific Congress of Nephrology. Beijing: International Academic Publishers; 1991. pp. 379-88.

19. Wald H, Scherzer P, Rasch R, Popovtzer MM. Renal tubular Na(+)-K(+)-ATPase in diabetes mellitus: relationship to metabolic abnormality. *Am J Physiol*. 1993;265(1 Pt 1):E96-101.

20. Scherzer P, Popovtzer MM, Segmental localization of mRNAs encoding Na(+)-K(+)-ATPase alpha(1)- and beta(1)-subunits in diabetic rat kidneys using RT-PCR. *Am J Physiol Renal Physiol*. 2002;282(3):F492-500.

21. Scherzer P, Katalan S, Got G, Pizov G, Londono I, Gal-Moscovici A, et al. Psammomys obesus, a particularly important animal model for the study of the human diabetic nephropathy. *Anat Cell Biol*. 2011;44(3):176-85.

22. Hostetter TH, Troy JL, Brenner BM. Glomerular hemodynamics in experimental diabetes mellitus. *Kidney Int*. 1981;19(3):410-5.

23. Hostetter TH, Rennke HG, Brenner BM. The case of intrarenal hypertension in the initiation and progression of diabetic and other glomerulopathies. *Am J Med*. 1982;72(3):375-80.

24. Hostetter TH, Rennke HG and Brenner BM. Compensatory renal hemodynamic injury: a final common pathway of residual nephron destruction. *Am J Kidney Dis*. 1982;1(5):310-4.

25. Béroniade VC, Lefebvre R, Falardeau P. Unilateral nodular diabetic glomerulosclerosis: recurrence of an experiment of nature. *Am J Nephrol*. 1987;7(1):55-9.

26. Mauer SM, Steffes MW, Azar S, Sandberg SK, Brown DM. The effect of Goldblatt hypertension on development of the glomerular lesion of diabetes mellitus in the rat. *Diabetes*. 1978;27(7):738-44.

27. Moriya T, Tsuchiya A, Okizaki S, Hayashi A, Tanaka K, Shichiri M. Glomerular hyperfiltration and increased glomerular filtration surface are associated with renal function decline in normo- and microalbuminuric type 2 diabetes. *Kidney Int*. 2012;81(5):486-93.

28. Christensen PK, Hansen HP, Parving HH. Impaired autoregulation of GFR in hypertensive non-insulin dependent diabetic patients. *Kidney Int*. 1997;52(5):1369-74.

29. Guyton AC. Renal function curve–a key to understanding the pathogenesis of hypertension. *Hypertension*. 1987;10(1):1-6.

30. Mogensen CE, Christensen CK. Blood pressure changes and renal function in incipient and overt diabetic nephropathy. *Hypertension*. 1985;7(6 Pt 2):1164-73.

31. Viberti GC, Earle K. Predisposition to essential hypertension and the development of diabetic nephropathy. *J Am Soc Nephrol.* 1992;3(4 Suppl):S27-33.

32. Dillon JJ. The quantitative relationship between treated between treated blood pressure and a progression of diabetic kidney disease. *Am J Kidney Dis.* 1993;22(6):798-802.

33. Bohlender JM, Franke S, Stein G, Wolf G. Advanced glycation end products and the kidney. *Am J Physiol Renal Physiol.* 2005;289(4):F645-59.

34. Yang CW, Vlassara H, Peten EP, He CJ, Striker GE, Striker LJ. Advanced glycation end products up-regulate gene expression found in diabetic glomerular disease. *Proc Natl Acad Sci USA.* 1994;91(20):9436-40.

35. Wendt TM, Tanji N, Guo J, Kislinger TR, Qu W, Lu Y, et al. RAGE drives the development of glomerulosclerosis and implicates podocyte activation in the pathogenesis of diabetic nephropathy. *Am J Pathol.* 2003;162(4):1123-37.

36. Chung ACK, Zhank H, Kong YZ, Tan JJ, Huang XR, Kopp JB, et al. Advanced glycation end-products induce tubular CTGF via TGF-beta-Independent Smad3 signaling. *J Am Soc Nephrol.* 2010;21(2):249-60.

37. Casarini DE. Upregulation of intrarenal angiotensinogen in diabetes. *Hypertens Res.* 2010;33(11):1106-7.

38. Lo CS, Liu F, Shi Y, Maachi H, Chenier I, Godin N, et al. Dual RAS blockade normalizes angiotensin-converting enzyme-2 expression and prevents hypertension and tubular apoptosis in Akita angiotensinogen-transgenic mice. *Am J Physiol Renal Physiol.* 2012; 302(7):F840-52.

39. Carey RM, Siragy HM. The intrarenal renin-angiotensin system and diabetic nephropathy. *Trends Endocrinol Metab.* 2003;14(6):274-81.

40. Singh R, Singh AK, Alavi N, Leehey DJ. Mechanism of increased angiotensin II levels in glomerular mesangial cells cultured in high glucose. *J Am Soc Nephrol.* 2003;14(4):873-80.

41. Vidotti DB, Casarini DE, Cristovam PC, Leite CA, Schor N, Boim MA. High glucose concentration stimulates intracellular renin activity and angiotensin II generation in rat mesangial cells. *Am J Physiol Renal Physiol.* 2004;286(6):F1039-45.

42. Yoo TH, Li JJ, Kim JJ, Jung DS, Kwak SJ, Ryu DR, et al. Activation of the renin-angiotensin system within podocytes in diabetes. *Kidney Int.* 2007;71(10):1019-27.

43. Müller DN, Luft FC. Direct renin inhibition with aliskiren in hypertension and target organ damage. *Clin J Am Soc Nephrol.* 2006;1(12):221-8.

44. Nguyen G, Delarue F, Burckle C, Bouzhir L, Giller T, Sraer JD. Pivotal role of the renin/prorenin receptor in angiotensin II production and cellular responses to renin. *J Clin Invest.* 2002;109(11):1417-27.

45. Véniant M, Ménard J, Bruneval P, et al. Vascular damage without hypertension in transgenic rats expressing prorenin exclusively in the liver. *J Clin Invest.* 1996;98(9): 1966-70.

46. Yuan W, Pan W, Kong J, Zheng W, Szeto FL, Wong KE, et al. 1,25-dihydroxyvitamin D3 suppresses renin gene transcription by blocking the activity of the cyclic AMP response element in the renin gene promoter. *J Biol Chem.* 2007;282(41):29821-30.

47. Deb DK, Chen Y, Zhang Z, Zhang Y, Szeto FL, Wong KE, et al. 1,25-Dihydroxyvitamin D3 suppresses high glucose-induced angiotensinogen expression in kidney cells by blocking the NF-{kappa}B pathway. *Am J Physiol Renal Physiol.* 2009;296(5):F1212-8.

48. Deb DK, Sun T, Wong KE, Zhang Z, Ning G, Zhang Y, et al. Combined vitamin D analog and AT1 receptor antagonists synergistically block the development of kidney disease in a model of type 2 diabetes. *Kidney Int.* 2010;77(11):1000-9.

49. Rüster C, Wolf G. Renin-angiotensin-aldosterone system and progression of renal disease. *J Am Soc Nephrol*. 2006;17(11):2985-91.

50. Bomback AS, Kshiragar AV, Amamoo MA, Klemmer PJ. Change in proteinuria after adding aldosterone blockers to ACE inhibitors or angiotensin receptor blockers in CKD: a systematic review. *Am J Kidney Dis*. 2008;51(2):199-211.

51. Xue C, Siragy HM. Local renal aldosterone system and its regulation by salt, diabetes, and angiotensin II type 1 receptor. *Hypertension*. 2005;46(3):584-90.

52. Lee SH, Yoo TH, Nam BY, Kim DK, Li JJ, Jung DS, et al. Activation of local aldosterone system within podocytes is involved in apoptosis under diabetic conditions. *Am J Physiol Renal Physiol*. 2009;297(5):F1381-90.

53. Brem AS, Morris DJ, Gong R. Aldosterone-induced fibrosis in kidney: questions and controversies. *Am J Kidney Dis*. 2011;58(3):471-9.

54. Yoshida H, Kuriyama S, Atsumi Y, Tomonari H, Mitarai T, Hamaguchi A, et al. Angiotensin I converting enzyme gene polymorphism in non-insulin dependent diabetes mellitus. *Kidney Int*. 1996;50(2):657-64.

55. Kuramoto N, Iizuka T, Ito H, Yagui K, Omura M, Nozaki O, et al. Effect of ACE gene on diabetic nephropathy in NIDDM patients with insulin resistance. *Am J Kidney Dis*. 1999; 33(2):276-81.

56. Kunz R, Bork JP, Fritsche L, Ringel J, Sharma AM. Association between the angiotensin converting enzyme-insertion/deletion polymorphism and diabetic nephropathy: a methodologic appraisal and systematic review. *J Am Soc Nephrol*. 1998;9(9):1653-63.

57. Pettersson-Ferenholm K, Frojdo S, Fagerudd J, Thomas MC, Forsblom C, Wessman M, et al. The AT2 gene may have a gender-specific effect on kidney function and pulse pressure in type 1 diabetic patients. *Kidney Int*. 2006;69(10):1880-4.

58. Shah VO, Scavini M, Nikolic J, Sun Y, Vai S, Griffith JK, et al. Z-2 microsattelite allele is linked to increased expression of the aldose reductases gene in diabetic nephropathy. *J Clin Endocrinol Metab*. 1998;83(8):2886-91.

59. Osternholm AM, He B, Pitkaniemi J, Albinsson L, Berg T, Sarti C, et al. Genome-wide scan for type 1 diabetic nephropathy in the Finnish population reveals suggestive linkage to a single locus on chromosome 3q. *Kidney Int*. 2007;71(2):140-5.

60. Ziyadeh FN, Wolf G. Pathogenesis of the podocypathy and proteinuria in diabetic glomerulopathy. *Curr Diabetes Rev*. 2008;4(1):39-45.

61. Diez-Sampedro A, Lenz O, Fornoni A. Pancytopathy in diabetes: a metabolic and endocrine disorder. *Am J Kidney Dis*. 2011;58(4):637-46.

62. Najafian B, Alpers CE, Fogo AB. Pathology of human diabetic nephropathy. *Contrib Nephrol*. 2011;170:36-47.

63. Weil EJ, Lemley KV, Yee B, Lovato T, Richardson M, Myers BD, et al. Podocyte detachment in type 2 diabetic nephropathy. *Am J Nephrol*. 2011;33 Suppl 1:21-4.

64. Welsh GI, Hale LJ, Eremina V, Jeansson M, Maezawa Y, Lennon R, et al. Insulin signaling to the glomerular podocyte is critical for normal kidney function. *Cell Metab*. 2010;12(4): 329-34.

65. Doublier S, Salvidio G, Lupia E, Ruotsalainen V, Verzola D, Deferrari G, et al. Nephrin expression is reduced in human diabetic nephropathy: evidence for a distinct role of glycated albumin and angiotensin II. *Diabetes*. 2003;52(4):1023-30.

66. Tervaert TW, Mooyaart AL, Amann K, Cohen AH, Cook HT, Drachenberg CB, et al. Pathologic classification of diabetic nephropathy. *J Am Soc Nephrol*. 2010;21(4):556-63.

67. Steffes MW, Brown DM, Basgen JM, Mauer SM. Amelioration of mesangial volume and surface alteration following islet transplantation in diabetic rats. *Diabetes*. 1980;29(7): 509-15.

68. Lee CS, Mauer SM, Brown DM, Southerland DE, Michael AF, Najarian JS. Renal transplantation in diabetes mellitus in rats. *J Exp Med*. 1974;139(4):793-800.

69. Abouna GM, Al-Adnani MS, Kremer GD, Kumar SA, Daddah SK, Kusma G. Reversal of diabetic nephropathy in human cadaveric kidneys after transplantation into non-diabetic recipients. *Lancet*. 1983;2(8362):1274-6.

70. Perkins BA, Ficociello LH, Silva KH, Finkelstein DM, Warram JH, Krolewski AS. Regression of microalbuminuria in type 1 diabetes. *N Engl J Med*. 2003;348(23):2285-93.

71. Van Stralen KJ, Stel VS, Reitsma JB, Dekker FW, Zoccali C, Jager KJ. Diagnostic methods I: sensitivity, specificity and other measures of accuracy. *Kidney Int*. 2009;75(12):1257-63.

72. Perkins BA, Ficociello LH, Roshan B, Warram JH, Krolewski AS. In patients with type 1 diabetes and new-onset microalbuminuria the development of advanced chronic kidney disease may not require progression to proteinuria. *Kidney Int*. 2010;77(1):57-64.

73. Araki S, Haneda M, Sugimoto T, Isono M, Isshiki K, Kashigawi A, et al. Factors associated with frequent remission of microalbuminuria in patients with type 2 diabetes. *Diabetes*. 2005;54(10):2983-7.

74. Retnakaran R, Cull CA, Thorn KI, Adler AI, Holman RR. Risk factors for renal dysfunction in type 2 diabetes. U.K. Prospective Diabetes Study 74. *Diabetes*. 2006;55(6):1832-9.

75. Budhiraja P, Popovtzer M. Diabetic glomerular lesions in type 2 diabetics with renal insufficiency and normoalbuminuria. *Nephrology Dialysis and Transplantation Plus*. 2011;4(Suppl 2):4s2.1-4s2.9.

76. Ritz E, Orth SR. Nephropathy in patients with type 2 diabetes mellitus. *N Engl J Med*. 1999; 341(15):1127-33.

77. Gall M, Nielsen FS, Smidt UM, Parving HH. The course of kidney function in type 2 (non-insulin-dependent) diabetic patients with diabetic nephropathy. *Diabetologia*. 1993;36(10):1071-8.

78. USRDS. (1999). Annual Data Report. Chapter 5. Patient mortality and survival. [online] Avaiable from: http://www.usrds.org/chapters/ch05.pdf [Accessed July, 2013].

79. USRDS. (1999). Annual Data Report. Chapter 7. Renal transplantation: access and outcomes. [online] Available from: http://www.usrds.org/chapters/ch07.pdf [Accessed July, 2013].

80. Keith DS, Nichols GA, Gullion CM, Brown JB, Smith DH. Longitudinal follow-up and outcomes among a population with chronic kidney disease in a large managed care organization. *Arch Intern Med*. 2004;164(6):659-63.

81. Adler AI, Stevens RJ, Manley SE, Bilous RW, Cull CA, Holman RR. Development and progression of nephropathy in type 2 diabetes: the United Kingdom Prospective Diabetes Study (UKPDS 64). *Kidney Int*. 2003;63(1):225-32.

82. Packham DK, Alves TP, Dwyer JP, Atkins R, de Zeeuw, Cooper M, et al. Relative incidence of ESRD versus cardiovascular mortality in proteinuric type 2 diabetes and nephropathy: results from DIAMETRIC (Diabetes Mellitus Treatment for Renal Insufficiency Consortium) database. *Am J Kidney Dis*. 2012;59(1):75-83.

83. Mogensen CE. Progression of nephropathy in long-term diabetics with proteinuria and effect of initial anti-hypertensive treatment. *Scand J Clin Lab Invest*. 1976;36(4):383-8.

84. Mogensen CE. Antihypertensive treatment inhibiting the progression of diabetic nephropathy. *Acta Endocrinol Suppl (Copenh)*. 1980;238:103-8.

85. Mogensen CE. Long-term antihypertensive treatment inhibiting progression of diabetic nephropathy. *Br Med J (Clin Res Ed)*. 1982;285(6343):685-8.

86. Parving HH, Smidt UM, Hommel E, Mathiesen ER, Rossing P, Nielsen F, et al. Effective antihypertensive treatment postpones renal insufficiency in diabetic nephropathy. *Am J Kidney Dis*. 1993;22(1):188-95.

87. Lewis EJ, Hunsicker LG, Bain RP, Rhode RD. The effect of angiotensin-converting-enzyme inhibition on diabetic nephropathy. The Collaborative Study Group. *N Engl J Med.* 1993; 329(20):1456-62.

88. Lewis EJ, Hunsicker LG, Clarke WR, Berl T, Pohl MA, Lewis JB, et al. Renopretective effect of the angiotensin receptor antagonist irbesartan in patients with nephropathy due to type 2 diabetes. *N Engl J Med.* 2001;345(12):851-60.

89. Brenner BM, Cooper ME, de Zeeuw D, Keane WF, Mitch WE, Parving HH, et al. Effects of losartan on renal and cardiovascular outcomes in patients with type 2 diabetes and nephropathy. *N Engl J Med.* 2001;345(12):861-9.

90. Mann JF, Schmieder RE, McQueen M, Dyal L, Schumacher H, Pogue J, et al. Renal outcomes with telmisartan, ramipril, or both, in people at high vascular risk (the ONTARGET Study): a multicentre, randomized, double blind, controlled trial. *Lancet.* 2008;372(9638):547-53.

91. Effects of ramipril on cardiovascular and microvascular outcomes in people with diabetes mellitus: results of the HOPE study and MICRO-HOPE substudy. Heart Outcomes Prevention Evaluation Study Investigators. *Lancet.* 2000;355(9200):253-9.

92. de Galan BE, Perkovic V, Ninomiya T, Pillai A, Patel A, Cass A, et al. Lowering blood pressure reduces renal events in type 2 diabetes. *J Am Soc Nephrol.* 2009;20(4):883-92.

93. Mancia G, De Backer G, Dominiczak A, Cifkova R, Fagard R, Germano G, et al. 2007 ESH-ESC practice guidelines for the management of arterial hypertension: ESH-ESC Task Force on the Management of Arterial Hypertension. *J Hypertens.* 2007;25(9):1751-62.

94. American Diabetes Association. Standards of medical care in diabetes–2008. *Diabetes Care.* 2008;31(Suppl 1):S12-54.

95. Chobanian AV, Bakris GL, Black HR, Cushman WC, Green LA, Izzo JL, et al. Seventh report of the Joint National Committee on Prevention, Detection, Evaluation, and Treatment of High Blood Pressure. *Hypertension.* 2003;42(6):1206-52.

96. Bakris GL, Williams M, Dworkin L, Elliott WJ, Epstein M, Toto R, et al. Preserving renal function in adults with hypertension and diabetes: a consensus approach. National Kidney Foundation Hypertension and Diabetes Executive Committee Working Group. *Am J Kidney Dis.* 2000;36(3):646-61.

97. Casas JP, Chua W, Loukogeorgakis S, Vallance P, Smeeth L, Hingorani AD, et al. Effects of inhibitors of the rennin-angiotensin system and other antihypertensive drugs on renal outcomes: systematic review and meta-analysis. *Lancet.* 2005;366(9502):2026-33.

98. Vejakama P, Thakkinstian A, Lertrattananon D, Ingsathit A, Ngarmukos C, Attia J. Reno-protective effects of renin-angiotensin system blockade in type 2 diabetic patients: a systematic review and network meta-analysis. *Diabetologia.* 2012;55(3):566-78.

99. Zhang MZ, Wang S, Yang S, Yang H, Fan X, Takahashi T, et al. Role of blood pressure and renin-angiotensin system in development of diabetic nephropathy (DN) in eNOS-/- db/ db mice. *Am J Physiol Renal Physiol.* 2012;302(4):F433-8.

100. Mauer M, Zinman B, Gardiner R, Suissa S, Sinaiko A, Strand T, et al. Renal and retinal effects of enalapril and losartan in type 1 diabetes. *N Engl J Med.* 2009;361(1):40-51.

101. Bilous R, Chaturvedi N, Sjolie AK, Fuller J, Klein R, Orchard T, et al. Effects of candesartan on microalbuminuria and albumin excretion rate in diabetes. three randomized trials. *Ann Intern Med.* 2009;151(1):11-20.

102. Desai A. Hyperkalemia associated with inhibitors of the renin-angiotensin-aldosterone system: balancing risk and benefit. *Circulation.* 2008;118(16):1609-11.

103. Takaichi K, Takemoto F, Ubara Y, Mori Y. Analysis of factors causing hyperkalemia. *Intern Med.* 2007;46(12):823-9.

104. Miao Y, Dobre D, Heerspink HJ, Brenner BM, Cooper ME, Parving HH, et al. Increased serum potassium affects renal outcomes: a post hoc analysis of the Reduction of Endpoints in NIDDM with the Angiotensin II Antagonist Losartan (RENAAL) trial. *Diabetologia.* 2011;54(1):44-50.

105. Mehdi UF, Adams-Huet B, Raskin B, Vega GL, Toto RD. Addition of angiotensin receptor blockade or mineralocorticoid antagonism to maximal angiotensin–converting enzyme inhibition in diabetic nephropathy. *J Am Soc Nephrol.* 2009;20(12):2641-50.

106. Navaneethan SD, Nigwekar SU, Seghal AR, Strippoli GF. Aldosterone antagonist for preventing progression of chronic kidney disease: a systematic review and meta-analysis. *Clin J Am Soc Nephrol.* 2009;4(3):542-51.

107. The Diabetes Control and Complications Trial Research Group. The effect of intensive treatment of diabetes on the development and progression of long-term complications in insulin dependent diabetes mellitus. *N Engl J Med.* 1993;329(14):977-86.

108. DCCT/EDIC Research Group, de Boer IH, Sun W, Cleary PA, Lachin JM, Molitch ME, et al. Intensive diabetes therapy and glomerular filtration rate in type 1 diabetes. *N Engl J Med.* 2011;365(25):2366-76.

109. UK Prospective Diabetes Study (UKPDS) Group. Intensive blood-glucose control with sulfonylureas or insulin compared with conventional treatment and risk of complications in patients with type 2 diabetes (UKPDS 33). *Lancet.* 1998;352(9131):837-53.

110. ADVANCE Collaborative Group, Patel A, MacMahon S, Chalmers J, Neal B, Billot L, et al. Intensive blood glucose control and vascular outcomes in patients with type 2 diabetes. *N Engl J Med.* 2008;358(24):2560-72.

111. Duckworth W, Abraira C, Moritz T, Reda D, Emanuele N, Reaven PD, et al. Glucose control and vascular complications in veterans with type 2 diabetes. *N Engl J Med.* 2009; 360(2):129-39.

112. Gaede P, Lund-Andersen H, Parving HH, Pedersen O. Effect of multifactorial intervention on mortality in type 2 diabetes. *N Engl J Med.* 2008;358(6):580-91.

113. Action to Control Cardiovascular Risk in Diabetes Study Group, Gerstein HC, Miller ME, Byington RP, Goff DC, Bigger JT, et al. Effects of intensive glucose lowering in type 2 diabetes. *N Engl J Med.* 2008;358(24):2545-59.

114. ACCORD Study Group, Gerstein HC, Miller ME, Genuth S, Ismail-Beigi F, Buse JB, et al. Long-term effects of intensive glucose lowering on cardiovascular outcomes. *N Engl J Med.* 2011;364(9):818-28.

115. Ismail-Beigi F. Action to Control Cardiovascular Risk in Diabetes (ACCORD) trial—clinical implications. *Clin Chem.* 2011;57(2):261-3.

116. Siegel D, Swislocki AL. The ACCORD Study: the devil is in the details. *Metab Syndr Relat Disord.* 2011;9(2):81-4.

117. Ismail-Beigi F, Craven TE, O'Connor PJ, Karl D, Calles-Escandon J, Hramiak I, et al. Combined intensive blood pressure and glycemic control does not produce and additive benefit on microvascular outcomes in type 2 diabetic patients. *Kidney Int.* 2012;81(6): 586-94.

118. Fabris B, Jackson B, Johnston CI. Salt blocks the renal benefits of ramipril in diabetic hypertensive rats. *Hypertension.* 1991;17(4):497-503.

119. Allen TJ, Waldron MJ, Casley D, Jerums G, Cooper ME. Salt restriction reduces hyper-filtration, renal enlargement, and albuminuria in experimental diabetes. *Diabetes.* 1997; 46(1):19-24.

120. Krikken JA, Laverman GD, Navis G. Benefits of sodium restriction in the management of chronic kidney disease. *Curr Opin Nephrol Hypertens.* 2009;18(6):531-8.

121. Vegter S, Perna A, Postma MJ, Navis G, Remuzzi G, Ruggenenti P. Sodium intake, ACE inhibition, and progression to ESRD. *J Am Soc Nephrol.* 2012;23(1):165-73.

122. Houlihan CA, Allen TJ, Baxter Al, Panangiotopoulos S, Casley DJ, Cooper ME, et al. A low-sodium diet potentiates the effects of losartan in type 2 diabetes. *Diabetes Care.* 2002;25(4):663-71.

123. de Zeeuw D, Agarval R, Amdahl M, Audhya P, Coyne D, Garimella T, et al. Selective vitamin D receptor activation with paricalcitol for reduction of albuminuria in patients with type 2 diabetes (VITAL study): a randomized controlled trial. *Lancet.* 2010;376(9752):1543-51.

124. Kim MJ, Frankel AH, Donaldson M, Darch SJ, Pusey CD, Hill PD, et al. Oral cholecalciferol decreases albuminuria and urinary TGF-beata-1 in patients with type 2 diabetic nephropathy on established renin-angiotensin-aldosterone system inhibition. *Kidney Int.* 2011;80(8):851-60.

125. Tang SC, Leung JC, Chan LY, Tsang AW, Lai KN. Activation of tubular epithelial cells in diabetic nephropathy and the role of peroxisome proliferator-activated receptor-gamma agonist. *J Am Soc Nephrol.* 2006;17(6):1633-43.

126. Imano E, Kanda T, Nakatani Y, Nishida T, Arai K, Motomura M, et al. Effect of troglitazone on microalbuminuria in patients with incipient diabetic nephropathy. *Diabetes Care.* 1998;21(12):2135-9.

127. Agarwal R, Saha C, Battiwala M, Vasavada N, Curley T, Chase SD, et al. A pilot randomized controlled trial of renal protection with pioglitazone in diabetic nephropathy. *Kidney Int.* 2005;68(1):285-92.

128. Bakris GL, Ruilope LM, McMorn SO, Weston WM, Heise MA, Freed MI, et al. Rosiglitazone reduces microalbuminuria and blood pressure independently of glycemia in type 2 diabetes patients with microalbuminuria. *J Hypertens.* 2006;24(10):2047-55.

129. de Boer IH, Sibley SD, Kestenbaum B, Sampson JN, Young B, Cleary PA, et al. Central obesity, incident microalbuminuria, and change in creatinine clearance in the epidemiology of diabetes interventions and complications study. *J Am Soc Nephrol.* 2007; 18(1):235-43.

130. Morales E, Valero MA, Leon M, Hernández E, Praga M. Beneficial effects of weight loss in overweight patients with chronic proteinuric nephropathies. *Am J Kidney Dis.* 2003; 41(2):319-27.

131. Saiki A, Nagayama D, Ohhira M, Endoh K, Ohtsuka M, Koide N, et al. Effect of weight loss using formula diet on renal function in obese patients with diabetic nephropathy. *Int J Obes (Lond).* 2005;29(9):1115-20.

132. United States Renal Data System. Excerpts from the USRDS 2009 annual data report: Atlas of end-stage renal disease in United States. *Am J Kidney Dis.* 2010;55(Suppl 1) S1.

133. United States Renal Data System. Excerpts from the USRDS 2005 annual data report: Atlas of end-stage renal disease in the United States. *Am J kidney Dis.* 2006;47(Suppl):S1.

134. Dikow R, Ritz E. Cardiovascular complications in the diabetic patient with renal disease: an update in 2003. *Nephrol Dial Transplant.* 2003;18(10):1993-8.

135. Khauli RB, Steinmuller DR, Novick AC, Buszta C, Goormastic M, Nakamoto S, et al. A critical look at survival of diabetics with end-stage renal disease. Transplantation versus dialysis therapy. *Transplantation.* 1986;41(5):598-602.

136. National Kidney Foundation. K/DOQI clinical practice guidelines for chronic kidney disease: evaluation, classification and stratification. *Am J Kidney Dis.* 2002;39(2 Suppl 1): S1-266.

137. Palder SB, Kirkman RL, Whittemore AD, Hakim RM, Lazarus JM, Tilney NL. Vascular access for hemodialysis patency rates and results of revision. *Ann Surg.* 1985;202(9):235-9.

138. Shideman JR, Buselmeier TJ, Kjellstrand CM. Hemodialysis in diabetics: complications in insulin-dependent patients accepted for renal transplantation. *Arch Intern Med.* 1976; 136(10):1126-30.

139. Shoji T, Tsubakihara Y, Fujii M, Imai E. Hemodialysis-associated hypotension as an independent risk factor for two-year mortality in hemodialysis patients. *Kidney Int.* 2004; 66(3):1212-20.

140. Daugirdas JT. Dialysis hypotension: a hemodynamic analysis. *Kidney Int.* 1991;39(2): 223-46.

141. Ritz E, Strumpf C, Katz F, Wing AJ, Quellhorst E. Hypertension and cardiovascular risk factors in hemodialyzed diabetic patients. *Hypertension.* 1985;7(6 Pt 2):II118-24.

142. Dorhout Mees EJ. Rise in blood pressure during hemodialysis-ultrafiltration: a "paradoxical" phenomenon? *Int J Artif Organs.* 1996;19(10):569-70.

143. Ifudu O. Diabetics manifest excess weight gain on maintenance hemodialysis. *Am Soc Artif Intern Organs.* 1991;38:85.

144. Jones R, Poston L, Hinestrosa H, Parsons V, Williams R. Weight gain between dialysis in diabetics: possible significance of raised intracellular sodium content. *Br Med J.* 1980; 280(6208):153.

145. Kimmel PL, Varela MP, Peterson RA, Weihs KL, Simmens SJ, Alleyne S, et al. Interdialytic weight gain and survival in hemodialysis patients: effects of duration of ESRD and diabetes mellitus. *Kidney Int.* 2000;57(3):1141-51.

146. Levin ME. Saving the diabetic foot. *Med Times.* 1980;108(5):56-64.

147. Lehto S, Rönnemaa T, Pyörälä K, Laakso M. Risk factors predicting lower extremity amputation in patients with NIDDM. *Diabetes Care.* 1996;19(6):607-13.

148. Vincenti F, Arnaud SB, Recker R, Genant H, Amend WJ, Feduska NJ, et al. Parathyroid and bone response of the diabetics to uremia. *Kidney Int.* 1984;25(4):677-82.

149. Popovtzer MM. Disorders of calcium, phosphorus, vitamin D, and parathyroid hormone activity. In: Schrier RW (Ed). Renal and Electrolyte Disorders, 7th edition. Philadelphia: Wolters Kluwer/Lippincott Williams & Wilkins; 2010. p. 220.

150. Pichaiwong W, Hudkins KL, Wietecha T, Nguyen TQ, Tachaudomdach C, Li W, et al. Reversibility of structural and functional damage in a model of advanced diabetic nephropathy. *J Am Soc Nephrol.* 2013;24(7):1088-102.

Management of Heart Failure in Diabetic Patients

Ryan K Crisel, Sanjiv J Shah

ABSTRACT

Heart failure (HF), defined as the inability of the heart to provide sufficient cardiac output to the body's tissues while maintaining normal filling pressures, can be further categorized as HF with preserved ejection fraction (HFpEF, previously termed diastolic HF) or HF with reduced ejection fraction (HFrEF; otherwise known as systolic HF). Diabetes mellitus is a major risk factor for HF, and contributes to HF through three central pathways: (1) diabetes is a major risk factor for coronary artery disease (CAD), which can lead to ischemic cardiomyopathy; (2) diabetes is often associated with other comorbidities, such as hypertension (HTN), obesity, and chronic kidney disease, all of which are known to be major HF risk factors; and (3) diabetes can cause direct myocardial toxicity (diabetic cardiomyopathy) which can occur in the absence of documented CAD or HTN. The significance of diabetes as a HF risk factor was highlighted in the HF staging system presented in the American College of Cardiology (ACC)/American Heart Association (AHA) guidelines for the management of chronic HF. The ACC/AHA guidelines argue that diabetes is such a potent risk factor for HF that it is a form of "pre-HF", and active efforts should be undertaken in diabetes to prevent the development of HF.

In this chapter, authors review (1) the epidemiology and early recognition of HF in diabetes; (2) the risks diabetes poses to the cardiovascular system, and how these changes relate to HF; (3) common HF syndromes that occur in diabetes patients; (4) the treatment of HF in diabetes (including pharmacologic and surgical options); and (5) summarize the important effects of HF therapies on diabetes and the effects of diabetes medications on HF.

OVERVIEW

Heart failure (HF), defined as the inability of the heart to provide sufficient cardiac output to the body tissues while maintaining normal filling pressures,[1] can be further categorized as HF with preserved ejection fraction (HFpEF, previously termed diastolic HF) or HF with reduced ejection fraction (HFrEF, otherwise known as systolic HF).[2] HF was originally thought to be a primary renal sodium and fluid retention syndrome, but with the advent of cardiac imaging techniques, HF was subsequently characterized by left ventricular (LV) systolic dysfunction, and a reduced EF was thought to be an essential diagnostic criteria. In the 1970s and 1980s, the occurrence of the HF syndrome in patients with preserved LVEF (HFpEF) was recognized,[3] and is now known to be the more common and increasingly prevalent form of HF, and a significant cause of morbidity and mortality.[4,5]

Diabetes mellitus is a major risk factor for HF and contributes to HF through three central pathways: (1) it is a major risk factor for coronary artery disease (CAD), which can lead to ischemic cardiomyopathy; (2) it is often associated with other comorbidities, such as hypertension (HTN), obesity, and chronic kidney disease (CKD), all of which are known to be major HF risk factors; and (3) it can cause direct myocardial toxicity (diabetic cardiomyopathy),[6] which can occur in the absence of documented CAD or HTN. The significance of diabetes as a HF risk factor was highlighted in the HF staging system presented in the American College of Cardiology (ACC)/American Heart Association (AHA) guidelines for the management of chronic HF.[7] In the ACC/AHA HF staging system (Figure 1), presence of diabetes alone is categorized as "Stage A HF"

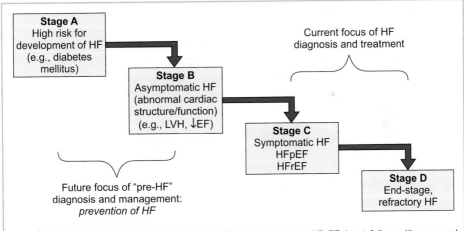

HF, heart failure; LVH, left ventricular hypertrophy; EF, ejection fraction; HFpEF, heart failure with preserved ejection fraction; HFrEF, heart failure with reduced ejection fraction.

FIGURE 1 The stages of heart failure. The staging system for heart failure was developed in 2006 as part of the American College of Cardiology/American Heart Association heart failure guidelines. The rationale behind the heart failure staging system is outlined in the Figure: the current focus of heart failure diagnosis and management (Stages C and D) occurs at a point in the HF syndrome when treatment is difficult, irreversible multiorgan damage has occurred, and the burden to the health care system and society is high. The future focus of heart failure should be the prevention of heart failure (i.e., Stages A and B). Diabetes is a major risk factor for HF and can be viewed as a form of "pre-heart failure". Thus, patients with diabetes with or without cardiac structural or functional abnormalities should be treated and monitored aggressively to prevent heart failure.

(the presence of a risk factor for HF). The ACC/AHA guidelines argue that diabetes is such a potent risk factor for HF that it is a form of "pre-HF", and active efforts should be undertaken in diabetes to prevent the development of HF.

In this chapter we describe (1) the epidemiology and early recognition of HF in diabetes; (2) the risks diabetes poses to the cardiovascular (CV) system and how these changes relate to HF; (3) common HF syndromes that occur in diabetes patients; (4) the treatment of HF in diabetes (including pharmacologic and surgical options); and (5) we summarize the important effects of HF therapies on diabetes and the effects of diabetes medications on HF.

EPIDEMIOLOGY OF HEART FAILURE IN DIABETIC PATIENTS

Data from the Framingham Study demonstrated the first well-established epidemiologic link between HF and diabetes. In diabetics, the risk of developing HF was 2.4-fold in men and 5-fold in women compared to age-matched controls.[8] The Cardiovascular Health Study also identified diabetes as an independent risk factor for HF in adults age >65 years, with a hazard ratio (HR) of 1.74 compared to non-diabetics.[9] Furthermore, large epidemiologic screening studies have demonstrated that LV systolic dysfunction is four times more prevalent in diabetics compared to nondiabetics.[10] Finally, although diabetes is a risk factor for HF in adults of all ages, the relationship between diabetes and HF is especially strong in the elderly. According to a study of patients enrolled in Medicare (age >65 years), the incidence of new HF in diabetics was 12.6% per year.[11] Other studies have confirmed that the risk of HF is alarmingly high in diabetics of all ages.[12,13] Table 1 outlines some key statistics summarizing the epidemiology of HF in patients with diabetes.

DIABETES AS A RISK FACTOR FOR HEART FAILURE

Diabetes is a multiorgan-system disease that often contributes to the development of clinical HF. In addition to the increased risk of developing incident (i.e., new-onset) HF,[14-16] the presence of diabetes appears to portend a worse prognosis in patients with

---

TABLE 1: Epidemiology of Heart Failure in Diabetic Patients

- Heart failure is twice as common in men with diabetes and five times as common in women with diabetes compared with age- and sex-matched individuals without diabetes
- The overall prevalence of diabetes (both type 1 and 2) in HF is approximately 20–25%
- The incidence of HF in diabetic patients over age 65 years is 12.6%/year
- Patients with diabetes have a nearly two-fold risk for HF hospitalization or death compared to those without diabetes
- A 1% rise in HbA1c is associated with a 12% increased risk of HF in elderly patients with diabetes

HF, heart failure, HbA1c, glycosylated hemoglobin.

previously diagnosed HF—the presence of diabetes is an independent risk factor for both HF hospitalization and mortality.[17]

Glycemic control appears to impact not only the risk of HF, but also the complications. In multiple reports, higher glycosylated hemoglobin (HbA1c) levels have been associated with progressively increased risk of HF.[18,19] This association between HbA1c and incident HF was also reported in type 1 diabetes.[20] Additionally, HF studies including both diabetic and nondiabetic patients found a direct correlation between fasting glucose and risk of HF hospitalization.[21] Diabetes is also a risk factor for hypercholesterolemia, HTN, and obesity. Adequate control of these risk factors via dietary measures and exercise could prevent HF, both directly and indirectly through the decrease in prevalence of CAD, which is described in detail below.

DIABETES AND CORONARY ARTERY DISEASE

Chronic ischemic heart disease is the most common cause of HF in the United States.[22] Diabetes accelerates atherosclerotic vascular events by approximately 15 years[23] and diabetics typically have more severe CAD at diagnosis[24] compared to nondiabetics. Thus, understanding the interaction of diabetes with CAD is of prime importance, given the synergy by which these two risk factors lead to incident HF and increase risk in patients with prevalent HF.

There have been multiple studies demonstrating the increased risk of myocardial infarction (MI) in diabetic patients.[25-27] Furthermore, diabetics with acute MI are more likely to present with more severe clinical manifestations, particularly pulmonary edema and HF, than are non-diabetics.[24,28,29] Diabetic patients with ST-elevation MI (STEMI) are more likely to develop HF and have a one-year mortality of 14.5% versus 9.8% in nondiabetics in the Global Utilization of Streptokinase and Tissue plasminogen activator for Occluded coronary arteries-1 (GUSTO-1) trial.[30] Of note, the GUSTO-1 trial was done in the era of thrombolysis, and the current pooled 1-year mortality for STEMI in the primary percutaneous coronary intervention (PCI) era is closer to 5%. A meta-analysis of 11 acute coronary syndrome (ACS) trials demonstrated a nearly 3-fold higher mortality for diabetics in both non-STEMI (NSTEMI) and STEMI. Additionally, the one-year mortality in diabetic patients with NSTEMI was approximately the same as a nondiabetic patient after a STEMI.[31] These data show that CAD is an important mediator of both acute and chronic HF in diabetics.

Several mechanisms may play roles in the increased risk of events in diabetic patients with CAD. In patients with diabetes who have an ACS, there is a greater frequency of other cardiac risk factors, hyperglycemia, inflammation, and a greater tendency toward thrombosis.[32,33] Diabetics commonly have persistent ST segment deviation despite having an open epicardial artery likely due to increased micro-vascular coronary dysfunction regardless of whether or not they are revascularized.[34] In addition to these factors, platelets in diabetic patients have increased reactivity and adhesion.[35] As such, the traditional antiplatelet agents used in CAD are less effective in diabetics.[36] Aspirin has an attenuated effect on platelets in diabetics,[37] and a Danish study found that diabetics benefited less from dual-antiplatelet therapy (aspirin plus clopidogrel) than nondiabetics.[38] More potent antiplatelet therapies (e.g., prasugrel and ticagrelor) have demonstrated a significant advantage over clopidogrel in ACS, and in diabetics, these drugs have been associated with better or similar outcomes when compared to nondiabetics.[39,40]

Mechanical coronary revascularization also has differential effects in diabetics. Revascularization as it relates to HF is primarily of two forms: revascularization after an ACS and revascularization of CAD that is contributing to HF. Early invasive revascularization has become the standard of care for patients with ACS of both NSTEMI and STEMI types. However, data over the past decade suggest the benefits of early revascularization after MI appears to be significantly diminished in diabetic patients.[41] The explanation of this difference is likely multifactorial and includes both the diabetic resistance to traditional antiplatelet therapies as well as the higher prevalence of diffuse CAD in diabetics. The method of revascularization of severe CAD in diabetics has long been a topic of study. In patients with diabetes, early trials of PCI versus coronary artery bypass grafting (CABG) demonstrated increased revascularization rates in the PCI arm but no mortality benefit for either.[42,43] The SYNergy between percutaneous coronary intervention with TAXus and cardiac surgery (SYNTAX) trial was the first to demonstrate the importance of the anatomic features of CAD and the role they play in treatment with PCI versus CABG by showing that the worse and more complex the CAD, the more likely CABG will be beneficial over PCI in diabetics.[44] The recently published Future REvascularization Evaluation in patients with Diabetes mellitus: optimal management of Multivessel disease (FREEDOM) randomized controlled trial extended these findings by showing that in diabetic patients with diffuse, three-vessel disease CABG was associated with lower mortality compared to PCI with first-generation drug eluting stents, whereas risk of stroke was slightly higher in the CABG group.[45]

Based on the data summarized above, diabetes is a major risk factor for CAD, and is associated with worse outcomes in the ACS setting (both of which are associated with increased risk for HF and worse HF-associated outcomes). Thus, diabetics should be treated aggressively to prevent CAD, and once present, CAD should be treated aggressively in order to prevent HF. The latest data suggests that in patients with multi-vessel CAD (the ones most likely to develop HF),[46] CABG is the preferred revascularization strategy.

DIAGNOSING HEART FAILURE IN THE DIABETIC PATIENT

Signs and symptoms of HF in the diabetic patient are largely similar to that of nondiabetics. However, since patients with diabetes are at higher risk for developing HF, clinicians who care for patients with diabetes should have a high index of suspicion for the HF syndrome. The earliest, albeit least specific symptom of HF is often fatigue. This is usually followed by symptoms due to elevated LV end-diastolic pressure (LVEDP) which leads to elevated left atrial and pulmonary venous pressure, paroxysmal nocturnal dyspnea (PND), orthopnea, and dyspnea. Signs of elevated LVEDP, which may or may not be present in the individual patient include rales, cardiac wheezes, and S3 and S4 heart sounds. Signs and symptoms of elevated right ventricular (RV) end-diastolic pressure include elevated jugular venous pressure, lower extremity edema, abdominal bloating due to ascites, early satiety, and right upper quadrant pain due to hepatic congestion. HF can also cause low cardiac output with symptoms of exercise intolerance (due to inability to augment cardiac output with activity), hypotension, and cool extremities. Besides symptoms and signs of HF, natriuretic peptides, specifically B-type natriuretic peptide (BNP) and N-terminal pro-BNP (NT-proBNP) are widely available biomarkers for HF screening and diagnosis. BNP is secreted from ventricular myocytes under stress and correlate with elevated cardiac filling pressures. A study in diabetic patients found that BNP was useful as a screening test for LV dysfunction.[47] When elevated, BNP and NT-proBNP levels point to a high likelihood of some type of cardiac dysfunction; however, normal values of these biomarkers, while associated with lower likelihood of HF, cannot fully exclude HF (especially in obese patients in whom natriuretic peptide levels may be low due to decreased production and enhanced clearance).[48]

The distinction between HFpEF and HFrEF is important when evaluating the diabetic patient with suspected HF. Compared to HFrEF, nearly all patients with HFpEF will typically have signs and symptoms due to elevated cardiac filling pressures and will only occasionally have signs and symptoms of decreased cardiac output at rest (although most HFpEF patients will have reduced ability to augment cardiac output with exercise).[49] Patients with HFrEF also usually have signs and symptoms of elevated cardiac filling pressures; however, low output syndromes in HFrEF are much more common than in HFpEF. Despite these differences in HFpEF and HFrEF, it is often difficult to distinguish the two entities by history, physical examination, electrocardiography, and chest radiography; thus, differentiating between the two and making a diagnosis of the sub-type of HF requires cardiac imaging (i.e., documentation of LVEF).[50]

Whereas the diagnosis of HFrEF simply requires the presence of HF symptoms and signs along with a reduced LVEF, the definitive diagnosis of HFpEF is much more challenging.[3] HFpEF is a heterogeneous syndrome that can occur both with and without significant LV diastolic dysfunction.[51] Furthermore, echocardiography, which is the most frequent test used to diagnose diastolic dysfunction, provides reliable information about impaired LV relaxation and elevated LV filling pressures, but is less able to provide insight into LV diastolic compliance. Finally, detailed echocardiographic studies have shown that despite a normal global LVEF, longitudinal systolic function is impaired in patients with HFpEF[52] and in patients with diabetes.[53] Thus, although the difference in LVEF clearly separates HFpEF from HFrEF, the distinction between HFpEF and HFrEF pathophysiology is not as concrete as previously recognized, which is not surprising given the tight coupling of myocyte calcium handling in systole and diastole.

For practical purposes, it is still important to make the clinical distinction between HFrEF and HFpEF, because management differs by sub-type of HF. Although HFpEF is a heterogeneous syndrome, it can be typically diagnosed using the following criteria: (1) signs and symptoms of HF; (2) documentation of normal or near-normal LV ejection fraction (EF >50%); and (3) evidence of elevated LV filling pressure [increased E/e' ratio on echocardiography (a noninvasive marker of LV filling pressure); elevated BNP or NT-proBNP; or elevated LVEDP or pulmonary capillary wedge pressure (measured invasively during cardiac catheterization)]. In our practice, we have found that patients require only one of the three criteria for evidence of elevated LV filling pressures. Although both BNP and NT-proBNP are very helpful for ruling in the HF syndrome, a normal BNP does not exclude HFpEF, especially in the outpatient setting.[54]

DIABETIC CARDIOMYOPATHY

Diabetic cardiomyopathy was first reported as a separate clinical entity in 1972 in a description of four patients who had diabetic glomerulosclerosis and LV failure with no other identifiable cause.[55] This association has now been supported by numerous epidemiologic studies.[56-58] These studies often focused on myocardial stiffness and hypertrophy in diabetics without demonstrable HTN. Hyperglycemia is considered to be a central driver in the pathophysiology of diabetic cardiomyopathy because it can trigger several maladaptive cardiac responses. Among these maladaptive responses are cytokine and renin-angiotensin-aldosterone system (RAAS) activation, free fatty acid metabolism disturbances, increased rate of apoptosis, fibrotic tissue deposition, and microvascular coronary dysfunction.[59-62] These pathologic alterations result in increased myocardial stiffness and may result in ventricular systolic dysfunction as well.

There are two important components in the clinical diagnosis of diabetic cardiomyopathy: the detection of myocardial abnormalities and the exclusion of other contributory causes of cardiomyopathy. Clinically, diabetic cardiomyopathy presents with signs and symptoms similar to other causes of HF as described above. However, diabetic cardiomyopathy is often subclinical for many years. In these cases, cardiac imaging is paramount. LV hypertrophy and evidence of diastolic dysfunction are hallmark changes on echocardiography in diabetic cardiomyopathy.[63] In cases of early diabetic cardiomyopathy, newer echocardiographic techniques, such as strain imaging (especially using speckle-tracking echocardiography) and diastolic stress testing (quantification of diastolic function at rest and peak exercise) have been used to increase the sensitivity for diagnosis but have yet to be implemented into regular clinical practice.[64,65] Cardiac magnetic resonance imaging (MRI) has also demonstrated utility in early diagnosis by demonstrating early focal cardiac fibrosis via late gadolinium enhancement.[66]

There is no specific treatment for diabetic cardiomyopathy other than treatment of underlying diabetes and HF. Strict glycemic control has demonstrated some mechanistic benefit in the early asymptomatic period of diabetic cardiomyopathy;[67,68] however, impact on clinical end-points once patients develop symptomatic HF have been disappointing.[69] Additionally, strict glycemic control in type 1 diabetes has been associated with a significant delay in the development (and possibly prevention) of diabetic cardiomyopathy.[70] Some studies have evaluated different antidiabetic medication regimens and found that clinical outcomes in diabetic patients with HF were better in groups treated with metformin.[71,72] Notably, this association was not present when a thiazolidinedione was added to this group of patients,[73-75] as will be discussed in more detail below. Treatment of patients with diabetic cardiomyopathy and symptomatic systolic dysfunction (HFrEF) should follow the ACC/AHA guidelines on treatment.[76] More detailed discussion on specific HFrEF and HFpEF treatment will be discussed below.

CARDIORENAL SYNDROME

Cardiorenal syndrome (CRS) in patients with HF is now recognized as an independent predictor of mortality, and one systematic review found that mortality increased by approximately 15% for every 10 mL/min reduction in estimated glomerular filtration rate (GFR).[77] CV and renal disease are involved in a complex relationship of a bidirectional association of kidney disease leading to CV disease and vice versa. Given the multiorgan nature of diabetes, it is important to assess its impact on cardio-renal interaction. The exact cause of CRS is not known but is likely multifactorial. The proposed pathophysiology is activation of the RAAS leading to vasoconstriction and sodium retention. This in turn leads to decreased renal perfusion and ischemia. These hormonal changes, as well as an acute or chronic elevation in renal venous pressure leading to a decreased perfusion pressure (especially in patients with low systemic blood pressure), are the most well-studied mechanisms.[78,79]

Heart failure and CKD are intimately associated. The prevalence of CKD, defined by a GFR less than 60 mL/min, is approximately 40% in HF. Furthermore, CKD has repeatedly been demonstrated as a poor prognostic indicator in HF with one recent study reporting a doubling of the mortality rate.[77] Additionally, CKD is a very common comorbidity in acute decompensated HF (ADHF): 30% of ADHF patients have a serum creatinine greater than 2.0 mg/dL and only 9% of ADHF patients have a normal GFR (>90 mL/min).[80] There is a significantly increased risk for CKD in diabetes; however there have been no prominent studies stratifying the incidence of CRS in diabetics with HF. Acute CRS, defined as acute worsening of renal function (an increase in serum creatinine by 0.3 mg/dL) during admission for ADHF occurs in 20–30% of admitted patients.[81-83] Diabetes has been recognized as one of the central risk factors for acute CRS in ADHF,[84,85] but there have been no studies on the impact of diabetes control on the incidence of acute CRS.

The treatment of CRS in diabetes is similar to the treatment of CRS in general. Improvement in cardiac function with resultant improvement in forward cardiac output has been associated with improved GFR.[86] Diuretics and ultrafiltration have a variable effect on short-term improvements in renal function in patients with acute CRS but do not affect long-term outcomes.[87–89] Dopamine has demonstrated an increased renal blood flow that is out of proportion to the increase in cardiac output, though most of these data are in animal studies.[90] The Dopamine in Acute Decompensated Heart Failure (DAD-HF) trial in patients with ADHF found that the combination of dopamine 5 µg/kg/min plus low-dose furosemide (5 mg/hour via continuous infusion) produced similar urine output as high-dose furosemide (20 mg/hour) with a reduced incidence of worsening of serum creatinine (>0.3 mg/dL).[91] These data have not yet been shown to have any effect on hard clinical endpoints and the combination of loop diuretic and dopamine infusion is not commonly used in the clinical setting. Finally, two investigational therapies antagonizing the vasopressin receptor 2 and the adenosine A1 receptor have been studied in acute CRS. Neither of these therapies had an impact on outcomes in CRS.[92,93]

Cardiorenal syndrome remains an elusive, complex clinical entity. Diabetes clearly increases the risk for development of acute CRS and likely often plays a role in CKD, which in turn increases the risk of development of HF. However, despite multiple studies into potential treatment strategies, only those that directly affect the forward cardiac output have ever had a sustainable effect on CRS. Unfortunately, there have been no studies demonstrating diabetic management has any role in preventing or resolving CRS.

PHARMACOLOGIC TREATMENT OF HEART FAILURE IN DIABETES

As discussed above, in general and in patients with diabetes, pharmacologic treatment of HF differs by the presence or preserved versus reduced LVEF. The following sections discuss the general treatment strategies for HFrEF and HFpEF, with a particular emphasis on the evidence for treatment options in diabetic patients.

Heart Failure with Reduced Ejection Fraction

Treatment of HFrEF in diabetic patients is similar to treatment of nondiabetic patients with HFrEF. No trial to date has included only diabetic patients with HFrEF. The pillar of treatment of symptomatic HFrEF is attenuation of the neurohormal pathway with blockade at multiple different sites. This can be achieved with beta-blockers and inhibition of the RAAS.

Beta-Blockers

In the past, there have been concerns that beta-blockers may be harmful to diabetics due to a blunting of the protective adrenergic response to hypoglycemia, despite the lack of compelling evidence of such a reaction. A review conducted in Australia demonstrated that HF patients with diabetes were less likely to receive a beta-blocker at discharge than their nondiabetic counterparts.[94] The CIBIS-II, MERIT-HF, COPERNICUS, and US Carvedilol Heart Failure Study randomized trials all demonstrated significant mortality benefits associated with beta-blocker use in diabetics with symptomatic HFrEF.[95-99] A meta-analysis of the six largest beta-blocker trials including 1,883 diabetics and 7,042 nondiabetics concluded that there was a significant survival benefit in the diabetic subgroup [relative risk (RR = 0.77)] though it was slightly lower than that of nondiabetics (RR = 0.65).[100] Based on these results, beta-blockers should be considered in all patients with stable HFrEF. Current ACC/AHA guidelines recommend carvedilol, metoprolol succinate (once daily, long-acting metoprolol), or bisoprolol as these three medications have the most robust data supporting their use in HFrEF.[76] As described below, of these agents, there may be added benefit with the use of carvedilol (especially over metoprolol) in diabetics.

Angiotensin Converting Enzyme Inhibitors

In a meta-analysis of six angiotensin converting enzyme inhibitor (ACEI) trials of patients with HFrEF, there was a significant reduction in mortality that was similar in diabetic and nondiabetic patients (RR = 0.85 and 0.84, respectively).[100] Similarly, in a community-based observational study of older patients hospitalized with HF, the prescription of ACEI at hospital discharge was associated with lower mortality at one year in patients with and without diabetes.[101]

Angiotensin converting enzyme inhibitor use in diabetics not only provides beneficial effect on CV outcomes, but has also demonstrated efficacy in renal protection and proteinuria in diabetes.[102] Thus, ACEI should be considered in all diabetic patients with symptomatic HFrEF. Often, ACEI are not started due to significant renal dysfunction. It has been demonstrated that with proper monitoring, ACEI therapy can be used safely in patients with advanced CKD.[103] Regardless, caution is advised given the fact that patients with diabetes and renal dysfunction can have renal tubular acidosis type IV, which increases the risk of hyperkalemia with concomitant ACEI therapy.

Angiotensin Receptor Blockers

Angiotensin receptor blockers (ARBs) provide an alternative to ACEI for antagonism of the renin-angiotensin system. The most common reason to change from ACEI to ARB is chronic cough, which occurs in approximately 10% of patients on chronic ACEI therapy. The cough associated with ACEI therapy results from accumulation of bradykinin.[104] The Val-HeFT (using valsartan) and candesartan in heart failure—assessment of reduction in mortality and morbidity (CHARM using candesartan) trials demonstrated significant mortality and morbidity benefit in patients with and without diabetes treated with either ARB.[105,106] A recent analysis of the Losartan Intervention For Endpoint (LIFE) and Reduction of Endpoints in non-insulin dependent diabetes mellitus (NIDDM) with the Angiotensin II Antagonist Losartan (RENAAL) clinical trials found losartan significantly reduced the incidence of first hospitalization for HF in patients without prior HF events.[14] Current HF guidelines recommend using ARBs in HFrEF if an ACEI is not tolerated due to intractable cough.

Aldosterone Antagonists

The initial trial demonstrating the ability of an aldosterone antagonist (spironolactone) to reduce mortality in severe HFrEF [New York Heart Association (NYHA) class III or IV HF] was the Randomized Aldactone Evaluation Study (RALES) trial.[107] A major criticism of the RALES trial is that it was done at a time prior standard beta-blocker use in HFrEF (indeed, the proportion of study patients on beta-blockers was 10% and 11% in the placebo and spironolactone groups, respectively, while ACEI use was greater than 90%). In addition, there have been no published diabetes subgroup analyses in RALES. The Eplerenone Post–Acute Myocardial Infarction Heart Failure Efficacy and Survival Study (EPHESUS) and Eplerenone in Patients with Systolic Heart Failure and Mild Symptoms (EMPHASIS-HF) trials evaluated the aldosterone antagonist eplerenone in HFrEF. Both trials were novel in that EPHESUS specifically included patients immediately post-MI, and EMPHASIS-HF included patients with mildly or moderately symptomatic (NYHA II or III) HF.[108,109] Both trials showed a mortality benefit associated with eplerenone use. Currently, the ACC/AHA guidelines recommend addition of an aldosterone antagonist in severely symptomatic patients (NYHA class III or IV) on optimal medical therapy with serum creatinine less than 2–2.5 mg/dL and serum potassium less than 5 mEq/L. However, based on the recently published EMPHASIS-HF trial this recommendation will likely be broadened to include NYHA class II patients. As with ACEIs and ARBs, diabetic patients on aldosterone antagonists must be monitored very closely for hyperkalemia given the high prevalence of type IV renal tubular acidosis and significant CKD (both of which increase the risk of hyperkalemia) in diabetics.

Heart Failure with Preserved Ejection Fraction

To date, most clinical trials specifically targeting HFpEF have been disappointing, as no pharmacologic treatment trials have shown a benefit in hard outcomes. Thus treatment of HFpEF remains largely empiric. The ACC/AHA HF guidelines state that treatment of HFpEF should focus on four main points: (1) control of systemic HTN; (2) control of ventricular rate in patients with atrial arrhythmias; (3) coronary revascularization in patients whom ischemia is thought to be playing a significant role in the pathophysiology of HFpEF; and (4) relief of congestive symptoms using loop and/or thiazide diuretics and/or nitrates.[76] The management of HFpEF in the diabetic patient is not different; however, the increased incidence of CAD, HTN, and atrial arrhythmias in diabetics often makes control of these entities vitally important in diabetic patients with HFpEF.

Management of Hypertension

Hypertension is extremely common in HFpEF, and often requires treatment with multiple antihypertensive agents. Treatment of HTN with carvedilol, an ACEI, and a thiazide diuretic (such as, chlorthalidone), along with optimization of fluid status with judicious use of loop diuretics, will result in adequate treatment of blood pressure in the majority of HFpEF patients. LV hypertrophy (LVH) is strongly associated with HFpEF. ARBs cause LVH to regress to a greater degree than other antihypertensive medications,[110] and regression of LVH using ARBs appears to improve diastolic function.[111] Despite the significant circumstantial data, ARBs have not demonstrated statistically significant reductions in HF hospitalization or death in two large randomized clinical trials of patients with HFpEF, [CHARM-Preserved and irbesartan in heart failure with preserved systolic function (I-PRESERVE)].[112,113]

Management of Heart Rate, Atrial Arrhythmias, and Beta-Blockers

In the past, it was thought that in patients with HFpEF (i.e., diastolic HF), slowing the heart rate would improve symptoms by increasing diastolic filling time, thereby allowing for improved emptying of the left atrium, resulting in decreased congestion and improved cardiac output. However, it is now known that the dynamics of heart rate and diastolic function in HFpEF are more complex.

The HFpEF patients who will likely benefit the most from slow heart rates are those in whom most of LV filling occurs in late diastole (i.e., those with E/A reversal on mitral inflow, in which case the majority of filling occurs during atrial contraction). These are the patients in whom atrial arrhythmias are poorly tolerated. However, patients with more advanced cardiomyopathy (including patients with advanced diabetic cardiomyopathy) have a restrictive filling pattern on mitral inflow (i.e., E/A ratio ≥1.5) with severely reduced e' and a' tissue Doppler velocities, indicative of severely impaired relaxation, a stiff LV, and poor left atrial function. In these patients, most of LV filling occurs in early diastole, and cardiac output is dependent primarily on heart rate because stroke volume is fixed (i.e., these patients cannot augment stroke volume during exertion or stress). In these patients, and in those HFpEF patients with chronotropic incompetence,[114] slowing the heart rate can be detrimental; in fact, these types of HFpEF patients may require pacemaker placement in order to augment heart rate appropriately with exercise and maintain heart rates high enough to provide adequate cardiac output.[115]

Regardless of type of HFpEF, we advocate a trial of attempting restoration of normal sinus rhythm (through cardioversion or electrophysiologic ablation) in all patients with HFpEF who suffer from an atrial arrhythmia because organized atrial contraction helps promote left atrial emptying and augmentation of cardiac output.

Only one randomized trial has evaluated beta-blockers in HFpEF. The Study of Effects of Nebivolol Intervention on Outcomes and Rehospitalization in Seniors with Heart Failure (SENIORS) trial, which evaluated nebivolol in elderly HF patients (age ≥70 years) and included a proportion of patients with relatively preserved LVEF, showed that nebivolol provided the modest benefit, a finding that was not dependent on underlying LVEF.[116,117] However, a subsequent analysis of SENIORS found that the benefits of nebivolol were less pronounced in diabetic patients.[117] In the COHERE observational registry, carvedilol was shown to be beneficial as compared to other beta-blockers in patients with chronic HF, regardless of underlying LVEF.[118]

Anti-Ischemic Therapy

Relief of ischemia with either medication or mechanical revascularization (i.e., PCI or CABG) can be beneficial in patients with HFpEF by improving cardiac function through improved coronary blood flow. Although there is a lack of high quality data associating relief of ischemia with improved outcomes in HFpEF, subendocardial ischemia is an important contributor to both diastolic dysfunction and longitudinal systolic dysfunction.[52,119] Treatment options for ischemia in diabetics with HFpEF include beta-blockers, nitrates, calcium-channel blockers, ranolazine, or revascularization (either CABG or PCI). Ranolazine, an inhibitor of the late inward sodium current (I_{Na}), which is accentuated in the setting of ischemia, has been shown to be an effective antianginal therapy, and may also be directly beneficial to patients with diabetes.[120-122] For example, in the Metabolic Efficiency With Ranolazine for Less Ischemia in Non–ST-Elevation Acute Coronary Syndrome (MERLIN)- Thrombolysis in Myocardial Infarction (TIMI)-36 randomized controlled trial, treatment with ranolazine in patients with ACS, and poorly controlled diabetes (HbA1c 8–10% at time of randomization) was associated with improved fasting glucose and HbA1c.[123] The mechanism underlying the beneficial effects of ranolazine in diabetes is unknown, but may involve enhanced glucose-induced insulin secretion. In MERLIN-TIMI-36 trial, ACS patients with the highest levels of BNP (i.e., those with the highest LV filling pressures), were also benefitted the most from ranolazine.[124] Taken together, these data suggest that diabetic patients with CAD and HF may benefit the most from ranolazine therapy.

Angiotensin Converting Enzyme Inhibitors

No trials have convincingly demonstrated efficacy of ACEI or ARBs in HFpEF. The perindopril in elderly people with chronic heart failure (PEP-CHF) trial was a randomized placebo-controlled trial evaluating clinical outcomes of perindopril in 850 patients age ≥70 years with HFpEF. At 1-year follow-up, combined mortality or unexpected HF hospitalization in the perindopril and placebo arms was 8.0% versus 12.4%, respectively (HR 0.69; 95% CI 0.47–1.01).[125] Perindopril did improve secondary end-points (functional class and six-minute walk distance).

Two major ARB trials have been performed in HFpEF. The CHARM-Preserved trial evaluated candesartan versus placebo in patients with symptomatic HF with an EF greater than 40%. This trial nearly missed a statistically significant reduction in the combined end-point of HF hospitalization or CV mortality (22% vs. 24%; adjusted HR 0.86; 95% CI 0.74–1.00).[126] Interestingly, candesartan resulted in a 40% reduction in new diabetes in this trial of HFpEF patients. Irbesartan was the most recent ARB studied in a randomized controlled trial in HFpEF. The I-PRESERVE trial demonstrated no significant overall difference in all-cause mortality or CV hospitalization in HFpEF.[112] In the diabetic subgroup of I-PRESERVE (N = 1,134), 44% of the irbesartan-treated patients versus 48% of the placebo-treated patients (HR 0.88, 95% CI 0.74–1.04) reached the primary end-point (all-cause mortality or CV hospitalization).

Aldosterone Antagonists

Enrollment in the large, multicenter Treatment of Preserved Cardiac function heart failure with an Aldosterone anTagonist (TOPCAT) randomized controlled trial of spironolactone in HFpEF is complete, but follow-up is still ongoing.[127] Diabetes was present in 32% of all TOPCAT patients at baseline (N = 1,114); thus, TOPCAT will provide helpful outcome data for the use of spironolactone in diabetics with HFpEF. In the smaller Aldosterone Receptor Blockade in Diastolic Heart Failure (Aldo-DHF) trial, which enrolled a much healthier population compared to TOPCAT, spironolactone improved diastolic function and structural LV remodeling but did not improve capacity, NYHA class, or quality of life.

In summary, pharmacologic treatment of diabetics with HFpEF is challenging. Treatment typically revolves around managing comorbidities[128] (HTN, ischemia, atrial arrhythmias, etc.) in addition to treatment of fluid overload. To date, no trials of pharmacologic therapies have demonstrated improved outcomes in HFpEF.

SURGICAL TREATMENT OF HEART FAILURE IN DIABETES

Several surgical treatment options, including device-based therapies and cardiac transplantation, are available for patients with HFrEF.

Defibrillators

Implantable cardioverter-defibrillators (ICDs) are intended to terminate life-threatening ventricular arrhythmias and, therefore, sudden cardiac death (SCD). There are no specific recommendations in diabetics related to ICDs. ICD indications in diabetic patients with HF should follow the current ACC/AHA guidelines.[76] For primary prevention of SCD, ICD indications include: (1) post-MI with reduced LVEF regardless of presence of HF (date of MI but be >40 days ago, the patient should be on optimal medical therapy, and LVEF <30%); and (2) persistent reduced LVEF (<35%) in a patient with NYHA class II or III symptoms of HF on optimal medical therapy for at least three months. For secondary prevention of SCD and ICD indications include: (1) a prior episode of resuscitated ventricular tachycardia (VT)/ventricular fibrillation (VF) or sustained, hemodynamically unstable VT in whom a completely reversible cause cannot be identified and (2) patients with episodes of spontaneous sustained VT in the presence of heart disease.

The only consideration specific to diabetics would be the possibility of a slightly increased risk of device infection at the time of implantation. However, the risk of device infection should not preclude the placement of an ICD in a diabetic patient who meets indications; rather, diabetic patients who require ICD should undergo ICD placement by a physician who performs a high volume of ICD placement procedures, and preferably the physician and facility at which the ICD is placed should have a history of low complication rates.

Cardiac Resynchronization Therapy

Cardiac resynchronization therapy (CRT) reduces symptoms, improves LV function, and reduces mortality in many patients who have systolic HF with reduced LVEF (<30–35%) and prolonged QRS on electrocardiography. Most initial CRT studies had varying cut off values of minimum QRS duration (usually ≥120–140 ms) as well as LVEF lesser than 30–35% and NYHA class III or IV HF.[129] However, based on the totality of CRT data,[130,131] the recently revised Heart Failure Society of America (HFSA), CRT guidelines stated that CRT is most beneficial in HFrEF patients who have (1) normal sinus rhythm; (2) a QRS duration of greater than 150 ms (in the absence of right bundle branch block); (3) NYHA functional class II or III symptoms despite optimal medical management; and (4) severe LV systolic dysfunction (EF <30–35%). Although diabetes is associated with an increased risk of mortality in patients receiving CRT, the degree to which diabetics benefit from CRT appears to be similar to those without diabetes.[132,133]

Ventricular Assist Devices

Left ventricular-assist devices (LVADs) refer to mechanical circulatory support (MCS) systems that are implanted surgically (or percutaneously) for the chronic (or acute) support of the LV in the setting of Stage DHF. The science of MCS and the types of VADs are expanding rapidly in an attempt to keep up with the increasing volume of patients with HFrEF. The two most common chronic VADs currently in use in the United States are the HeartMate II and the HeartWare continuous flow pumps. The indications for LVAD therapy are similar to those for cardiac transplantation; however, VAD therapy may be appropriate for certain patients in whom cardiac transplantation may be contraindicated due to age or multiple comorbidities. Studies evaluating LVAD outcomes in patients with diabetes have found conflicting results (one study found increased mortality in diabetics compared to nondiabetics;[49] whereas another found similar mortality rates after LVAD placement but worse mortality in diabetics postcardiac transplantation[46]). Whereas the primary purpose of LVADs is to increase cardiac output and relieve congestion in patients with advanced HF, these devices may have noncardiac benefits as well. Indeed, in diabetics, a provocative study found that LVAD placement (with consequential increase in cardiac output) resulted in improved control of diabetes through mechanisms that have yet to be fully elucidated.[54]

Cardiac Transplantation

Cardiac transplantation offers substantial benefits to patients with end-stage HF.[134,135] However, the most recent guidelines from the International Society for Heart and Lung Transplantation (ISHLT), currently lists diabetes as a relative contraindication for orthotopic heart transplantation (OHT).[134] The appropriateness of OHT in diabetic patients remains controversial. One single-center study found that the incidence of acute rejection in the first year, allograft vasculopathy, and infection was similar in diabetics compared to nondiabetics.[136] A subsequent analysis of the United Network of Organ Sharing (UNOS) database found that while severe diabetes did impact survival post-OHT, well-selected patients with diabetes and minimal diabetes-related complications had a similar survival to those without diabetes.[137] In the same study, it was reported that the greater the number of diabetes-related complications pretransplant, the worse the post-transplant survival.[137] Another concern post-transplant has been worsening renal function in diabetics who are taking calcineurin inhibitors (e.g., cyclosporine and tacrolimus). However, another single-center retrospective study demonstrated that during three years of follow-up, there was no significant difference in the GFR between diabetics and nondiabetics taking calcineurin inhibitors.[138] It does appear likely that infection rates post-transplant are more likely in diabetics. Thus, at the present time, OHT should only be considered in highly selected diabetic patients who do not have multiple diabetes-related complications.

PRO-HEART FAILURE EFFECTS OF DIABETES MEDICATIONS

Thiazolidinediones

Thiazolidinediones (TZDs), which increase insulin sensitivity by activating the peroxisome proliferator-activated receptor-gamma (PPAR-gamma) receptor, have pleiotropic effects that are germane to the management of HF in diabetics. For example, PPAR-gamma receptors are present in the nephron, and treatment with TZDs can lead to sodium (and subsequent fluid) retention with worsening of edema.[139] The different TZDs (rosiglitazone and pioglitazone) appear to have different CV effects as demonstrated by multiple subgroup analyses of clinical trials of these agents. Rosiglitazone results in a significant increase in the risk of MI and, therefore, is no longer approved by the US Food and Drug Administration and the European Medicines Agency.[140]

Dyslipidemia is one mechanism proposed to link the use of rosiglitazone with increased risk for MI. A meta-analysis of TZD trials found that pioglitazone did not change low density lipoprotein (LDL) cholesterol levels (as opposed to rosiglitazone, which increased LDL) and it increased high density lipoprotein (HDL) by approximately 10% and resulted in mildly decreased triglycerides.[141] The PROactive trial found that pioglitazone was associated with a reduction in all-cause mortality,

MI (excluding silent MI), and stroke among patients at high risk for macrovascular events.[142] However, HF events were more common compared to placebo (16.0% vs. 11.5%, respectively). In a pooled analysis, peripheral edema occurs in 4–6% of patients on TZDs compared to 1–2% of placebo.[141] This effect appears to be especially common in the combination of insulin and TZDs. In fact, one study found that the frequency of symptomatic HF was 2.5 times higher with combination therapy with insulin and TZDs compared with insulin alone.[143]

In summary, TZDs have been associated with sodium and fluid retention and worsening of HF, especially when they are used in combination with insulin. Accordingly, the AHA and American Diabetes Association both recommend avoiding use of TZDs in NYHA class III or IV HF.[144]

Metformin

There are conflicting data and views on the use of metformin in HF. Historically, the primary concern has been an increased risk of lactic acidosis as a side effect of treatment with metformin in patients with prevalent HF. However, the risk of metformin-induced lactic acidosis is quite rare.[145] At least two studies have demonstrated the benefit and safety of metformin in HF,[74,146] and a Cochrane systematic review of all prospective studies evaluating metformin use in all patient populations found zero cases of fatal or nonfatal lactic acidosis in over 70,000 patient-years of data.[147] Given the available evidence, metformin can be safely used in diabetic patients with HF.

PRO-DIABETIC EFFECTS OF HEART FAILURE MEDICATIONS

Diuretics

Both loop and thiazide diuretics have been associated with an increase in fasting glucose, and thiazide diuretics have been associated with increased risk of developing type 2 diabetes.[148] However, the clinical significance of diuretic-induced hyperglycemia has been questioned, since subjects who had diabetes associated with chlorthalidone had no significant increase in CV events and had a better prognosis than did those who had preexisting diabetes.[149] In the doses typically used to treat HTN and fluid overload (e.g., hydrochlorothiazide or chlorthalidone 12.5–25 mg daily); there is minimal effect on fasting glucose.[150] The effect of diuretics on fasting glucose appears to be mediated by hypokalemia.[151,152] Each 0.5 mEq/L decrease in serum potassium is associated with a 45% higher risk of new diabetes. The mechanism of this association is a failure of potassium channels to close in response to rising plasma glucose concentrations, with a resultant decrease in insulin secretion. This close association of diuretic-induced hypokalemia leading to diabetes is substantiated by a small trial that demonstrated no effect on serum glucose if patients were given potassium replacement concomitantly with a thiazide diuretic.[153] Additionally, correcting serum hypokalemia appears to have a small further reduction in blood pressure.[154] Given the available evidence, it seems reasonable to continue the use of thiazide and loop diuretics for treatment of HTN or volume management in patients with diabetes, with the caveat that potassium should be monitored closely and supplemented as needed.

Beta-Blockers

As reviewed above, beta-blockers are a mainstay of therapy for patients with reduced LVEF (both in those with asymptomatic LV systolic dysfunction and in those with symptomatic HFrEF). However, these drugs must be used with caution in patients with diabetes and in those who are at risk for developing diabetes. This appears to be specific to certain types of beta-blockers and not an overall class effect.

Metoprolol has been associated with a modest worsening of glycemic control.[155,156] This effect appears to be mediated by detrimental effects primarily on insulin sensitivity.[157] Metoprolol has also been associated with an increased incidence of diabetes in patients who have not been diagnosed prior to the administration.[156] The epidemiologic Atherosclerosis Risk In Communities (ARIC) study found that beta-blockers therapy (but not carvedilol) was associated with a 28% increased risk of developing type 2 diabetes compared to no antihypertensive therapy. Interestingly, this relationship was not seen with thiazides, calcium-channel blockers, or ACEI. The Glycemic Effects in diabetes Mellitus: carvedilol-Metoprolol comparison In hypertensives (GEMINI) trial included 1,235 type 2 diabetes patients with HTN (>130/80 mmHg) randomized to carvedilol or metoprolol. After 5 months, the metoprolol group (compared to the carvedilol group) had a significantly higher HbA1c, reduced insulin sensitivity, higher rates of microalbuminuria, and had a higher rate of withdrawal from the trial due to worsened glycemic control. Unfortunately, the GEMINI trial was not powered to detect clinical events between the two groups. These data suggests that in diabetic patients, if a beta-blocker is necessary (i.e., LV systolic dysfunction or control of BP), carvedilol is the beta-blocker of choice.

The other major concern of beta-blocker use in diabetes is blunting the adrenergic surge in cases of significant hypoglycemia. However, it is now well accepted that this risk is most likely theoretical rather than clinically significant since no prior studies have demonstrated an association between beta-blocker use and worse clinical events in the setting of hypoglycemia.

CONCLUSIONS AND RECOMMENDATIONS

Diabetes is a highly morbid condition and relates to HF in multiple ways; thus, clinicians who care for diabetic patients should have a high index of suspicion for the presence of HF. Figure 2 summarizes the diagnostic and treatment algorithm for the prevention and management of HF in the diabetic patient, but several key points will be summarized here.

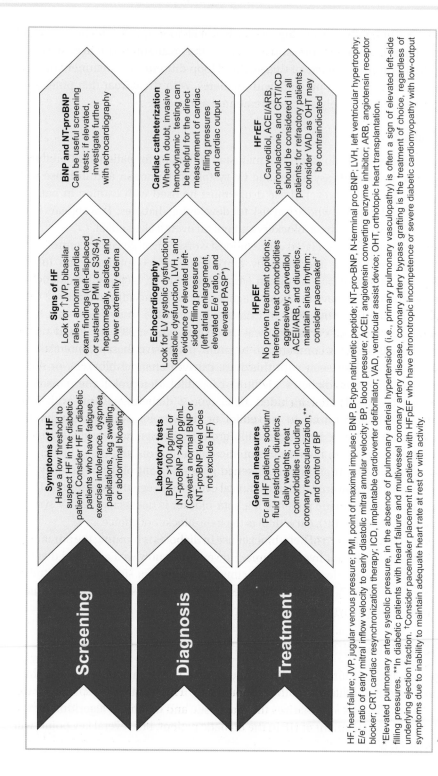

Screening

Symptoms of HF
Have a low threshold to suspect HF in the diabetic patient. Consider HF in diabetic patients who have fatigue, exercise intolerance, dyspnea, palpitations, leg swelling, or abdominal bloating

Signs of HF
Look for ↑JVP, bibasilar rales, abnormal cardiac exam findings (left-displaced or sustained PMI, or S3/S4), hepatomegaly, ascites, and lower extremity edema

BNP and NT-proBNP
Can be useful screening tests; if elevated, investigate further with echocardiography

Diagnosis

Laboratory tests
BNP >100 pg/mL or NT-proBNP >400 pg/mL (Caveat: a normal BNP or NT-proBNP level does not exclude HF)

Echocardiography
Look for LV systolic dysfunction, diastolic dysfunction, LVH, and evidence of elevated left-sided filling pressures (left atrial enlargement, elevated E/e′ ratio, and elevated PASP*)

Cardiac catheterization
When in doubt, invasive hemodynamic testing can be helpful for the direct measurement of cardiac filling pressures and cardiac output

Treatment

General measures
For all HF patients, sodium/fluid restriction, diuretics, daily weights; treat comorbidities including coronary revascularization,** and control of BP

HFpEF
No proven treatment options; therefore, treat comorbidities aggressively; carvedilol, ACEI/ARB, and diuretics, maintain sinus rhythm; consider pacemaker†

HFrEF
Carvedilol, ACEI/ARB, spironolactone, and CRT/ICD should be considered in all patients; for refractory patients, consider VAD as OHT may be contraindicated

HF, heart failure; JVP, jugular venous pressure; PMI, point of maximal impulse; BNP, B-type natriuretic peptide; NT-pro-BNP, N-terminal pro-BNP; LVH, left ventricular hypertrophy; E/e′, ratio of early mitral inflow velocity to early diastolic mitral annular velocity; BP, blood pressure; ACEI, angiotensin converting enzyme inhibitor; ARB, angiotensin receptor blocker; CRT, cardiac resynchronization therapy; ICD, implantable cardioverter defibrillator; VAD, ventricular assist device; OHT, orthotopic heart transplantation.

*Elevated pulmonary artery systolic pressure, in the absence of pulmonary arterial hypertension (i.e., primary pulmonary vasculopathy) is often a sign of elevated left-side filling pressures. **In diabetic patients with heart failure and multivessel coronary artery disease, coronary artery bypass grafting is the treatment of choice, regardless of underlying ejection fraction. †Consider pacemaker placement in patients with HFpEF who have chronotropic incompetence or severe diabetic cardiomyopathy with low-output symptoms due to inability to maintain adequate heart rate at rest or with activity.

FIGURE 2 Algorithm for the screening, diagnosis and treatment of heart failure in diabetes.

In diabetic patients with new or worsening dyspnea or exercise intolerance, the presence of HF should be suspected. Diabetes is a major risk factor for all forms of HF, including HFpEF and HFrEF, and patients with diabetes can develop a cardiomyopathy independent of the association of diabetes with risk factors, such as CAD, HTN, and obesity. Treatment of HF in diabetes includes (1) aggressive management of HF risk factors, especially CAD; (2) categorizing patients as having HFrEF versus HFpEF through the use of cardiac imaging and formulating a treatment plan appropriate to the type of HF; and (3) understanding the pro-HF risks of antidiabetic medications and the pro-diabetes effects of HF medications in order to tailor therapy adequately in the individual diabetic patient.

Specific pearls for treatment include: (1) consideration of newer anti-platelet agents (e.g., prasugrel and ticagrelor) in diabetic patients with ACS given their association with better outcomes in diabetes compared to clopidogrel; (2) a preference for treating multivessel CAD with CABG instead of PCI in the diabetic patient given the recent results of the FREEDOM trial; (3) the use of carvedilol instead of metoprolol when treating either HTN or HFrEF given its superiority over metoprolol in preventing worsening of diabetes; (4) cautious use of TZDs in diabetic HF patients given the propensity for sodium and fluid retention; and (5) the potential expanding utility of LVADs in diabetics with Stage D HFrEF given the difficulties with cardiac transplantation in diabetic patients, and the possibility that LVAD therapy is associated with improved control of diabetes in diabetic patients with advanced HF.

Given the dual epidemics of diabetes and HF, the need for clinicians to fully understand and recognize the interaction between diabetes and HF will continue to grow. Whether or not the development of novel therapeutic strategies for the prevention and treatment of HF in diabetic patients will also continue to grow remains to be seen.

REFERENCES

1. Denolin H, Kuhn H, Krayenbuehl HP, Loogen F, Reale A. The definition of heart failure. *Eur Heart J.* 1983;4(7):445-8.
2. Aurigemma GP. Diastolic heart failure—a common and lethal condition by any name. *N Engl J Med.* 2006;355(3):308-10.
3. Redfield MM. Heart failure with normal ejection fraction. In: Bonow RO, Mann DP, Zipes DL, Libby P, (Eds). Braunwald's Heart Disease - A Textbook of Cardiovascular Medicine, 9th edition. Philadelphia: Saunders; 2011. pp. 586-99.
4. Owan TE, Hodge DO, Herges RM, Jacobsen SJ, Roger VL, Redfield MM. Trends in prevalence and outcome of heart failure with preserved ejection fraction. *N Engl J Med.* 2006;355(3):251-9.
5. Steinberg BA, Zhao X, Heidenreich PA, Peterson ED, Bhatt DL, Cannon CP, et al. Trends in patients hospitalized with heart failure and preserved left ventricular ejection fraction: prevalence, therapies, and outcomes. *Circulation.* 2012;126(1):65-75.
6. Boudina S, Abel ED. Diabetic cardiomyopathy revisited. *Circulation.* 2007;115(25):3213-23.

7. Hunt SA, Abraham WT, Chin MH, Feldman AM, Francis GS, Ganiats TG, et al. ACC/AHA 2005 Guideline Update for the Diagnosis and Management of Chronic Heart Failure in the Adult: a report of the American College of Cardiology/American Heart Association Task Force on Practice Guidelines (Writing Committee to Update the 2001 Guidelines for the Evaluation and Management of Heart Failure): developed in collaboration with the American College of Chest Physicians and the International Society for Heart and Lung Transplantation: endorsed by the Heart Rhythm Society. *Circulation.* 2005; 112(12):e154-235.

8. Kannel WB, Hjortland M, Castelli WP. Role of diabetes in congestive heart failure: the Framingham study. *Am J Cardiol.* 1974;34(1):29-34.

9. Gottdiener JS, Arnold AM, Aurigemma GP, Polak JF, Tracy RP, Kitzman DW, et al. Predictors of congestive heart failure in the elderly: the Cardiovascular Health Study. *J Am Coll Cardiol.* 2000;35(6):1628-37.

10. Davies M, Hobbs F, Davis R, Kenkre J, Roalfe AK, Hare R, et al. Prevalence of left-ventricular systolic dysfunction and heart failure in the Echocardiographic Heart of England Screening study: a population based study. *Lancet.* 2001;358(9280):439-44.

11. Bertoni AG, Hundley WG, Massing MW, Bonds DE, Burke GL, Goff DC. Heart failure prevalence, incidence, and mortality in the elderly with diabetes. *Diabetes Care.* 2004; 27(3):699-703.

12. Thrainsdottir IS, Aspelund T, Thorgeirsson G, Gudnason V, Hardarson T, Malmberg K, et al. The association between glucose abnormalities and heart failure in the population-based Reykjavik study. *Diabetes Care.* 2005;28(3):612-6.

13. Amato L, Paolisso G, Cacciatore F, Ferrara N, Ferrara P, Canonico S, et al. Congestive heart failure predicts the development of non-insulin-dependent diabetes mellitus in the elderly. The Osservatorio Geriatrico Regione Campania Group. *Diabetes Metab.* 1997;23(3):213-8.

14. Carr AA, Kowey PR, Devereux RB, Brenner BM, Dahlof B, Ibsen H, et al. Hospitalizations for new heart failure among subjects with diabetes mellitus in the RENAAL and LIFE studies. *Am J Cardiol.* 2005;96(11):1530-6.

15. Mosterd A, Cost B, Hoes AW, de Bruijne MC, Deckers JW, Hofman A, et al. The prognosis of heart failure in the general population: The Rotterdam Study. *Eur Heart J.* 2001;22(15):1318-27.

16. Halon DA, Merdler A, Flugelman MY, Rennert HS, Weisz G, Shahla J, et al. Late-onset heart failure as a mechanism for adverse long-term outcome in diabetic patients undergoing revascularization (a 13-year report from the Lady Davis Carmel Medical Center registry). *Am J Cardiol.* 2000;85(12):1420-6.

17. Romero SP, Garcia-Egido A, Escobar MA, Andrey JL, Corzo R, Perez V, et al. Impact of new-onset diabetes mellitus and glycemic control on the prognosis of heart failure patients: A propensity-matched study in the community. *Int J Cardiol.* 2012. Epub ahead of print.

18. Erqou S, Lee CT, Suffoletto M, Echouffo-Tcheugui JB, de Boer RA, van Melle JP, et al. Association between glycated haemoglobin and the risk of congestive heart failure in diabetes mellitus: systematic review and meta-analysis. *Eur J Heart Fail.* 2013;15(2): 185-93.

19. Iribarren C, Karter AJ, Go AS, Ferrara A, Liu JY, Sidney S, et al. Glycemic control and heart failure among adult patients with diabetes. *Circulation.* 2001;103(22):2668-73.

20. Lind M, Bounias I, Olsson M, Gudbjornsdottir S, Svensson AM, Rosengren A. Glycaemic control and incidence of heart failure in 20,985 patients with type 1 diabetes: an observational study. *Lancet.* 2011;378(9786):140-6.

21. Held C, Gerstein HC, Yusuf S, Zhao F, Hilbrich L, Anderson C, et al. Glucose levels predict hospitalization for congestive heart failure in patients at high cardiovascular risk. *Circulation.* 2007;115(11):1371-5.

22. He J, Ogden LG, Bazzano LA, Vupputuri S, Loria C, Whelton PK. Risk factors for congestive heart failure in US men and women: NHANES I epidemiologic follow-up study. *Arch Intern Med.* 2001;161(7):996-1002.

23. Booth GL, Kapral MK, Fung K, Tu JV. Relation between age and cardiovascular disease in men and women with diabetes compared with non-diabetic people: a population-based retrospective cohort study. *Lancet.* 2006;368(9529):29-36.

24. Granger CB, Califf RM, Young S, Candela R, Samaha J, Worley S, et al. Outcome of patients with diabetes mellitus and acute myocardial infarction treated with thrombolytic agents. The Thrombolysis and Angioplasty in Myocardial Infarction (TAMI) Study Group. *J Am Coll Cardiol.* 1993;21(4):920-5.

25. Haffner SM, Lehto S, Ronnemaa T, Pyorala K, Laakso M. Mortality from coronary heart disease in subjects with type 2 diabetes and in nondiabetic subjects with and without prior myocardial infarction. *N Engl J Med.* 1998;339(4):229-34.

26. Gu K, Cowie CC, Harris MI. Diabetes and decline in heart disease mortality in US adults. *JAMA.* 1999;281(14):1291-7.

27. Yusuf S, Hawken S, Ounpuu S, Dans T, Avezum A, Lanas F, et al. Effect of potentially modifiable risk factors associated with myocardial infarction in 52 countries (the INTERHEART study): case-control study. *Lancet.* 2004;364(9438):937-52.

28. Stone PH, Muller JE, Hartwell T, York BJ, Rutherford JD, Parker CB, et al. The effect of diabetes mellitus on prognosis and serial left ventricular function after acute myocardial infarction: contribution of both coronary disease and diastolic left ventricular dysfunction to the adverse prognosis. The MILIS Study Group. *J Am Coll Cardiol.* 1989; 14(1):49-57.

29. Jaffe AS, Spadaro JJ, Schechtman K, Roberts R, Geltman EM, Sobel BE. Increased congestive heart failure after myocardial infarction of modest extent in patients with diabetes mellitus. *Am Heart J.* 1984;108(1):31-7.

30. Mak KH, Moliterno DJ, Granger CB, Miller DP, White HD, Wilcox RG, et al. Influence of diabetes mellitus on clinical outcome in the thrombolytic era of acute myocardial infarction. GUSTO-I Investigators. Global Utilization of Streptokinase and Tissue Plasminogen Activator for Occluded Coronary Arteries. *J Am Coll Cardiol.* 1997;30(1):171-9.

31. Donahoe SM, Stewart GC, McCabe CH, Mohanavelu S, Murphy SA, Cannon CP, et al. Diabetes and mortality following acute coronary syndromes. *JAMA.* 2007;298(5):765-75.

32. Angiolillo DJ. Antiplatelet therapy in type 2 diabetes mellitus. *Curr Opin Endocrinol Diabetes Obes.* 2007;14(2):124-31.

33. Sobel BE. Optimizing cardiovascular outcomes in diabetes mellitus. *Am J Med.* 2007;120 (9 Suppl 2):S3-11.

34. Timmer JR, van der Horst IC, de Luca G, Ottervanger JP, Hoorntje JC, de Boer MJ, et al. Comparison of myocardial perfusion after successful primary percutaneous coronary intervention in patients with ST-elevation myocardial infarction with versus without diabetes mellitus. Am J Cardiol. 2005;95(11):1375-7.

35. Ferroni P, Basili S, Falco A, Davi G. Platelet activation in type 2 diabetes mellitus. *J Thromb Haemost.* 2004;2(8):1282-91.

36. Ferreiro JL, Angiolillo DJ. Diabetes and antiplatelet therapy in acute coronary syndrome. *Circulation.* 2011;123(7):798-813.

37. Sacco M, Pellegrini F, Roncaglioni MC, Avanzini F, Tognoni G, Nicolucci A. Primary prevention of cardiovascular events with low-dose aspirin and vitamin E in type 2 diabetic patients: results of the Primary Prevention Project (PPP) trial. *Diabetes Care.* 2003;26(12):3264-72.

38. Andersson C, Lyngbaek S, Nguyen CD, Nielsen M, Gislason GH, Kober L, et al. Association of clopidogrel treatment with risk of mortality and cardiovascular events following myocardial infarction in patients with and without diabetes. *JAMA.* 2012;308(9):882-9.

39. Wiviott SD, Braunwald E, Angiolillo DJ, Meisel S, Dalby AJ, Verheugt FW, et al. Greater clinical benefit of more intensive oral antiplatelet therapy with prasugrel in patients with diabetes mellitus in the trial to assess improvement in therapeutic outcomes by optimizing platelet inhibition with prasugrel-Thrombolysis in Myocardial Infarction 38. *Circulation.* 2008;118(16):1626-36.

40. James S, Angiolillo DJ, Cornel JH, Erlinge D, Husted S, Kontny F, et al. Ticagrelor vs. clopidogrel in patients with acute coronary syndromes and diabetes: a substudy from the PLATelet inhibition and patient Outcomes (PLATO) trial. *Eur Heart J.* 2010;31(24):3006-16.

41. Cubbon RM, Wheatcroft SB, Grant PJ, Gale CP, Barth JH, Sapsford RJ, et al. Temporal trends in mortality of patients with diabetes mellitus suffering acute myocardial infarction: a comparison of over 3000 patients between 1995 and 2003. *Eur Heart J.* 2007;28(5):540-5.

42. Serruys PW, Unger F, Sousa JE, Jatene A, Bonnier HJ, Schonberger JP, et al. Comparison of coronary-artery bypass surgery and stenting for the treatment of multivessel disease. *N Engl J Med.* 2001;344(15):1117-24.

43. Sedlis SP, Morrison DA, Lorin JD, Esposito R, Sethi G, Sacks J, et al. Percutaneous coronary intervention versus coronary bypass graft surgery for diabetic patients with unstable angina and risk factors for adverse outcomes with bypass: outcome of diabetic patients in the AWESOME randomized trial and registry. *J Am Coll Cardiol.* 2002;40(9):1555-66.

44. Banning AP, Westaby S, Morice MC, Kappetein AP, Mohr FW, Berti S, et al. Diabetic and nondiabetic patients with left main and/or 3-vessel coronary artery disease: comparison of outcomes with cardiac surgery and paclitaxel-eluting stents. *J Am Coll Cardiol.* 2010;55(11):1067-75.

45. Farkouh ME, Domanski M, Sleeper LA, Siami FS, Dangas G, Mack M, et al. Strategies for Multivessel Revascularization in Patients with Diabetes. *N Engl J Med.* 2012;367(25):2375-84.

46. Topkara VK, Dang NC, Martens TP, Cheema FH, Liu JF, Liang LM, et al. Effect of diabetes on short- and long-term outcomes after left ventricular assist device implantation. *J Heart Lung Transplant.* 2005;24(12):2048-53.

47. Epshteyn V, Morrison K, Krishnaswamy P, Kazanegra R, Clopton P, Mudaliar S, et al. Utility of B-type natriuretic peptide (BNP) as a screen for left ventricular dysfunction in patients with diabetes. *Diabetes Care.* 2003;26(7):2081-7.

48. Clerico A, Giannoni A, Vittorini S, Emdin M. The paradox of low BNP levels in obesity. *Heart Fail Rev.* 2012;17(1):81-96.

49. Butler J, Howser R, Portner PM, Pierson RN, 3rd. Diabetes and outcomes after left ventricular assist device placement. *J Card Fail.* 2005;11(7):510-5.

50. Kitzman DW, Little WC, Brubaker PH, Anderson RT, Hundley WG, Marburger CT, et al. Pathophysiological characterization of isolated diastolic heart failure in comparison to systolic heart failure. *JAMA.* 2002;288(17):2144-50.

51. Bench T, Burkhoff D, O'Connell JB, Costanzo MR, Abraham WT, St John Sutton M, et al. Heart failure with normal ejection fraction: consideration of mechanisms other than diastolic dysfunction. *Curr Heart Fail Rep.* 2009;6(1):57-64.

52. Shah SJ. Evolving approaches to the management of heart failure with preserved ejection fraction in patients with coronary artery disease. *Curr Treat Options Cardiovasc Med.* 2010;12(1):58-75.

53. Fonseca CG, Dissanayake AM, Doughty RN, Whalley GA, Gamble GD, Cowan BR, et al. Three-dimensional assessment of left ventricular systolic strain in patients with type 2 diabetes mellitus, diastolic dysfunction, and normal ejection fraction. *Am J Cardiol.* 2004;94(11):1391-5.

54. Anjan VY, Loftus TM, Burke MA, Akhter N, Fonarow GC, Gheorghiade M, et al. Prevalence, clinical phenotype, and outcomes associated with normal B-type natriuretic Peptide levels in heart failure with preserved ejection fraction. *Am J Cardiol.* 2012;110(6):870-6.

55. Rubler S, Dlugash J, Yuceoglu YZ, Kumral T, Branwood AW, Grishman A. New type of cardiomyopathy associated with diabetic glomerulosclerosis. *Am J Cardiol.* 1972;30(6):595-602.

56. Devereux RB, Roman MJ, Paranicas M, O'Grady MJ, Lee ET, Welty TK, et al. Impact of diabetes on cardiac structure and function: the strong heart study. *Circulation.* 2000;101(19):2271-6.

57. Palmieri V, Bella JN, Arnett DK, Liu JE, Oberman A, Schuck MY, et al. Effect of type 2 diabetes mellitus on left ventricular geometry and systolic function in hypertensive subjects: Hypertension Genetic Epidemiology Network (HyperGEN) study. *Circulation.* 2001;103(1):102-7.

58. Rutter MK, Parise H, Benjamin EJ, Levy D, Larson MG, Meigs JB, et al. Impact of glucose intolerance and insulin resistance on cardiac structure and function: sex-related differences in the Framingham Heart Study. *Circulation.* 2003;107(3):448-54

59. Hattori Y, Kawasaki H, Abe K, Kanno M. Superoxide dismutase recovers altered endothelium-dependent relaxation in diabetic rat aorta. *Am J Physiol.* 1991;261 (4 Pt 2):H1086-94.

60. Fiordaliso F, Leri A, Cesselli D, Limana F, Safai B, Nadal-Ginard B, et al. Hyperglycemia activates p53 and p53-regulated genes leading to myocyte cell death. *Diabetes.* 2001;50(10):2363-75.

61. Rodrigues B, Cam MC, McNeill JH. Metabolic disturbances in diabetic cardiomyopathy. *Mol Cell Biochem.* 1998;180(1-2):53-7.

62. Frustaci A, Kajstura J, Chimenti C, Jakoniuk I, Leri A, Maseri A, et al. Myocardial cell death in human diabetes. *Circ Res.* 2000;87(12):1123-32.

63. Perez JE, McGill JB, Santiago JV, Schechtman KB, Waggoner AD, Miller JG, et al. Abnormal myocardial acoustic properties in diabetic patients and their correlation with the severity of disease. *J Am Coll Cardiol.* 1992;19(6):1154-62.

64. Ernande L, Bergerot C, Rietzschel ER, De Buyzere ML, Thibault H, Pignonblanc PG, et al. Diastolic dysfunction in patients with type 2 diabetes mellitus: is it really the first marker of diabetic cardiomyopathy? *J Am Soc Echocardiogr.* 2011;24(11):1268-75.

65. Ernande L, Rietzschel ER, Bergerot C, De Buyzere ML, Schnell F, Groisne L, et al. Impaired myocardial radial function in asymptomatic patients with type 2 diabetes mellitus: a speckle-tracking imaging study. *J Am Soc Echocardiogr.* 2010; 23(12):1266-72.

66. Kwong RY, Sattar H, Wu H, Vorobiof G, Gandla V, Steel K, et al. Incidence and prognostic implication of unrecognized myocardial scar characterized by cardiac magnetic resonance in diabetic patients without clinical evidence of myocardial infarction. *Circulation.* 2008;118(10):1011-20.

67. von Bibra H, Hansen A, Dounis V, Bystedt T, Malmberg K, Ryden L. Augmented metabolic control improves myocardial diastolic function and perfusion in patients with non-insulin dependent diabetes. *Heart.* 2004;90(12):1483-4.

68. von Bibra H, Siegmund T, Hansen A, Jensen J, Schumm-Draeger PM. [Augmentation of myocardial function by improved glycemic control in patients with type 2 diabetes mellitus]. *Dtsch Med Wochenschr.* 2007(14);132:729-34.

69. Turnbull FM, Abraira C, Anderson RJ, Byington RP, Chalmers JP, Duckworth WC, et al. Intensive glucose control and macrovascular outcomes in type 2 diabetes. *Diabetologia.* 2009;52(11):2288-98.

70. Konduracka E, Gackowski A, Rostoff P, Galicka-Latala D, Frasik W, Piwowarska W. Diabetes-specific cardiomyopathy in type 1 diabetes mellitus: no evidence for its occurrence in the era of intensive insulin therapy. *Eur Heart J.* 2007;28(20):2465-71.

71. Aguilar D, Chan W, Bozkurt B, Ramasubbu K, Deswal A. Metformin use and mortality in ambulatory patients with diabetes and heart failure. *Circ Heart Fail.* 2011;4(1):53-8.

72. Andersson C, Olesen JB, Hansen PR, Weeke P, Norgaard ML, Jorgensen CH, et al. Metformin treatment is associated with a low risk of mortality in diabetic patients with heart failure: a retrospective nationwide cohort study. *Diabetologia.* 2010;53(12):2546-53.

73. Tang WH, Francis GS, Hoogwerf BJ, Young JB. Fluid retention after initiation of thiazolidinedione therapy in diabetic patients with established chronic heart failure. *J Am Coll Cardiol.* 2003;41(8):1394-8.

74. Masoudi FA, Inzucchi SE, Wang Y, Havranek EP, Foody JM, Krumholz HM. Thiazolidinediones, metformin, and outcomes in older patients with diabetes and heart failure: an observational study. *Circulation.* 2005;111(5):583-90.

75. Aguilar D, Bozkurt B, Pritchett A, Petersen NJ, Deswal A. The impact of thiazolidinedione use on outcomes in ambulatory patients with diabetes mellitus and heart failure. *J Am Coll Cardiol.* 2007;50(1):32-6.

76. Hunt SA, Abraham WT, Chin MH, Feldman AM, Francis GS, Ganiats TG, et al. 2009 focused update incorporated into the ACC/AHA 2005 Guidelines for the Diagnosis and Management of Heart Failure in Adults: a report of the American College of Cardiology Foundation/American Heart Association Task Force on Practice Guidelines: developed in collaboration with the International Society for Heart and Lung Transplantation. *Circulation.* 2009;119(14):e391-479.

77. Smith GL, Lichtman JH, Bracken MB, Shlipak MG, Phillips CO, DiCapua P, et al. Renal impairment and outcomes in heart failure: systematic review and meta-analysis. *J Am Coll Cardiol.* 2006;47(10):1987-96.

78. Bock JS, Gottlieb SS. Cardiorenal syndrome: new perspectives. *Circulation.* 2010;121(23):2592-600.

79. Shamseddin MK, Parfrey PS. Mechanisms of the cardiorenal syndromes. *Nat Rev Nephrol.* 2009;5(11):641-9.

80. Heywood JT, Fonarow GC, Costanzo MR, Mathur VS, Wigneswaran JR, Wynne J. High prevalence of renal dysfunction and its impact on outcome in 118,465 patients hospitalized with acute decompensated heart failure: a report from the ADHERE database. *J Card Fail.* 2007;13(6):422-30.

81. Forman DE, Butler J, Wang Y, Abraham WT, O'Connor CM, Gottlieb SS, et al. Incidence, predictors at admission, and impact of worsening renal function among patients hospitalized with heart failure. *J Am Coll Cardiol.* 2004;43(1):61-7.

82. Smith GL, Vaccarino V, Kosiborod M, Lichtman JH, Cheng S, Watnick SG, et al. Worsening renal function: what is a clinically meaningful change in creatinine during hospitalization with heart failure? *J Card Fail.* 2003;9(1):13-25.

83. Damman K, Navis G, Voors AA, Asselbergs FW, Smilde TD, Cleland JG, et al. Worsening renal function and prognosis in heart failure: systematic review and meta-analysis. *J Card Fail.* 2007;13(8):599-608.

84. Krumholz HM, Chen YT, Vaccarino V, Wang Y, Radford MJ, Bradford WD, et al. Correlates and impact on outcomes of worsening renal function in patients > or = 65 years of age with heart failure. *Am J Cardiol.* 2000;85(9):1110-3.

85. Butler J, Forman DE, Abraham WT, Gottlieb SS, Loh E, Massie BM, et al. Relationship between heart failure treatment and development of worsening renal function among hospitalized patients. *Am Heart J.* 2004;147(2):331-8.

86. Boerrigter G, Costello-Boerrigter LC, Abraham WT, Sutton MG, Heublein DM, Kruger KM, . Cardiac resynchronization therapy improves renal function in human heart failure with reduced glomerular filtration rate. *J Card Fail.* 2008;14(7):539-46.

87. Testani JM, Chen J, McCauley BD, Kimmel SE, Shannon RP. Potential effects of aggressive decongestion during the treatment of decompensated heart failure on renal function and survival. *Circulation.* 2010;122(3):265-72.

88. Costanzo MR, Guglin ME, Saltzberg MT, Jessup ML, Bart BA, Teerlink JR, et al. Ultra-filtration versus intravenous diuretics for patients hospitalized for acute decompensated heart failure. *J Am Coll Cardiol.* 2007;49(6):675-83.

89. Bart BA, Boyle A, Bank AJ, Anand I, Olivari MT, Kraemer M, et al. Ultrafiltration versus usual care for hospitalized patients with heart failure: the Relief for Acutely Fluid-Overloaded Patients With Decompensated Congestive Heart Failure (RAPID-CHF) trial. *J Am Coll Cardiol.* 2005;46(11):2043-6.

90. Ungar A, Fumagalli S, Marini M, Di Serio C, Tarantini F, Boncinelli L, et al. Renal, but not systemic, hemodynamic effects of dopamine are influenced by the severity of congestive heart failure. *Crit Care Med.* 2004;32(5):1125-9.

91. Giamouzis G, Butler J, Starling RC, Karayannis G, Nastas J, Parisis C, et al. Impact of dopamine infusion on renal function in hospitalized heart failure patients: results of the Dopamine in Acute Decompensated Heart Failure (DAD-HF) Trial. *J Card Fail.* 2010;16(12):922-30.

92. Konstam MA, Gheorghiade M, Burnett JC Jr., Grinfeld L, Maggioni AP, Swedberg K, et al. Effects of oral tolvaptan in patients hospitalized for worsening heart failure: the EVEREST Outcome Trial. *JAMA.* 2007;297(12):1319-31.

93. Massie BM, O'Connor CM, Metra M, Ponikowski P, Teerlink JR, Cotter G, et al. Rolofylline, an adenosine A1-receptor antagonist, in acute heart failure. *N Engl J Med.* 2010;363(15):1419-28.

94. Wlodarczyk JH, Keogh A, Smith K, McCosker C. CHART: congestive cardiac failure in hospitals, an Australian review of treatment. *Heart Lung Circ.* 2003;12(2):94-102.

95. Colucci WS, Packer M, Bristow MR, Gilbert EM, Cohn JN, Fowler MB, et al. Carvedilol inhibits clinical progression in patients with mild symptoms of heart failure. US Carvedilol Heart Failure Study Group. *Circulation.* 1996;94(11):2800-6.

96. The Cardiac Insufficiency Bisoprolol Study II (CIBIS-II): a randomised trial. *Lancet.* 1999;353(9146):9-13.

97. Packer M, Coats AJ, Fowler MB, Katus HA, Krum H, Mohacsi P, et al. Effect of carvedilol on survival in severe chronic heart failure. *N Engl J Med.* 2001;344(22):1651-8.

98. Fowler MB, Vera-Llonch M, Oster G, Bristow MR, Cohn JN, Colucci WS, et al. Influence of carvedilol on hospitalizations in heart failure: incidence, resource utilization and costs. U.S. Carvedilol Heart Failure Study Group. *J Am Coll Cardiol.* 2001;37(6):1692-9.

99. Effect of metoprolol CR/XL in chronic heart failure: Metoprolol CR/XL Randomised Intervention Trial in Congestive Heart Failure (MERIT-HF). *Lancet.* 1999;353(9169):2001-7.

100. Shekelle PG, Rich MW, Morton SC, Atkinson CS, Tu W, Maglione M, et al. Efficacy of angiotensin-converting enzyme inhibitors and beta-blockers in the management of left

ventricular systolic dysfunction according to race, gender, and diabetic status: a meta-analysis of major clinical trials. *J Am Coll Cardiol.* 2003;41(9):1529-38.

101. Masoudi FA, Rathore SS, Wang Y, Havranek EP, Curtis JP, Foody JM, et al. National patterns of use and effectiveness of angiotensin-converting enzyme inhibitors in older patients with heart failure and left ventricular systolic dysfunction. *Circulation.* 2004;110(6):724-31.

102. Patel A, MacMahon S, Chalmers J, Neal B, Woodward M, Billot L, et al. Effects of a fixed combination of perindopril and indapamide on macrovascular and microvascular outcomes in patients with type 2 diabetes mellitus (the ADVANCE trial): a randomised controlled trial. *Lancet.* 2007;370(9590):829-40.

103. Hou FF, Zhang X, Zhang GH, Xie D, Chen PY, Zhang WR, et al. Efficacy and safety of benazepril for advanced chronic renal insufficiency. *N Engl J Med.* 2006;354(2):131-40.

104. Bangalore S, Kumar S, Messerli FH. Angiotensin-converting enzyme inhibitor associated cough: deceptive information from the Physicians' Desk Reference. *Am J Med.* 2010; 123(11):1016-30.

105. Cohn JN, Tognoni G. A randomized trial of the angiotensin-receptor blocker valsartan in chronic heart failure. *N Engl J Med.* 2001;345(23):1667-75.

106. Young JB, Dunlap ME, Pfeffer MA, Probstfield JL, Cohen-Solal A, Dietz R, et al. Mortality and morbidity reduction with Candesartan in patients with chronic heart failure and left ventricular systolic dysfunction: results of the CHARM low-left ventricular ejection fraction trials. *Circulation.* 2004;110(17):2618-26.

107. Pitt B, Zannad F, Remme WJ, Cody R, Castaigne A, Perez A, et al. The effect of spironolactone on morbidity and mortality in patients with severe heart failure. Randomized Aldactone Evaluation Study Investigators. *N Engl J Med.* 1999;341(10):709-17.

108. Zannad F, McMurray JJ, Krum H, van Veldhuisen DJ, Swedberg K, Shi H, et al. Eplerenone in patients with systolic heart failure and mild symptoms. *N Engl J Med.* 2011;364(1):11-21.

109. Pitt B, Remme W, Zannad F, Neaton J, Martinez F, Roniker B, et al. Eplerenone, a selective aldosterone blocker, in patients with left ventricular dysfunction after myocardial infarction. *N Engl J Med.* 2003;348(14):1309-21.

110. Klingbeil AU, Schneider M, Martus P, Messerli FH, Schmieder RE. A meta-analysis of the effects of treatment on left ventricular mass in essential hypertension. *Am J Med.* 2003;115(1):41-6.

111. Wachtell K, Bella JN, Rokkedal J, Palmieri V, Papademetriou V, Dahlof B, et al. Change in diastolic left ventricular filling after one year of antihypertensive treatment: The Losartan Intervention For Endpoint Reduction in Hypertension (LIFE) Study. *Circulation.* 2002; 105(9):1071-6.

112. Massie BM, Carson PE, McMurray JJ, Komajda M, McKelvie R, Zile MR, et al. Irbesartan in patients with heart failure and preserved ejection fraction. *N Engl J Med.* 2008;359(23): 2456-67.

113. Solomon SD, Janardhanan R, Verma A, Bourgoun M, Daley WL, Purkayastha D, et al. Effect of angiotensin receptor blockade and antihypertensive drugs on diastolic function in patients with hypertension and diastolic dysfunction: a randomised trial. *Lancet.* 2007; 369(9579):2079-87.

114. Borlaug BA, Melenovsky V, Russell SD, Kessler K, Pacak K, Becker LC, et al. Impaired chronotropic and vasodilator reserves limit exercise capacity in patients with heart failure and a preserved ejection fraction. *Circulation.* 2006;114(20):2138-47.

115. Kass DA, Kitzman DW, Alvarez GE. The restoration of chronotropic competence in heart failure patients with normal ejection fraction (RESET) study: rationale and design. *J Card Fail.* 2010;16(1):17-24.

116. Flather MD, Shibata MC, Coats AJ, Van Veldhuisen DJ, Parkhomenko A, Borbola J, et al. Randomized trial to determine the effect of nebivolol on mortality and cardiovascular hospital admission in elderly patients with heart failure (SENIORS). *Eur Heart J.* 2005; 26(3):215-25.

117. de Boer RA, Doehner W, van der Horst IC, Anker SD, Babalis D, Roughton M, et al. Influence of diabetes mellitus and hyperglycemia on prognosis in patients > or =70 years old with heart failure and effects of nebivolol (data from the Study of Effects of Nebivolol Intervention on Outcomes and Rehospitalization in Seniors with heart failure [SENIORS]). *Am J Cardiol.* 2010;106(1):78-86.

118. Massie BM, Nelson JJ, Lukas MA, Greenberg B, Fowler MB, Gilbert EM, et al. Comparison of outcomes and usefulness of carvedilol across a spectrum of left ventricular ejection fractions in patients with heart failure in clinical practice. *Am J Cardiol.* 2007;99(9):1263-8.

119. Gaasch WH. Diagnosis and treatment of heart failure based on left ventricular systolic or diastolic dysfunction. *JAMA.* 1994;271(16):1276-80.

120. Sossalla S, Maier LS. Role of ranolazine in angina, heart failure, arrhythmias, and diabetes. *Pharmacol Ther.* 2012;133(3):311-23.

121. Cooper-DeHoff R, Pepine CJ. Ranolazine is associated with cardiovascular and metabolic improvement: a win-win for patients with diabetes. *Eur Heart J.* 2006;27(1):5-6

122. Timmis AD, Chaitman BR, Crager M. Effects of ranolazine on exercise tolerance and HbA1c in patients with chronic angina and diabetes. *Eur Heart J.* 2006;27(1):42-8.

123. Morrow DA, Scirica BM, Chaitman BR, McGuire DK, Murphy SA, Karwatowska-Prokopczuk E, et al. Evaluation of the glycometabolic effects of ranolazine in patients with and without diabetes mellitus in the MERLIN-TIMI 36 randomized controlled trial. *Circulation.* 2009;119(15):2032-9.

124. Morrow DA, Scirica BM, Sabatine MS, de Lemos JA, Murphy SA, Jarolim P, et al. B-type natriuretic peptide and the effect of ranolazine in patients with non-ST-segment elevation acute coronary syndromes: observations from the MERLIN-TIMI 36 (Metabolic Efficiency With Ranolazine for Less Ischemia in Non-ST Elevation Acute Coronary-Thrombolysis In Myocardial Infarction 36) trial. *J Am Coll Cardiol.* 2010;55(12):1189-96.

125. Cleland JG, Tendera M, Adamus J, Freemantle N, Polonski L, Taylor J. The perindopril in elderly people with chronic heart failure (PEP-CHF) study. *Eur Heart J.* 2006;27(19): 2338-45.

126. Yusuf S, Pfeffer MA, Swedberg K, Granger CB, Held P, McMurray JJ, et al. Effects of candesartan in patients with chronic heart failure and preserved left-ventricular ejection fraction: the CHARM-Preserved Trial. *Lancet.* 2003;362(9386):777-81.

127. Desai AS, Lewis EF, Li R, Solomon SD, Assmann SF, Boineau R, et al. Rationale and design of the treatment of preserved cardiac function heart failure with an aldosterone antagonist trial: a randomized, controlled study of spironolactone in patients with symptomatic heart failure and preserved ejection fraction. *Am Heart J.* 2011;162(6):966-72.

128. Shah SJ, Gheorghiade M. Heart failure with preserved ejection fraction: treat now by treating comorbidities. *JAMA.* 2008;300(4):431-3.

129. McAlister FA, Ezekowitz J, Hooton N, Vandermeer B, Spooner C, Dryden DM, et al. Cardiac resynchronization therapy for patients with left ventricular systolic dysfunction: a systematic review. *JAMA.* 2007;297(22):2502-14.

130. Nery PB, Ha AC, Keren A, Birnie DH. Cardiac resynchronization therapy in patients with left ventricular systolic dysfunction and right bundle branch block: a systematic review. *Heart Rhythm.* 2011;8(7):1083-7.

131. Sipahi I, Carrigan TP, Rowland DY, Stambler BS, Fang JC. Impact of QRS duration on clinical event reduction with cardiac resynchronization therapy: meta-analysis of randomized controlled trials. *Arch Intern Med.* 2011;171(16):1454-62.

132. Hoppe UC, Freemantle N, Cleland JG, Marijianowski M, Erdmann E. Effect of cardiac resynchronization on morbidity and mortality of diabetic patients with severe heart failure. *Diabetes Care.* 2007;30(3):722-4.

133. Fantoni C, Regoli F, Ghanem A, Raffa S, Klersy C, Sorgente A, et al. Long-term outcome in diabetic heart failure patients treated with cardiac resynchronization therapy. *Eur J Heart Fail.* 2008;10(3):298-307.

134. Mehra MR, Kobashigawa J, Starling R, Russell S, Uber PA, Parameshwar J, et al. Listing criteria for heart transplantation: International Society for Heart and Lung Transplantation guidelines for the care of cardiac transplant candidates—2006. *J Heart Lung Transplant.* 2006;25(9):1024-42.

135. Levy WC, Mozaffarian D, Linker DT, Sutradhar SC, Anker SD, et al. The Seattle Heart Failure Model: prediction of survival in heart failure. *Circulation.* 2006;113(11):1424-33.

136. Lang CC, Beniaminovitz A, Edwards N, Mancini DM. Morbidity and mortality in diabetic patients following cardiac transplantation. *J Heart Lung Transplant.* 2003;22(3):244-9.

137. Russo MJ, Chen JM, Hong KN, Stewart AS, Ascheim DD, Argenziano M, et al. Survival after heart transplantation is not diminished among recipients with uncomplicated diabetes mellitus: an analysis of the United Network of Organ Sharing database. *Circulation.* 2006;114(21):2280-7.

138. Almuti K, Haythe J, Tsao L, Naka Y, Mancini D. Does renal function deteriorate more rapidly in diabetic cardiac transplant recipients? *Transplantation.* 2007;83(5):550-3.

139. Guan Y, Hao C, Cha DR, Rao R, Lu W, Kohan DE, et al. Thiazolidinediones expand body fluid volume through PPARgamma stimulation of ENaC-mediated renal salt absorption. *Nat Med.* 2005;11(8):861-6.

140. Nissen SE, Wolski K. Effect of rosiglitazone on the risk of myocardial infarction and death from cardiovascular causes. *N Engl J Med.* 2007;356(24):2457-71.

141. Yki-Jarvinen H. Thiazolidinediones. *N Engl J Med.* 2004;351(11):1106-18.

142. Dormandy JA, Charbonnel B, Eckland DJ, Erdmann E, Massi-Benedetti M, Moules IK, et al. Secondary prevention of macrovascular events in patients with type 2 diabetes in the PROactive Study (PROspective pioglitAzone Clinical Trial In macroVascular Events): a randomised controlled trial. *Lancet.* 2005;366(9493):1279-89.

143. Czoski-Murray C, Warren E, Chilcott J, Beverley C, Psyllaki MA, Cowan J. Clinical effectiveness and cost-effectiveness of pioglitazone and rosiglitazone in the treatment of type 2 diabetes: a systematic review and economic evaluation. Health Technol Assess. 2004;8(13):iii, ix-x, 1-91.

144. Nesto RW, Bell D, Bonow RO, Fonseca V, Grundy SM, Horton ES, et al. Thiazolidinedione use, fluid retention, and congestive heart failure: a consensus statement from the American Heart Association and American Diabetes Association. October 7, 2003. *Circulation.* 2003;108(23):2941-8.

145. Misbin RI. The phantom of lactic acidosis due to metformin in patients with diabetes. *Diabetes Care.* 2004;27(7):1791-3.

146. Eurich DT, Majumdar SR, McAlister FA, Tsuyuki RT, Johnson JA. Improved clinical outcomes associated with metformin in patients with diabetes and heart failure. *Diabetes Care.* 2005;28(10):2345-51.

147. Salpeter SR, Greyber E, Pasternak GA, Salpeter EE. Risk of fatal and nonfatal lactic acidosis with metformin use in type 2 diabetes mellitus. *Cochrane Database Syst Rev.* 2010;14(4):CD002967.

148. Major outcomes in high-risk hypertensive patients randomized to angiotensin-converting enzyme inhibitor or calcium channel blocker vs diuretic: The Antihypertensive and Lipid-Lowering Treatment to Prevent Heart Attack Trial (ALLHAT). *JAMA*. 2002;288(23):2981-97.

149. Kostis JB, Wilson AC, Freudenberger RS, Cosgrove NM, Pressel SL, Davis BR. Long-term effect of diuretic-based therapy on fatal outcomes in subjects with isolated systolic hypertension with and without diabetes. *Am J Cardiol*. 2005;95(1):29-35.

150. Harper R, Ennis CN, Heaney AP, Sheridan B, Gormley M, Atkinson AB, et al. A comparison of the effects of low- and conventional-dose thiazide diuretic on insulin action in hyper-tensive patients with NIDDM. *Diabetologia*. 1995;38(7):853-9.

151. Shafi T, Appel LJ, Miller ER, 3rd, Klag MJ, Parekh RS. Changes in serum potassium mediate thiazide-induced diabetes. *Hypertension*. 2008;52(6):1022-9.

152. Zillich AJ, Garg J, Basu S, Bakris GL, Carter BL. Thiazide diuretics, potassium, and the development of diabetes: a quantitative review. *Hypertension*. 2006;48(2):219-24.

153. Helderman JH, Elahi D, Andersen DK, Raizes GS, Tobin JD, Shocken D, et al. Prevention of the glucose intolerance of thiazide diuretics by maintenance of body potassium. *Diabetes*. 1983;32(2):106-11.

154. Kaplan NM, Carnegie A, Raskin P, Heller JA, Simmons M. Potassium supplementation in hypertensive patients with diuretic-induced hypokalemia. *N Engl J Med*. 1985;312(12):746-9.

155. Gress TW, Nieto FJ, Shahar E, Wofford MR, Brancati FL. Hypertension and antihypertensive therapy as risk factors for type 2 diabetes mellitus. Atherosclerosis Risk in Communities Study. *N Engl J Med*. 2000;342(13):905-12.

156. Messerli FH, Bangalore S, Julius S. Risk/benefit assessment of beta-blockers and diuretics precludes their use for first-line therapy in hypertension. *Circulation*. 2008;117(20):2706-15.

157. Sarafidis PA, Bakris GL. Antihypertensive treatment with beta-blockers and the spectrum of glycaemic control. *QJM*. 2006;99(7):431-6.

Sexual Dysfunction in Diabetes

18
Chapter

Vikram Kamdar, Jayendra H Shah

ABSTRACT

The sexual dysfunction is a common symptom in patients with diabetes. In male diabetic patient, the sexual dysfunction presents as erectile dysfunction (ED). In female diabetic patient, the sexual dysfunction mainly presents as dyspareunia. The sexual dysfunction in female diabetic patients is reported less commonly than erectile dysfunction in diabetic male. ED is also strongly associated with concurrent, silent, and future coronary artery disease. Therefore, a thorough cardiac evaluation in every patient with ED is encouraged. Endothelial dysfunction is the common factor present in diabetes, metabolic syndrome, hypertension, cardiovascular disease, and obesity. The chapter discusses the pathophysiology of sexual dysfunction in diabetic patients and how improvement in lifestyle, adequate control of hyperglycemia, treatment of hypertension, and hyperlipidemia can postpone or prevent this quality of life disturbing and depressing complication in male population with diabetes. The chapter further discusses various modes of therapy for sexual dysfunction in male and female diabetic patients. A detail assessment is also given on various phosphodiesterase-5 inhibitors in the management of ED and further discussed how their positive effect on endothelial function may have a protective effect in cardiovascular disease in diabetic patients.

INTRODUCTION

Sexual dysfunction is a common symptom in patients with diabetes. In a male diabetic patient, sexual dysfunction presents as erectile dysfunction (ED). In a female diabetic patient, sexual dysfunction mainly presents as dyspareunia. Sexual dysfunction in female diabetic patients is reported less commonly than ED in diabetic males.

ERECTILE DYSFUNCTION IN DIABETES MELLITUS

The US National Institute of Health has defined ED as the inability to achieve, maintain, or sustain a penile erection, firm enough for sexual intercourse.[1] ED has been reported in ancient Egyptian scriptures over 5000 years old.[2-3] In 10th century, Avicenna described the "collapse of sexual function" as a complication of diabetes.[4] In India, today, a cultural/religious tradition is practiced where a couple voluntarily takes the vow of celibacy after the age of 60 which is publicly hailed and celebrated, perhaps a step toward a commonly encountered ED with aging. ED is a common disorder which essentially affects men above the age of 40. International Consultation Committee for Sexual Medicine published a report in 2010 showing 1–10% prevalence of ED before the age of 40, increasing to 2–9% between ages of 40 and 49 years, 20–40% between ages 60 and 69 years and reaching 50–100% above the age of 70 years.[5-10] It is estimated that the worldwide prevalence of ED may reach 322 million by year 2025.[11-12] Cross-sectional and longitudinal studies have linked ED to diabetes mellitus (DM), hypertension, dyslipidemia, metabolic syndrome, depression, and lower urinary tract disorders.[13-19] A meta-analysis published in 2011 which included over 36,000 participants from 12 prospective studies noted a significant risk for increase in cardiovascular disease (CVD), coronary heart disease, stroke, and all-cause mortality with ED. Nineteen other studies have noted relationship of smoking, obesity, and lack of exercise to ED and improvement in ED with life style changes.[20-27]

Patients with diabetes who share many of the above risk factors have been noted to suffer from ED disproportionately. The prevalence of ED has been reported from various studies done internationally in various countries between 35% and 75% above the age of 40.[28-34] Massachusetts Male Aging Study has reported age-adjusted prevalence of 28% of ED in patients with DM as compared to 10% in general population.[35] The diabetic patients develop ED a decade earlier than the control population. Earlier reports had noted similar prevalence in both type 1 and type 2 diabetic patients.[29,31] In unselected patients with diabetes, the prevalence was noted to be 6% between age 20 and 24 yeras, 52% between age 55 and 59 years, and 55–95% above the age of 60 years.[36] It can be summarized that diabetes associated ED increases with age, duration of diabetes, poor metabolic control, untreated hypertension, neuropathy, micro- and macroalbuminuria, retinopathy, CVD, diuretic and beta-blocker therapy, low testosterone, and psychological vulnerability. Prospectively, a link between elevated glycosylated hemoglobin (HbA1c) and ED has been noted.

PHYSIOLOGY OF ERECTILE FUNCTION

A normal erection occurs with the erectile cavernous smooth muscle relaxation brought about by the release of nitric oxide (NO) from endothelium and the parasympathetic nerve terminals leading to the filling of arterial blood in the normal cavernous tissue from penile artery, and also the filling of erectile tissue leading to the compression of the subtunical small veins thereby preventing the simultaneous venous return. Stimulation of adrenergic receptors of the cavernous arteries and trabecular smooth muscles leads to diminished arterial blood supply and a fall of lacunar spaces, decompression of the subtunical veins leading to detumescence. Thus to have a normal erectile function, one needs a normal erectile tissue, normal arterial blood supply, normal endothelial function, normal autonomic nerves, and normal venous drainage system.[37,38] Normal sexual activity involves the coordination of psychological, endocrine, vascular, and neurological functions of the body. ED is generally classified as psychogenic or organic (endothelial dysfunction, arterial, venous leak, hormonal, cavernous, neurogenic, or drug induced) or mixed type, which is generally the case.

PATHOPHYSIOLOGY OF THE DIABETIC ERECTILE DYSFUNCTION

There are several causes of ED in patients with diabetes, which are depicted in figure 1. The pathophysiology of ED in patients with diabetes is multifactorial and is shared by other conditions like hypertension, metabolic syndrome, obesity, dyslipidemia, and CVD and highly associated with poor life style (Table 1). Multiple recent meta-analysis suggests that ED may be the marker for future development of metabolic syndrome, DM, and CVDs.[19]

Psychological Factors

The most common psychological factor is the performance anxiety but the factors can be multiple (developmental, cognitive, affective, and interpersonal) and can be predisposing, precipitating, and maintaining ED.[28] ED affects quality of life of an individual with poor self-esteem, sexual dissatisfaction, and strain in the interpersonal relationship. Both the meta-analysis and longitudinal studies have noted depression

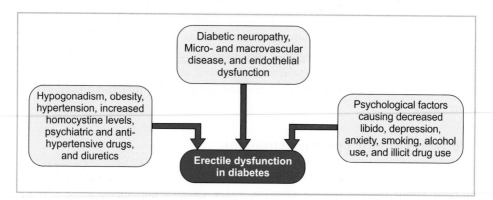

FIGURE 1 Causes of erectile dysfunction in diabetes.

TABLE 1: Pathophysiology of Erectile Dysfunction in Medical Conditions					
Medical conditions	Pathophysiology				
	Altered erectile tissue	Compromised arterial blood supply	Endothelial dysfunction	Autonomic and somatic neuropathy	Hypo-gonadism
Ageing	Yes	Yes	–	–	Yes
Metabolic syndrome	–	–	Yes	–	–
Hypertension	Yes	Yes	Yes	–	–
Cardiovascular disease	–	Yes	Yes	–	–
Diabetes mellitus	Yes	Yes	Yes	Yes	Yes
Drugs	–	–	Yes	Yes	Yes
Smoking	–	–	Yes	Yes	–

being the common predisposing as well as precipitating factor.[39-41] It is important to note that some of the antidepressant drugs can cause ED.

Endothelial Dysfunction

In diabetic patient, impaired NO and cyclic guanosine monophosphate (cGMP) synthesis along with increased superoxide radicals affects the synthesis of both NO synthase and guanylyl cyclase.[42,43] Oxidative stress and free-radical interferes with NO production.[43] In diabetic patients, advanced glycation end-products (AGEs) are developed nonenzymatically with sustained hyperglycemia. AGEs form covalent bonds with vascular collagen causing increased vascular permeability, procoagulant expression, reactive oxygen species, and endothelial expression of adhesion molecules which in turn lead to oxidative cell damage and decrease NO production.[44] Hyperglycemia in diabetic patients causes increased levels of endothelin-I and endothelin-B receptor binding sites both of which lead to vasoconstriction of cavernous tissue leading to ED. RhoA/Rho-kinase pathway which is up-regulated in patients with diabetes leads to decrease production of NO in penile tissue and ultimately causes ED.[45,46]

Vasculogenic Erectile Dysfunction

Multiple factors accelerate the atherosclerotic process in the patients with diabetes leading to atherosclerotic penile arterial insufficiency. These factors include dyslipidemia, hypertension, cigarette smoking, obesity, and metabolic syndrome. However, the prevalence of this vasculogenic ED is very small.[47-49]

Diabetic Microangiopathy and Neuropathy

There is a strong relationship between ED and the presence of retinopathy and proteinuria in diabetic patient. These two complications are correlated with the glycemic control of diabetes as well as duration of diabetes.[30,50]

Both peripheral and autonomic neuropathies are associated with ED. Peripheral neuropathy leads to impaired sensation transmission from penis to the reflexogenic erectile center. The center governs the tone of bulbocavernosus and ischiocavernosus muscle which in turn maintains the compression on subtunical venues in the corpora cavernosa, thereby sustaining the erection. The autonomic neurons are carried by dorsal penile and perineal nerves. The autonomic neuropathy is highly correlated with ED.[51] The reduced or absent parasympathetic neuronal activity reduces neuronal isoform of NO synthase (nNOs) generation brought about by increased acetylcholine levels and decreased norepinephrine levels.[52] Clinically, it is correlated in diabetic patients with cardiac autonomic neuropathy, silent ischemia, and painless myocardial infarctions.[53]

Endocrinological Causes

Androgen has been recognized as a responsible hormone for libido and adequacy of sleep-related erections. It is also an important hormone for the expression of NOs and phosphodiesterase-5 (PDE-5) in penile erectile tissue. Hypogonadism and ED have been well-correlated and so is metabolic syndrome and type 2 diabetes.[54] Men with ED and type 2 diabetes have a higher prevalence of hypogonadism, low testosterone, and ED; all worsen with poor glycemic control. Metabolic syndrome with central obesity is also associated with low testosterone.[54-56]

There are several explanations for low testosterone levels in these individuals and a true hypogonadal state is still being debated. In patients with diabetes, central obesity, and metabolic syndrome, insulin resistance causes a decrease in plasma sex hormone binding globulin that leads to low total testosterone levels. Increased aromatase activity associated with central obesity can convert testosterone to estradiol which results into low testosterone level. It is also suggested that there may be insulin resistance at the hypothalamus resulting into hypogonadotropic hypogonadism.[57] Hyperprolactinemia associated with drugs used for the treatment of comorbidities (hypertension, depression, gastroparesis, etc.) in patients with DM can lead to hypogonadotropic hypogonadism.

Drug-induced Erectile Dysfunction

Antiandrogens, antihypertensives, antiarrhythmics, statins, psychotropic drugs, and recreational drugs (Table 2) can cause ED in the diabetics.[58,59] Of the many hypertensive drugs causing ED, angiotensin converting enzyme (ACE) inhibitors, alpha blockers and angiotensin receptor blockers (ARB) are least likely to have ED.[58] Unhealthy lifestyle, aging, and systemic diseases are well known causes of ED.

TABLE 2: Drugs Associated with Erectile Dysfunction

Drug class	Name of drug
Antiandrogens	Gonadotropin-releasing hormone agonists (leuprolide, goserelin, lupron, and zoladex), chemotherapeutic agents—cyclophosphamide and busulfan; flutamide, ketoconazole, spironolactone, H2 blockers, and cimetidine
Antihypertensive	Thiazide diuretics, beta-blockers, and calcium channel blockers
Antiarrhythmic	Digoxin, amioderone, and disopyramide
Statins	Atorvastatin
Psychotropic drugs	Tricyclic antidepressants, selective serotonin reuptake inhibitors, phenothiazines, and butyrophenones
Recreational agents	Marijuana, opiates, cocaine, nicotine, and alcohol

DIAGNOSIS

Evaluation and management of a diabetic patient with ED is a great challenge in clinical medicine because of overlapping and multiple etiologies. A patient with diabetes is the harbinger of those multiple etiologies as discussed above and continues to evolve with the duration of the disease state as well as the progression of the number of diabetes-related complications. A comprehensive history taking, physical examination, laboratory, and other investigations are integral in the management of ED (Figure 2).

History Taking

After ascertaining the presence of ED in an individual, a comprehensive sexual and medical history to include risk factors for ED, DM, CVD, and medications is the essential initial step (Figure 2). The presence of night or morning erection or sexual thoughts related erection rules out organic ED. ED with sudden onset and intermittent progress points toward psychological ED. The gradual onset with progressive decline and long duration suggest organic ED. Relevant drug history for hypertension, depression, and antiandrogens is essential. The history of the use of alcohol in excess, tobacco, and recreational drugs is important. A use of standardized questionnaire for ED is highly recommended. Since ED is considered to be an important risk factor for overt as well as silent coronary artery disease (CAD), a thorough risk assessment of CVD should be undertaken. Taking the history with the partner may be important to estimate the severity and if interpersonal issues are predominant factors (Figure 2).

Physical Examination

Physical examination should include secondary sex characteristics, blood pressure, pulses, and neurological examination to rule out peripheral and autonomic

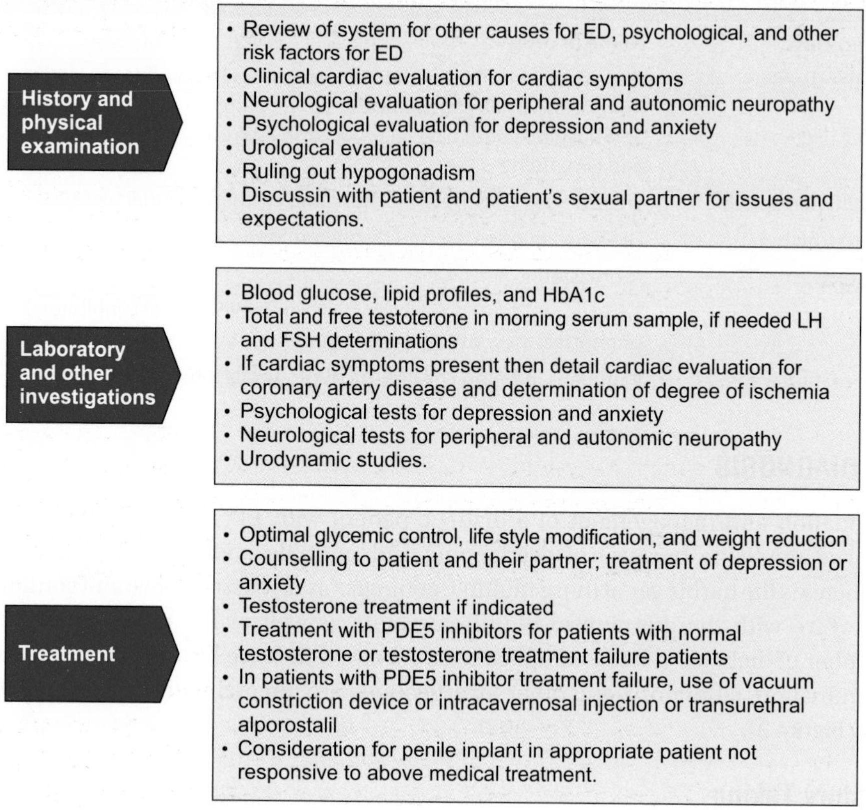

History and physical examination	• Review of system for other causes for ED, psychological, and other risk factors for ED • Clinical cardiac evaluation for cardiac symptoms • Neurological evaluation for peripheral and autonomic neuropathy • Psychological evaluation for depression and anxiety • Urological evaluation • Ruling out hypogonadism • Discussin with patient and patient's sexual partner for issues and expectations.
Laboratory and other investigations	• Blood glucose, lipid profiles, and HbA1c • Total and free testoterone in morning serum sample, if needed LH and FSH determinations • If cardiac symptoms present then detail cardiac evaluation for coronary artery disease and determination of degree of ischemia • Psychological tests for depression and anxiety • Neurological tests for peripheral and autonomic neuropathy • Urodynamic studies.
Treatment	• Optimal glycemic control, life style modification, and weight reduction • Counselling to patient and their partner; treatment of depression or anxiety • Testosterone treatment if indicated • Treatment with PDE5 inhibitors for patients with normal testosterone or testosterone treatment failure patients • In patients with PDE5 inhibitor treatment failure, use of vacuum constriction device or intracavernosal injection or transurethral alporostalil • Consideration for penile inplant in appropriate patient not responsive to above medical treatment.

ED, erectile dysfunction; HbA1c, glycosylated hemoglobin; LH, luteinizing hormone; FSH, follicular-stimulating hormone; PDE, phosphodiesterase.

FIGURE 2 Management of diabeteic patients with erectile dysfunction.

neuropathy. In patents with diabetes, a retinal examination to rule out retinopathy is important. Local genital examination should be undertaken to determine the size of penis, presence of scars, fibrosis, and poor elasticity. The size and consistency of testes should be examined. The rectal examination should include the prostatic size and the tone of the rectal sphincter. Evaluation of bulbocavernosus reflex may be needed if neurological examination indicates the presence of peripheral and/or autonomic neuropathy.

Laboratory Evaluation

Fasting blood glucose, lipid profile, HbA1c, and morning total serum testosterone are the initial tests to be obtained. The next step is to estimate luteinizing hormone, prolactin, and free (bio available) testosterone if initial test shows low total testosterone level. In the patients with diabetes, presence of microalbuminuria should be ruled out (Figure 2).

Specialized Investigations

Intracavernosal injection, color Doppler ultrasound, arteriography, cavernosometry, cavernosography, neurological evaluation, and nocturnal penile tumescence testing can be undertaken by the urologists or the respective specialists trained to undertake these investigations.

▍MANAGEMENT

Since 1998, use of selective PDE-5 inhibitors (PDE-5Is) have become the first line of treatment in the management of ED. Other treatments include lifestyle modification; penile injection therapies, hormone replacement therapy, and surgical implantation of penile devices have taken the subsequent seats in the management. Psychosexual, couple counseling, and psychotherapy are options for appropriate patients.

Lifestyle Intervention

Lifestyle modification with weight reduction by diet and exercise, reduced alcohol consumption, and smoking cessation have led to improvement in ED as noted in both basic and clinical research. Lifestyle interventions and associated weight loss are responsible with improved endothelial dysfunction and NO generation, decreased markers of inflammation, increased testosterone levels, and improved self-esteem.[60,61] Smoking is a well-established cause for ED and stoppage has been shown to improve ED.[62,63] A simultaneous use of PDE-5Is and lifestyle modification can improve the ED relatively rapidly and one need not wait to have the effects of nonpharmacological therapy.[64,65]

Control of Diabetes

Poor metabolic control in patients with diabetes has been associated with increased prevalence as well as the incidence of ED. With improved glycemic control, various pathophysiological mechanisms get ameliorated but there is a paucity of data in clinical trials. In the Uro-EDIC study of the longitudinal follow-up of type 1 diabetic patients recruited in Diabetes Control and Complication Trial showed secondary prevention of ED in patients assigned to intensive control. Recently, it was shown that glycemic control was independently and inversely associated with ED in patients with type 2 diabetes. In the Look AHEAD (Action for Health in Diabetes) trial, cardiorespiratory fitness was associated with improved or preserved erectile function and 39% lower risk of ED in 373 diabetic men.[66]

Management of Comorbid Conditions

Hypertension and dyslipidemia are the common comorbid conditions associated with diabetes and appropriate selections of medications for treatment of them can prevent further contributions toward ED. Avoiding hydrochlorothiazides, beta blockers except nebivolol, alpha blockers, aldosterone antagonists, and instead using ACE inhibitors and ARBs may be the prudent choices for the treatment of hypertension in diabetic patients with ED. There are controversies regarding the effect of statins and their effects on ED. In the management of depression in diabetic patients, use of medications with least side-effects on erectile functions should be the goal of clinicians.

Cardiovascular Disease, Diabetes, and Erectile Dysfunction

The prevalence of ED and CVD is high in patients with diabetes. Several studies have shown strong association of CVD and ED, and ED is considered a predictor for both diabetes and CVD.[67] ED is a powerful predictor of all causes of death, cardiovascular death, myocardial infarction, stroke, and heart failure. The severity of ED is also correlated with severity of CAD. The prevalence and severity of CAD is higher in patients with diabetes and ED than without ED. In the recent prospective studies, it was proven that history of ED was a strong predictor of CAD in the diabetic patients and it was suggested that a diabetic patients with ED should undergo comprehensive cardiovascular assessment before a pharmacological therapy as well as sexual activity are advised.

FIRST LINE OF THERAPY

Oral PDE-5Is inhibit the PDE-5 enzyme responsible for the degradation of cGMP in the cavernous smooth muscles essential for erection, thereby prolonging their relaxed status to accommodate arterial blood needed for erection. The inhibitor slows the degradation of cGMP, thereby prolonging the smooth muscle relaxation and allowing the penile rigidity to be prolonged. They do not initiate the erection but facilitate the sexually aroused stimulatory status to end up into a satisfactory erection. Sildenafil, vardenafil, tadalafil (available in the USA), udenafil, and mirodenafil are the first choice of medications for ED (Table 3). The onset of action is between 30 minutes to 60 minutes and duration from 4 hours to 8 hours except tadalafil which can have effects up to 36 hours. The response rate in the nondiabetics is from 65% to 83%. They are reasonably safe and the common side-effects are headache, flushing, dyspepsia, nasal congestion, abnormal vision, and diarrhea. Sildenafil can lead to hearing impairment. They are contraindicated with simultaneous use of nitrate containing compounds and alpha blockers. Vardenafil is contraindicated with type 1 (quinine and procainamide) or type 3 (sotalol or amioderone) antiarrhythmatics and patients with congenital prolonged QT syndrome. The sildenafil and vardenafil interact with food but not tadalafil. Tadalafil also comes in a smaller dose for single use. If a person fails on the

TABLE 3: Phosphodiesterase-5 Inhibitors—Dosage, Action, and Adverse Effects				
Name of drug	Dosage	Action	Adverse effects	Comments
Sildenafil	Starting 25 mg and maximum 100 mg	Starts in 30–60 minutes and lasts 4–8 hour	Headache, dyspepsia, and flushing	Administer while fasting
Vardenafil	Starting 10 mg and maximum 20 mg	Starts in 30 minutes and lasts 4–8 hour	Headache, flushing, and dyspepsia	Contraindicated in type 1 or 3 antiarrhythmic drugs and in patients with congenital prolonged QT syndrome
Tadalafil	Starting 10 mg and maximum 20 mg once a day	Starts in 45 minutes and lasts 4–36 hour	Flushing, myalgia, and back pain	10 mg available for prior to sexual activity
Mirodenafil	Starting 50 mg and maximum 100 mg	Starts in 30–60 minutes and lasts 6–12 hour	Facial flushing, nausea, headache, and redness of eyes	Not available in USA
Udenafil	Starting 100 mg and maximum 200 mg	Starts in 30–60 minutes and lasts 12 hour	Facial flushing, headache, nasal congestion, and redness of eyes	Not available in USA

Note: All the drugs, are contraindicated with simultaneous use of nitrates, alpha blockers, recent cardiovascular events and optic neuropathy.

first drug then the other should be tried after the failure of the first drug tried for four times. The drugs should be used with cautions with serious CVDs, unstable angina, and uncontrolled hypertension. The next generations of PDE-5Is are available outside the USA and are namely udenafil and mirodenafil (Table 3).

The response rate of PDE-5Is in patients with diabetes is between 57% and 74% in two major trials.[68,69] If there is a failure to respond, it is essential to rule out hypogonadal state in which case testosterone replacement may facilitate the response. Another meta-analysis noted lower response to sildenafil in the type 2 diabetics as compared to nondiabetics (63% vs. 83%).[70] It has been suggested that the daily use of these drugs may improve the performance in diabetic patients. Tadalafil 20 mg taken on demand or three times a week is safe for ED in diabetic patients.[71,72]

Cardioprotective effects of PDE-5Is have been investigated recently as the drug was originally developed to improve the endothelial dysfunction. The recent studies have recognized their cardioprotective effects, improved myocardial perfusion, reduced ischemic cell death, inhibition of platelet activation, and dilatation of epicardial coronary arteries.[73] It is speculated that the drug group may reduce cardiovascular events and deaths.[74-76]

SECOND LINE OF THERAPY

Testosterone Replacement Therapy

Testosterone has been important for adequate erectile function. Low testosterone has been noted in patients with obesity, metabolic syndrome, and DM.[54-56] However, its role in the treatment of ED is limited. Testosterone replacement therapy is recommended in patients with confirmed low free testosterone and ED.[77] In a meta-analysis of 16 studies, improvement in erectile function was noted in testosterone treated hypogonadal patients.[78] In elderly patients who have failed PDE-5I therapy may be tried with testosterone replacement.[79]

The diagnosis of androgen deficiency should be made in men with consistent signs and symptoms and serum testosterone levels that are below the lower limit of the normal range for healthy young men. Normative ranges for testosterone vary. In many research laboratories, the lower limit of the normal for testosterone is 300 ng/dL (10.5 nmol/L). Clinicians should use the normative range established in their own reference laboratory.

Intracavernous Injections

Intracavernous Injection of Alprastodil

Intracavernous injection of alprastodil (Prostaglandin E1) which stimulates adenylate cyclase and in turn generates cyclic adenosine monophosphate (cAMP). cAMP leads to smooth muscle relaxation and vasodilatation. Erection happens in 5–15 minutes after the injection and the efficacy is above 70%. This modality of treatment requires training of the patient and has a high dropout rate. The complications include penile discomfort, prolonged erection, priapism, and fibrosis. The drug can be mixed with other vasodilator agents like papaverine, phentolamine, and vasoactive intestinal polypeptide. Intraurethral prostaglandin suppositories can lead to similar effect on corpus cavernosum thereby allowing an erection.

Intraurethral Prostaglandin Suppositories

Prostaglandin E1 delivered in the urethral suppository is absorbed by urethral epithelium and reaches corpus cavernosum. The vasodilatation and relaxation of smooth muscle through prostacyclin receptor stimulation leads to successful erection.

Yohimbine, an alpha-adrenergic receptor antagonist, taken in the dosage of 5–10 mg three times a day can have a modest success rate of 30% in patients with diabetes and ED.[80]

Vacuum Constriction Devices

Vacuum constrictive device (VCD) works by applying negative pressure to the shaft of penis, drawing venous blood into the penis that is retained by a visible elastic constricting band at the base of the penis. These devices are inexpensive and suitable for elderly patients and achieve satisfactory erection in over 70% of men with diabetes.[81] There is 30% failure rate because of pain caused by the constricting ring, lack of spontaneity, cold penile sensation, inadequate orgasm, and discomfort with ejaculation.[82]

THIRD-LINE OF THERAPY

Penile Prosthesis

Implantation of penile prosthesis by surgical procedure is the last resort for treatment of ED. There are two types of prosthesis: (1) malleable (semi-rigid) which is difficult to hide and (2) inflatable (two or three- piece) with two penile cylinders with a scrotal pump. After the implantation surgery, the penile structure is irreversibly changed, hence a careful selection is important. The hydraulic three piece implant is the most popular with the satisfaction rate up to 70%. This method has reliable and predictable erection and hence has a high degree of satisfaction. The most common complication of the procedure is infection which has been reduced dramatically with antibiotic-impregnated implant. The clinical data on the diabetic patients have suggested higher rates of infections but recent experience suggests no difference with nondiabetics.[83,84]

SEXUAL DYSFUNCTION IN FEMALE DIABETIC PATIENTS

Sexual dysfunction in women with diabetes is an inadequately explored area in clinical medicine.[85] Although dyspareunia is a common presenting symptom in female diabetics, these patients may also present with decrease in libido, arousal, orgasm, or resolution.

The measurement of vaginal congestion with erotic stimuli has noted reduced reflexive engorgement in diabetic patients compared to nondiabetics though there was no difference in subjective arousal.[86] Patients with reduced vibratory sense of genitalia did not correlate with sexual dysfunction. The available data, though sparse, noted increased prevalence of dyspareunia in both type 1 and type 2 diabetics as compared to nondiabetics.[87] Dyspareunia can be related to reduced lubrication and highly prevalent vaginal candidiasis in the diabetic patients.

Therapy for Women with Sexual Dysfunction

After ruling out or treating vaginal candida infections, using estrogen cream locally for vaginal dryness is recommended.[88,89] For the persistent sexual dysfunction, vibrostimulatory therapy or treatment with PDE-5Is may be tried.[90]

FUTURE DEVELOPMENTS

Newer and safer PDE-5 are being developed. Several guanylate cyclase activators, potassium-channel inhibitors, Rho kinase inhibitors, and melanocortin system activators are being extensively researched.[91] Since the penile artery mirrors coronary arterial system and successful treatment of CAD by angioplasty and stent placement has led to the exploration of similar evaluation and treatment of stenosed pudendal artery. Some preliminary data and early studies have shown promising results.[92] Recently, gene therapy to incorporate vasodilatory molecules for penile tissue has shown some promises.[93] Another area of therapy stimulating neuropathic factors in the penile tissue is being explored.[94]

CONCLUSION

Sexual dysfunction in diabetic patients is commonly manifested as ED in males and dyspareunia in female patients. ED is a common symptom encountered in clinical practice and more so with the male patients suffering from diabetes and it's chronic complications. ED is also strongly associated with concurrent, silent, and future CAD. Therefore, a thorough cardiac evaluation in every patient with ED is encouraged. Endothelial dysfunction is a common factor present in diabetes, metabolic syndrome, hypertension, CVD, and obesity. PDE-5Is are the greatest medical advancement in the management of ED and with their positive effect on endothelial function may have a protective effect in CVD. There is enough evidence that improvement in life style, adequate control of hyperglycemia, treatment of hypertension, and hyperlipidemia can postpone or prevent this quality of life disturbing and depressing complication in male population with diabetes. Although decrease in libido, arousal, orgasm, and resolution can occur in female diabetic patients, the most common symptoms reported are dyspareunia. Symptomatic treatment with vaginal estrogen cream and treatment of vaginal candidiasis if present is recommended.

REFERENCES

1. Consensus development conference statement. National Institute of Health. Impotence. December 7-9, 1992. *Int J Impot Res.* 1993;5(4):181-284.
2. Smith GE. Papyrus Ebers. English translation. Chicago: Ares Publishers;1974.
3. Shah J. Erectile dysfunction through the ages. *BJU Int.* 2002;90(4):433-41.
4. Macfarlane I, Bliss M, Jackson JGL, Williams G. The history of diabetes. In: Pickup J, Williams G, editors. Textbook of Diabetes, 2nd edition. Oxford: Blackwell Science; 1997. pp. 1-19.
5. Lewis RW, Fugl-Meyer KS, Corona G, Hayes RD, Laumann EO, Moreira ED, et al. Definitions/epidemiology/risk factors for sexual dysfunction. *J Sex Med.* 2010;7(4 Pt 2): 1598-607.
6. Bejin A. The epidemiology of premature ejaculation and of its association with erectile dysfunction. *Andrologie.* 1999;9:211-25.

7. Braun M, Wassmer G, Klotz T, Reifenrath B, Mathers M, Engelmann U. Epidemiology of erectile dysfunction: results of the 'Cologne Male Survey'. *Int J Impot Res*. 2000;12(6): 305-11.

8. Pinnock CB, Stapleton AM, Marshall VR. Erectile dysfunction in the community: a prevalence study. *Med J Aust*. 1999;171(7):353-7.

9. Nicolosi A, Glasser DB, Kim SC, Marumo K, Laumann EO; GSSAB Investors' group. Sexual behavior and dysfunction and help-seeking patterns in adults aged 40-80 years in the urban population in Asian countries. *BJU int*. 2005;95(4):609-14.

10. Nicolosi A, Moreira ED, Shirai M, Bin Mohd Tambi MI, Glasser DB. Epidemiology of erectile function in four countries: cross-national study of the prevalence and correlates of erectile dysfunction. *Urology*. 2003;61(1):201-6.

11. Bacon CG, Mittleman MA, Kawachi I, Giovannucci E, Glasser DB, Rimm EB. Sexual functioning in men older than 50 years of age: results from the health professionals follow-up study. *Ann Intern Med*. 2003;139(3):161-8.

12. Ayta IA, McKinlay JB, Krane RJ. The likely worldwide increase in erectile dysfunction between 1995 and 2025 and some possible policy consequences. *BJU Int*. 1999;84(1):50-6.

13. Rosen RC, Link CL, O'Leary MP, Giuliano F, Aiyer LP, Mollon P. Lower urinary tract symptoms and sexual health: the role of gender, lifestyle and medical comorbidities. *BJU Int*. 2009;103(Suppl 3):42-7.

14. Inman BA, Sauver JL, Jacobson DJ, McGree ME, Nehra A, Lieber MM, et al. A population-based, longitudinal study of erectile dysfunction and future of coronary artery disease. *Mayo Clin Proc*. 2009;84(2):108-13.

15. Thompson IM, Tangen CM, Goodman PJ, Probstfield JL, Moinpour CM, Coltman CA. Erectile dysfunction and subsequent cardiovascular disease. *JAMA*. 2005;294(23):2996-3002.

16. Quek KF, Sallam AA, Ng CH, Chua CB. Prevalence of sexual problems and it's association with social, psychological and physical factors among men in Malaysian population: a crosses-sectional study. *J Sex Med*. 2998;5(1):70-6.

17. Clark NG, Fox KM, Grandy S; SHIELD Study Group. Symptoms of diabetes and their association with the risk and presence of diabetes: findings from the Study to Help Improve Early evaluation and management of risk factors Leading to Diabetes (SHIELD). *Diabetes Care*. 2007;30(11):2868-73.

18. Ponholzer A, Gutjahr G, Temml C, Madersbacher S. Is erectile dysfunction a predictor of cardiovascular events or stroke? A prospective study using a validated questionnaire. *Int J Impot Res*. 2010;22(1):25-9.

19. Chung SD, Chen YK, Lin HC. Increased risk of stroke among men with erectile dysfunction: a nationwide population-based study. *J Sex Med*. 2011;8(1):240-6.

20. Dong JY, Zhang YH, Quin LQ. Erectile dysfunction and risk of cardiovascular disease: meta-analysis of prospective cohort studies. *J Am Coll Cardiol*. 2011;58(13):1378-85.

21. Cheng JY, Ng EM. Body mass index, physical activity and erectile dysfunction: an U-shaped relationship from population-based study. *Int J Obes (Lond)*. 2007;31(10):1571-8.

22. Rosen RC, Wing R, Schneider S, Gendrano N 3rd. Epidemiology of erectile dysfunction: the role of medical comorbidities and lifestyle factors. *Urol Clin North Am*. 2005;32(4): 403-17.

23. Esposito K, Giugliano F, Di Palo C, Giugliano G, Marfella R, D'Andrea F, et al. Effect of lifestyle changes on erectile dysfunction in obese men: a randomized controlled trial. *JAMA*. 2004;291(24):2978-84.

24. Esposito K, Ciotola M, Giugliano F, Maiorino MI, Autorino R, De Sio M, et al. Effects of intensive lifestyle changes on erectile dysfunction in men. *J Sex Med*. 2009;6(1):243-50.

25. Esposito K, Giugliano D. Lifestyle/dietary recommendations for erectile dysfunction and female sexual dysfunction. *Urol Clin North Am.* 2011;38(3):293-301.

26. Esposito K, Giugliano F, De Sio M, Carleo D, Di Palo C, D'Armiento M, et al. Dietary factors in erectile dysfunction. *Int J Impot Res.* 2006;18(4):370-4.

27. Esposito K, Ciotola M, Giugliano F, De Sio M, Giugliano G, D'armiento M, et al. Mediterranean diet improves erectile function in subjects with the metabolic syndrome. *Int J Impot Res.* 2006;18(4):405-10.

28. De Berardis G, Franciosi M, Belfiglio M, Nardo B, Greenfield S, Kaplan SH, et al. Erectile dysfunction and quality of life in type 2 diabetic patients: a serious problem too often overlooked. *Diabetes Care.* 2002;25(2):284-91.

29. Kalter-Leibovici O, Weinstein J, Ziv A, Harman-Bohem I, Murad H, Raz I; Israel Diabetes Research Group (IDRG) Investigators. Clinical, socioeconomic, and lifestyle parameters associated with erectile dysfunction among diabetic men. *Diabetes Care.* 2005;28(7): 1739-44.

30. Siu SC, Lo SK, Wong KW, Ip KM, Wong YS. Prevalence of and risk factors for erectile dysfunction in Hong Kong diabetic patients. *Diabet Med.* 2001;18(9):732-8.

31. Bacon CG, Hu FB, Giovannucci E, Glasser DB, Mittleman MA, Rimm EB. Association of type and duration of diabetes with erectile dysfunction in a large cohort of men. *Diabetes Care.* 2002;25(8):1458-63.

32. Fedele D, Coscelli C, Santeusanio F, Bortolotti A, Chatenoud L, Colli E, et al. Erectile dysfunction in diabetic subjects in Italy. Gruppo Italiano Studio Deficit Erettile nei Diabetici. *Diabetes Care.* 1998;21(11):1973-7.

33. Sasaki H, Yamasaki H, Ogawa K, Nanjo K, Kawamori R, Iwamoto Y, et al. Prevalence and risk factors for erectile dysfunction in Japanese diabetics. *Diabetes Res Clin Pract.* 2005; 70(1):81-9.

34. Cho NH, Ahn CW, Park JY, Ahn TY, Lee HW, Park TS, et al. Prevalence of erectile dysfunction in Korean men with type 2 diabetes mellitus. *Diabet Med.* 2006;23(2): 198-203.

35. Feldman HA, Goldstein I, Hatzichristou DG, Krane RJ, McKinlay JB. Impotence and its medical and psychosocial correlates: results of the Massachusetts Male Aging Study. *J Urol.* 1994;151(1):54-61.

36. McCulloch DK, Campbell IW, Wu FC, Prescott RJ, Clarke BF. The prevalence of diabetic importance. *Diabetologia.* 1980;18(4):279-83.

37. Lue TF. Erectile dysfunction. *N Engl J Med.* 2000;342(24):1802-13.

38. Prieto D. Physiological regulation of penile arteries and veins. *Int J Impot Res.* 2008; 20(1):17-29.

39. Anderson RJ, Freedland KE, Clouse RE, Lustman PJ. The prevalence of comorbid depression in adults with diabetes: a meta-analysis. *Diabetes Care.* 2001;24(6):1069-78.

40. De Beradis G, Pellegrini F, Franciosi M, Belfiglio M, Di Nardo B, Greenfield S, et al. Clinical and psychological predictors of incidence of self-reported erectile dysfunction in patients with type 2 diabetes. *J Urol.* 2007;177(1):252-7.

41. De Beradis G, Pellegrini F, Franciosi M, Belfiglio M, Di Nardo B, Greenfield S, et al. Longitudinal assessment of quality of life in patients with type 2 diabetes and self-reported erectile dysfunction. *Diabetes Care.* 2005;28(11):2637-43.

42. Solomon H, Man JW, Jackson G. Erectile dysfunction and the cardiovascular patient: endothelial dysfunction is the common denominator. *Heart.* 2003;89(3):251-3.

43. Cellek S, Rodrigo J, Lobos E, Fernandez P, Serrano J, Moncada S. Selective nitrergic neurodegeneration in diabetes mellitus - a nitric oxide-dependent phenomenon. *Br J Pharmacol.* 1999;128(8):1804-12.

44. Wen Y, Skidmore JC, Porter-Turner MM, Rea CA, Khokher MA, Singh BM. Relationship of glycation, antioxidant status and oxidative stress to vascular endothelial damage in diabetes. *Diabetes Obes Metab*. 2002;4(5):305-8.

45. Takahashi K, Ghatei MA, Lam HC, O'Halloran DJ, Bloom SR. Elevated plasma endothelin in patients with diabetes mellitus. *Diabetologia*. 1990;33(5):306-10.

46. Rees RW, Ziessen T, Ralph DJ, Kell P, Moncada S, Cellek S. Human and rabbit cavernosal smooth muscle cells express Rho-kinase. *Int J Impot Res*. 2002;14(1):1-7.

47. Foresta C, Caretta N, Aversa A, Bettocchi C, Corona G, Mariani S, et al. Erectile dysfunction: symptom or disease? *J Endocrinol Invest*. 2004;27(1):80-95.

48. Foresta C, Caretta N, Corona G, Fabbri A, Francavilla S, Jannini E, et al. Clinical and metabolic evaluation of subjects with erectile dysfunction: a review with a proposal flowchart. *Int J Androl*. 2009;32(3):198-211.

49. Fung MM, Bettencourt R, Barrett-Connor E. Heart disease risk factors predict erectile dysfunction 25 years later: the Rancho Bernardo Study. *J Am Coll Cardiol*. 2004;43(8): 1405-11.

50. Yamasaki H, Ogawa K, Sasaki H, Nakato T, Wakasaki H, Matsumoto E, et al. Prevalence and risk factors of erectile dysfunction in Japanese men with type 2 diabetes. *Diabetes Res Clin Pract*. 2004;66 Suppl 1: S173-7.

51. Hecht MJ, Neundörfer B, Kiesewetter F, Hilz MJ. Neuropathy is a major contributing factor to diabetic erectile dysfunction. *Neurol Res*. 2001;23(6):651-4.

52. Pegge NC, Twomey AM, Vaughton K, Gravenor MB, Ramsey MW, Price DE. The role of endothelial dysfunction in the pathophysiology of erectile dysfunction in diabetes and in determining response to treatment. *Diabet Med*. 2006;23(8):651-4.

53. Debono M, Cachia E, Cassar A, Calleja N, Mallia M, Vassallo J. Is erectile dysfunction a sentinel symptom for cardiovascular autonomic neuropathy in patients with type 2 diabetes? *Andrologia*. 2008;40(1):1-6.

54. Corona G, Mannucci E, Petrone L, Ricca V, Balercia G, Mansani R, et al. Association of hypogonadism and type 2 diabetes in men attending an outpatient erectile dysfunction clinic. *Int J Impot Res*. 2006;18(2):190-7.

55. Kapoor D, Aldred H, Clark S, Channer KS, Jones TH. Clinical and biochemical assessment of hypogonadism in men with type 2 diabetes: correlations with bioavailable testosterone and visceral adiposity. *Diabetes Care*. 2007;30(4):911-7.

56. Kapoor D, Clarke S, Channer KS, Jones TH. Erectile dysfunction is associated with low bioactive testosterone levels and visceral adiposity in men with type 2 diabetes. *Int J Androl*. 2007;30(6):500-7.

57. Burning JC, Gautam D, Burks DJ, Gillette J, Schubert M, Orban PC, et al. Role of brain insulin receptor in control of body weight and reproduction. *Science*. 2000;289(5487):2122-5.

58. Thomas A, Woodard C, Rovner ES, Wein AJ. Urologic complications of nonurologic medications. *Urol Clin North Am*. 2003;30(1):123-31.

59. Baumhäkel M, Schlimmer N, Kratz M, Hackett G, Jackson G, Böhm M. Cardiovascular risk, drugs and erectile dysfunction–a systematic analysis. *Int J Clin Pract*. 2011;65(3):289-98.

60. Derby CA, Mohr BA, Goldstein I, Feldman HA, Johannes CB, McKinlay JB. Modifiable risk factors and erectile dysfunction: can lifestyle changes modify risk? *Urology*. 2000; 56(2):302-6.

61. Hannan JL, Maio MT, Komolova M, Adams MA. Beneficial impact of exercise and obesity interventions on erectile dysfunction and its risk factors. *J Sex Med*. 2009;6 Suppl 3:254-61.

62. Manning DM, Klevens RM, Flanders WD. Cigarette smoking: an independent risk factor for impotence? *Am J Epidemiol*. 1994;140(11):1003-8.

63. Guay AT, Perez JB, Heatley GJ. Cessation of smoking rapidly decrease erectile dysfunction. *Endocr Pract.* 1998;4(1):23-6.

64. Maio G, Saraeb S, Marchiori A. Physical activity and PDE5 inhibitors in the treatment of erectile dysfunction: results of a randomized controlled study. *J Sex Med.* 2010;7(6):2201-8.

65. Gupta BP, Murad MH, Clifton MM, Prokop L, Nehra A, Kopecky SL. The effect of lifestyle modification and cardiovascular risk factor reduction on erectile dysfunction: a systematic review and meta-analysis. *Arch Intern Med.* 2011;171(20):1297-803.

66. Wing RR, Rosen RC, Fava JL, Bahnson J, Brancati F, Gendrano Iii IN, et al. Effects of weight loss intervention on erectile function in older men with type 2 diabetes in the Look AHEAD trial. *J Sex Med.* 2010;7(1 Pt 1):156-65.

67. Montorsi P, Ravagnani PM, Galli S, Salonia A, Briganti A, Werba JP, et al. Association between erectile dysfunction and coronary artery disease: Matching the right target with the right test in the right patient. *Eur Urol.* 2006;50(4):721-31.

68. Goldstein I, Young JM, Fischer J, Bangerter K, Segerson T, Taylor T; Vardenafil Diabetes Study Group. Vardenafil, a new phosphodiesterase type 5 inhibitor, in the treatment of erectile dysfunction in men with diabetes: a multicenter double-blind placebo-controlled fixed-dose study. *Diabetes Care.* 2003;26(3):777-83.

69. Rendell MS, Rajfer J, Wicker PA, Smith MD. Sildenafil for treatment of erectile dysfunction in men with diabetes: a randomized controlled trial. Sildenafil Diabetes Study Group. *JAMA.* 1999;281(5):421-6.

70. Fink HA, Mac Donald R, Rutks IR, Nelson DB, Wilt TJ. Sildenafil for male erectile dysfunction: a systematic review and meta-analysis. *Arch Intern Med.* 2002;162(12): 1349-60.

71. Fonseca V, Seftel A, Denne J, Fredlund P. Impact of diabetes mellitus on the severity of erectile dysfunction and response to treatment: analysis of data from tadalafil clinical trials. *Diabetologia.* 2004;47(11):1914-23.

72. Buvat J, van Ahlen H, Schmitt H, Chan M, Kuepfer C, Varanese L. Efficacy and safety of two dosing regimens of tadalafil and patterns of sexual activity in men with diabetes mellitus and erectile dysfunction: Scheduled use vs. on-demand regimen evaluation (SURE) study in European countries. *J Sex Med.* 2006;3(3):512-20.

73. Weinsaft JW, Hickey K, Bokhari S, Shahzad A, Bedding A, Costigan TM, et al. Effects of tadalafil on myocardial blood flow in patients with coronary artery disease. *Coron Artery Dis.* 2006;17(6):493-9.

74. Reffelmann T, Kloner RA. Cardiovascular effects of phosphodiesterase 5 inhibitors. *Curr Pharm Des.* 2006;12(27):3485-94.

75. Sesti C, Florio V, Johnson EG, Kloner RA. The phosphodiesterase-5 inhibitor tadalafil reduces myocardial infarct size. *Int J Impot Res.* 2007;19(1):55-61.

76. Bocchio M, Pelliccione F, Passaquale G, Mihalca R, Necozione S, Desideri G, et al. Inhibition of phosphodiesterase type 5 with tadalafil is associated to an improved activity of circulating angiogenic cells in men with cardiovascular risk factors and erectile dysfunction. *Atherosclerosis.* 2008;196(1):313-9.

77. Traish AM, Guay A, Feeley R, Saad F. The dark side of testosterone deficiency: I. Metabolic syndrome and erectile dysfunction. *J Androl.* 2009;30(1):10-22.

78. Jain P, Rademaker AW, McVary KT. Testosterone supplementation for erectile dysfunction: results of a mete-analysis. *J Urol.* 2000;164(2):371-5.

79. Shabsigh R, Kaufman JM, Steidle C, Padma-Nathan H. Randomized study of testosterone gel as adjunctive therapy to sildenafil in hypogonadal men with erectile dysfunction who do not respond to sildenafil alone. *J Urol.* 2008;179(5 Suppl):S97-S102.

80. Susset JG, Tessier CD, Wincze J, Bansal S, Malhotra C, Schwacha MG. Effect of yombine hydrochloride on erectile impotence: a double-blind study. *J Urol.* 1989;141(6):1360-3.

81. Price DE, Cooksey G, Jehu D, Bentley S, Hearnshaw JR, Osborn DE. The management of impotence in diabetic men by vacuum tumescence therapy. *Diabet Med.* 1991;8(10): 964-7.

82. Glina S, Porst H. Vacuum constriction devices. In: Porst H, Buvat J, editors. Standard practice in sexual medicine. Malden, MA: Blackwell/ISSM; 2006. pp. 121-5.

83. Bettocchi C, Palumbo F, Spilotros M, Lucarelli G, Palazzo S, Battaglia M, et al. Patient and partner satisfaction after AMS inflatable penile prosthesis implant. *J Sex Med.* 2010;7 (1 Pt 1):304-9.

84. Montague DK, Angermeier KW, Lakin MM. Penile prosthesis infections. *Int J Impot Res.* 2001;13(6):326-8.

85. Althof SE, Dean J, Derogates LR, Rosen RC, Sisson M. Current perspectives on the clinical assessment and diagnosis of female sexual dysfunction and clinical studies of potential therapies: a statement of concern. *J Sex Med.* 2005;2 Suppl 3:146-53.

86. Erol B, Tefekli A, Sanli O, Ziylan O, Armagan A, Kendirci M, et al. Does sexual dysfunction correlates with deterioration of somatic sensory system in diabetic women? *Int J Impot Res.* 2003;15(3):198-202.

87. Errol B, Tefekli A, Ozbey I, Salman F, Dincag N, Kadioglu A, et al. Sexual dysfunction in type 2 diabetic females: a comparative study. *J Sex Marital Ther.* 2002;28 Suppl1:55-62.

88. Enzlin P, Mathieu C, Van den Bruel A, Bosteels J, Vanderschueren D, Demyttenaere K. Sexual dysfunction in women with type 1 diabetes: a controlled study. *Diabetes Care.* 2002;25(4):672-7.

89. Sobel JD, Chaim W, Nagapan V, Leaman D. Treatment of vaginitis caused by Candida glabrata: use of topical boric acid and flucytosine. *Am J Obstet Gynecol.* 2003;189(5): 1297-300.

90. Caruso S, Rugolo S, Agnello C, Intelisano G, Di Mari L, Cianci A. Sildenafil improves sexual functioning in premenopausal women with type 1 diabetes who are affected by sexual arousal disorder: a double-blind, crossover, placebo-controlled pilot study. *Fertil Steril.* 2006;85(5):1496-501.

91. Shamloul R, Ghanem H. Erectile dysfunction. *Lancet.* 2013;381:153-165.

92. Babaev A, Jhaveri RR. Angiography and endovascular revascularization of pudendal artery atherosclerotic disease in patients with medically refractory erectile dysfunction. *J Invasive Cardiol.* 2012;24(5):236-40.

93. Melman A, Bar-Chama N, McCullough A, Davies K, Christ G. hMaxi-K gene transfer in males with erectile dysfunction: results of the first human trial. *Hum Gene Ther.* 2006; 17(12):1165-76.

94. Xie D, Annex BH, Donatucci CF. Growth factors for therapeutic angiogenesis in hyper-cholesterolemic erectile dysfunction. *Asian J Androl.* 2008;10(1):23-7.

Management of Diabetes During Special Situations

19

Jayendra H Shah

ABSTRACT

Fasting of various degrees has been observed in many religions in the world as fasting is considered to provide spiritual upliftment and purification. The people following Jain religion in India is known to observe one day to one week of continuous fasting during religious days of "Per-u-shan". In Jewish religion people fast for 24 hours during Yom Kippur and Tisha B'Av, the Jewish calendar's holiest days. Some followers of Mormon religion (Latter Days Saints) fast one weekend day every month. People of Muslim faith fast during day time (sunrise to sunset) during holy month of Ramadan which is ninth month of Islamic lunar calendar. The fast of various degrees has implication on the management of diabetic patients, especially those who are managed with pharmacologic agents. Many diabetic patients disregard physician's advice not to participate in religious fasting. Furthermore, many of these diabetic patients are reluctant in taking their medications during fasting. Therefore, when patients insist on participating in religious fast, physician will be required to provide proper guideline to manage the patient's diabetes.

The jet age has created easy travel from continents to continents. For type 1 and type 2 diabetic patients taking insulin to manage hyperglycemia, long travel across the time zones may create confusion and difficulties in the management of their diabetes. Since traveling across the time zones either extends or shorten the hours (some times a day), travelling diabetics may need to adjust the medications to manage their diabetes. Preplanning and consultation with their health care providers may help diabetic patients in the management of their diabetes.

Working in irregular shift can create difficulties in management of patient with type 1 and 2 diabetes. A significant deterioration glycemic control and hypoglycemia has been observed in those diabetic patients who were assigned to a more rapidly rotating shift pattern.

In this chapter, the author reviews the important aspects of patient education, diet planning, adjustment of oral hypoglycemic agents and insulin dosage, and timing in the management of diabetic patients during the religious fasting, traveling through multiple time zones, and the shift changes.

Management of Diabetes During Religious Fasting

INTRODUCTION

Fasting of various degrees has been observed in many religions in the world as fasting is considered to provide spiritual upliftment and purification. The people following Jain religion in India are known to observe one day to one week of continuous fasting during religious days of *"Per-u-shan"*. In Jewish religion, people fast for 24 hours during *Yom Kippur* and *Tish B'Av*, the Jewish calendar's holiest days. Some followers of Mormon religion (Latter-Day Saint) fast one weekend day every month. People of Muslim faith fast during day time (sunrise to sunset) during holy month of *Ramadan* which is 9th month of Islamic lunar calendar. Because of the lunar calendar, *Ramadan* month precedes approximately 10 days every year and, therefore, it appears in different seasons of the year.[1] When *Ramadan* falls in summer, in the Western countries daylight may last longer (15–17 hours) and in winter shorter (8–10 hours). This has implication on diabetic patients, especially those who are managed with pharmacologic agents.

Most physicians would recommend diabetic patient (especially type 1) not to participate in the religious fast. Also, religious authorities of all religions have made exception and exempted diabetic and other ill persons for not fasting due to medical reasons.[2] However, many diabetic patients disregard this advice and participate in religious fasting. Furthermore, many of these diabetic patients are reluctant in taking their medications during fasting. Therefore, when patients insist on participating in religious fast, physician will be required to provide proper guideline to manage the patients diabetes. There are few controlled studies conducted to examine implication of religious fasting in diabetic patients. Many published reports are survey oriented and mainly provided review and guidelines for fasting during *Ramadan*.[2-6]

PATHOPHYSIOLOGY OF FASTING

During fasting, insulin levels are decreased and an increase in counter-regulatory hormones, such as glucagon and catecholamines occur which cause glycogenolysis, gluconeogenesis, and lipolysis. Once glycogen stores are depleted, the increased gluconeogenesis and lipolysis results in increased free fatty acids and ketones which are used as alternative energy source by various tissues in the body. In healthy persons, significant rise in high-density lipoprotein (HDL) cholesterol has been observed during *Ramadan* fasting which is reverted to its previous level after the fast.[7,8] The period of 6–24 hours after initiation of fast, can be described as postabsorptive phase; the period of 2–10 days since beginning of fast can be described as gluconeogenic phase and the period beyond 10 days of fasting can be described as protein conservation phase.[9] In healthy individuals without diabetes, a balance between insulin and counter-regulatory hormones help maintain glucose levels in physiological range. In type 1 diabetic patients and insulin requiring type 2 diabetic patients, fasting may further exacerbate gluconeogenesis, lipolysis, and ketosis if patient refrains from taking any exogenous insulin. This may precipitate hyperglycemia and ketoacidosis along with dehydration.[10] On the other hand, if type 1 and insulin requiring type 2 diabetic patients continue to take insulin and/ or oral hypoglycemic agents, they may experience significant hypoglycemia.[10,11] Furthermore, in diabetic patients, especially in type 1, counter-regulatory hormone response due to autonomic neuropathy may not occur appropriately causing hypoglycemia.

In obese type 2 diabetic patients who are managed on diet alone actually may benefit by fasting. These patients have insulin resistance with elevated levels of circulating insulin. Fasting may actually reduce insulin resistance in such patients.[12] It is interesting to note that Horne et al. in their study on the followers of Latter-Day Saint showed that those who followed routine periodic fast have a lower risk of coronary artery disease.[13] However, in a population-based study of *Ramadan* fasting showed no difference in acute coronary syndrome during *Ramadan* when compared with other months.[14]

MANAGEMENT OF TYPE 1 DIABETES DURING FASTING

It is advisable that patients with type 1 diabetes should not participate in religious fasting. If patient insist on fasting, then it is essential to clearly educate and explain the patient and family members about how to manage diabetes during fasting, importance of taking basal insulin, and potential risks of hypo- and hyperglycemia while fasting. Basal insulin will prevent hyperglycemia by controlling glycogenolysis, gluconeogenesis, and ketosis. Longer-acting insulin like glargine or detemir dose should be reduced to one-half or one-third the daily dose patient has been taking prior to fasting (Table 1). Since patient would not be eating during the fast, there will be no need to administer prandial doses of rapid-acting insulin. Those patients who are taking intermediate-acting insulin or 70/30 mix insulin should be switched to long-acting insulin during the fast. The patients on insulin pump should reduce the basal rate by 20% with further adjustment and reduction in the basal rate as fasting progresses. The type 1 diabetic patients are advised not to participate in more than 24 hours of continuous fasting.

Patient participating in *Ramadan* fast may reduce the basal insulin dose and continue to take prandial, fast-acting insulin at meal time appropriately. We recommend that those patients who are on 70/30 mix or intermediate insulin regimen should decrease their insulin dose by 20% initially (Table 1). The insulin dosing should be taken in relation to night meals. It is imperative that frequent SMBG is essential for glycemic management and detecting hypoglycemia especially in those who have difficulty in perceiving hypoglycemic symptoms. It is important to note that tachycardia and hypotension caused by dehydration can be mistaken

TABLE 1: Guidelines for Management of Diabetic Patients Treated with Insulin During Religious Fasting

Prefasting treatment	During 24-hour fasting	During Ramadan fasting
Long-acting (basal) insulin (e.g., glargine or levemir) and fast-acting (prandial) insulin (e.g., aspart)	One-third usual dose of long-acting (basal) insulin at the same time. Since patient is fasting no need to take prandial (fast acting) insulin	Take 80% of usual long-acting (basal) insulin and appropriate dose of prandial (fast-acting) insulin for sunset meal (slightly reduced dose for sunrise meal)
Intermediate-acting insulin (e.g., NPH)	One-third usual morning dose or once a day dose in morning	• For patient taking once a day dose of NPH take 80% of usual dose before sunset meal • For patient taking NPH twice a day, take usual morning dose prior to sunset meal and one-half usual evening dose prior to sunrise meal
70/30 mix insulin twice a day	One-third dose of long acting portion of insulin in the morning*	Take usual 70/30 insulin morning dose before sunset meal and half of usual evening dose before sunrise meal. Or, if possible, switch insulin regimen to basal (long-acting) and prandial (fast-acting) insulin

NHP, neutral protamine hagedorn.
*For example if patient is taking 30 units of 70/30 insulin in morning then 70% long acting is 21 units. One third dose of 21 units is 7 units.

as hypoglycemia. Therefore, proper hydration of the patient is also essential during the fast. Obviously, fasting should be aborted if significant hypoglycemia ensues. Also, in any type of religious fasting, if monitored blood glucose level cannot be kept under 300 mg/dL (16.7 mmol/L) or at occurrence of hypoglycemia, the fast should be terminated.[2]

It is recommended that pregnant patients with type 1 diabetes should not fast due to deleterious effect on the fetus due to hypo- and hyperglycemia. Infection with fever in diabetic patients may precipitate sever hyperglycemia and even ketoacidosis and, therefore, advised to refrain from fasting. The diabetic patient with significant renal impairment (stage-4 chronic renal disease) is prone to hyperglycemia and hypoglycemia and, therefore, advised to refrain from religious fasting. Furthermore, in these patients, clearance of oral hypoglycemic agent is often delayed and unpredictable making it difficult to provide appropriate advice on taking medications. Diabetic patients who have recently suffered acute illness (e.g., cerebrovascular accident, acute myocardial infarction, major surgical procedure, etc.) are also advised not to participate in the religious fasting.

MANAGEMENT OF TYPE 2 DIABETES DURING FASTING

Type 2 diabetic patients who are managed by diet therapy only may continue to participate in the fast without much concern. The type 2 diabetic patients who are observing one day fast and taking sulfonylureas (glyburide, glipizide, and glimepiride), long-acting incretin mimetics (liraglutide), and dipeptidyl peptidase-4 (DPP-4) inhibitor (sitagliptin and saxagliptin) should be advised not to take the medication 24 hour before and on the day of fast (Table 2). Patients who are taking thiazolidinediones (TZD) (pioglitazone and rosiglitazone), metformin, short-acting incretin mimetic (exenatide), and meglitinides (repaglinide and nateglinide) should be advised not to take these medications on the day of fast. Patients who are taking insulin to control hyperglycemia should be advised to take one-third dose of the long-acting or intermediate-acting insulin to prevent hyperglycemia. Patients should refrain on taking fast-acting insulin on the day of fast. More than 24 hour fast is not advisable for these patients.

The patients observing *Ramadan* should be advised to switch the dosing of medication to be effective during night. In general, for metformin, two-thirds of the metformin dose should be taken at sunset and one-third dose taken at sunrise (Table 2), coinciding with the meals taken around those times.[2,5] No adjustment in the doses of TZD is needed during the *Ramadan* fast, if the medications are taken alone. If TZDs are taken with other oral agents (sulfonylureas and metformin) then the dose should be divided to be taken at sunset and sunrise, coinciding with the meals. Long-acting sulfonylurea drugs (glyburide and glipizide) should be used with caution as patients may become hypoglycemic during fasting hours. In general, it is recommended taking daily dose or decrease the dose to 75% of daily dose taken at sunset before meal. If patient is taking twice a day dose of sulfonylurea, then daily morning dose should be taken prior to sunset meal and one-half of the daily evening dose should be taken prior to sunrise meal during *Ramadan* fasting (Table 2). Alternatively, patients can be switched to short-acting prandial medications, such as repaglinide during the fasting days of *Ramadan*. Type 2 diabetic patients who are managed on insulin are advised to decrease the dose to 80% of daily dose coinciding with meals taken after sunset and prior to sunrise (Table 1). In type 2 diabetic patients also, if blood glucose cannot be maintained under 300 mg/dL (16.7 mmol/L) or at the occurrence of hypoglycemia, the fast should be terminated.[2]

It is important that appropriate self-monitoring of blood glucose (SMBG) should be done in type 2 diabetic patients during the fast. Also, proper hydration during the fasting is a must to prevent postural hypotension, which may mimic symptoms of hypoglycemia.

The diabetic patients may be taking medication to manage other diseases, such as heart disease and hypertension. It is advisable not to take any medications on the day of 24 hour fast unless it is unsafe to avoid those medications (such as anticoagulants).[4] Other exception are beta blockers and clonidine taken to manage

TABLE 2: Guidelines for Management of Type 2 Diabetic Patients Treated with Oral Agents During Religious Fasting

Prefasting treatment	During 24-hour fasting	During Ramadan fasting
Biguanide (metformin)	Last dose at meal prior to fasting. No dose on the day of fasting	Two-thirds or three-fourths daily dose with sunset meal and rest with sunrise meal
Incretin mimetic short-acting (exenatide)	Last dose at meal prior to fasting. No dose on the day of fasting	Usual main meal dose coinciding with sunset meal. Consider reducing dose with sunrise meal if exenatide is taken twice a day
Incretin mimetic long-acting (liraglutide)	Last dose at meal prior to fasting. No dose on the day of fasting	No clear guideline is available. Consider switching to short-acting drug
Dipeptidyl peptidase-4 inhibitors (e.g., sitagliptin, saxagliptin)	Last dose at meal prior to fasting. No dose on the day of fasting	No clear guideline is available. Use with caution. Consider decreasing the dose
Thiazolidinediones (rosiglitazone, pioglitazone)	Last dose at meal prior to fasting. No dose on the day of fasting	Continue prefasting treatment
Sulfonylurea (glyburide, glimepiride, glipizide)	Last dose 24–48 hours before starting fasting depending on renal function and patient's age. No dose on the day of fasting	• Take once a day dose (or 75% of daily dose) before sunset meal and adjust the dose according to glycemic control • For twice a day dose, take usual morning dose before sunset meal and one-half usual evening dose before sunrise meal
Meglitinides (repaglinide, nateglinide)	Last dose at meal prior to fasting. No dose on the day of fasting	No change in premeal dose for sunset meal. Adjust sunrise meal dose to prevent hypoglycemia during daytime
Alpha glucosidase inhibitors (e.g., acarbose, miglitol)	Last dose at meal prior to fasting. No dose on the day of fasting	Continue prefasting treatment

hypertension as rebound hypertension may ensue if these medications are not taken. It is recommended to reduce the dose of these drugs during the fast to prevent precipitation of hypotension caused by dehydration during fasting.[4] The diabetic patients taking medications for arrhythmias, angina, and congestive heart failure should continue their medications. The patients should be advised the need for proper hydration to prevent hypoglycemia.

CONCLUSION

Religious fasting is recommended in many religions for spiritual upliftment and purification. For these reasons, many patients with diabetes want to participate in the religious fasting. It is important for physicians and other health care providers to make assessment of these patients prior to the fast and provide them proper guidance. In order to provide appropriate guidelines to the patients, health care providers should have good understanding of the pathophysiology of fasting in healthy people and in patients with type 1 and 2 diabetes. In general, patients with type 1 diabetes should be advised not to participate in continuous religious fasting beyond 24 hours. Pregnant type 1 diabetic patient, diabetic patient with marked renal failure, patients with concurrent infection with fever and those with recent serious illness (cerebrovascular accident, acute myocardial infarction, etc.) or those who have undergone major surgical procedure must not participate in the religious fasting. It is relatively easy to manage the patients who participate in "day light" fasting during the religious month of *Ramadan* as patients are permitted to eat from sunset to sunrise. With appropriate guidelines, most of the diabetic patients can be managed during the *Ramadan* fasting. The diabetic patients observing the fast should maintain hydration to prevent orthostatic hypotension and tachycardia mimicking the symptoms of hypoglycemia. Physicians and other health care providers should be aware of coexisting conditions in diabetic patient to provide proper management guidelines. Appropriate patient education, diet planning, hydration, oral adjustment of hypoglycemic agents, and insulin dosage and timing are important aspects in the management of diabetic patients during religious fasting.

Management of Diabetes During Travel Through Multiple Time Zones

The jet age has created easy traveling from continent to continent. For type 1 and type 2 diabetic patients taking insulin to manage hyperglycemia, long travel across the time zones may create confusion and difficulties in the management of their diabetes. Driessen et al. in their survey of insulin-taking diabetic patients showed that only 36% of the patients increased SMBG to help manage their diabetes and majority of patients (68%) experienced metabolic derangements.[15] Since traveling across the time zones either extend or shorten the hours (some times a day), travelling diabetic may need to adjust the management of their diabetes. Preplanning and consultation with their health care providers may help diabetic patients in the management of their diabetes.

In general, a reduction in insulin dose is required during eastward travel across several time zones which shorten the day; and an increase in the insulin dose is required during westward travel which extends the day. However, a significant change in the insulin dose may not be required if travel is confined to less than five time zones.

In patients who are taking basal, long-acting, and multiple doses of prandial, fast-acting insulin, an adjustment in the dose and timing is flexible and easy. However, patients on twice a day regimen of 70/30 mix insulin, it may pose some difficulties in the glycemic management of diabetes because the time and number of meal may vary during the air travel. Some relaxation in the glycemic control is better than risking hypoglycemia under such situation. Usually a patient taking once a day sulfonylurea, metformin, or other oral diabetic medication does not require any special adjustment as long as they eat the meals following ingestion of medication. An adjustment in the dose of twice a day sulfonylurea medication may require to prevent hypoglycemia.

The diabetic traveler should be advised to pack in carry-on handbag glucose meter, adequate number of strips and lancets, enough insulin in cold bag, insulin syringes with needles or insulin pen, rapid acting carbohydrates (glucose tablets), complex carbohydrates (cereal bars, crackers) and ideally duplicate supplies in another (companion's) carry-on bag. The patient should be advised that it is essential to prevent hypoglycemia and intensive glycemic control should be relaxed. The patient should be advised to SMBG every 4–6 hours to maintain blood glucose between 150 and 200 mg/dL (8.3 and 11.1 mmol/L). In temperate countries, insulin is stable at room temperature. However, in tropical climate, it is advisable to keep insulin in refrigerator or carry it in the cool bag. Patients should be advised that insulin is absorbed more rapidly in hot weather as well as during outdoor physical activity increasing risk of hypoglycemia.

The patients with diabetes may become ill with gastroenteritis or upper respiratory infections during foreign travel, which is not uncommon. Frequently, when diabetic patients are ill they stop taking insulin. In diabetic patients with gastroenteritis, if unable to keep food and fluid intake, leads to dehydration. Not taking insulin further complicates the diabetic state and may precipitate ketoacidosis and/or hyperosmolar state. Therefore, diabetic patients should be advised that under such circumstances insulin, in the reduced dose, must be taken to prevent ketosis and ketoacidosis. Proper hydration is also essential to prevent dehydration and its consequences.

Management of Diabetes During Shift Work

It has been postulated that shift work in an individual may precipitate type 2 diabetes and metabolic syndrome.[16] A long-term longitudinal Japanese study in 2,426 male workers performing alternating shift work and 3,203 male workers performing day shift work revealed that alternating shift work is an independent risk for development of diabetes, defined as increase in HbA1c.[17] Pan et al. followed 69,269 women (age 42–67 years) in Nurses' Health Study (NHS)-I (1988–2008) and 107,915 women (age 25–42 years) in NHS-II without diabetes, cardiovascular disease and cancer at baseline.[18] They observed increased risk of type 2 diabetes in women with extended period of night shift work. It was hypothesized that disruption of circadian rhythm associated obesity, insulin resistance and lack of exercise may have played a role in the development of diabetes in these women.[18,19]

Working in irregular shift can create difficulties in management of the disease in patient with type 1 and 2 diabetes. A significant deterioration glycemic control has been observed in those diabetic patients who were assigned to a more rapidly rotating shift pattern.[20] Under these circumstances, in type 1 diabetic patients and insulin requiring type 2 diabetes, the treatment with basal (long-acting) insulin and prandial (fast-acting) insulin would be useful. The basal insulin can be taken in the morning or in the evening regardless of shift pattern. The prandial insulin can coincide with the meals taken during the shift. The patient should be advised to perform frequent SMBG to assess blood glucose pattern to adjust the insulin dose. Meal planning is also important during shift work. During the shift, a consistent meal type which is spaced at 4–5 hours apart is essential to match physical activity during work. Insulin dose should be matched accordingly. If the work during the shift demands much physical activities then adjustment of food intake (meals and snacks) and the insulin dose is required to prevent hypoglycemia. It is difficult to manage diabetes during the shift work with 70/30 mix insulin and, therefore, we recommend switching such patients to long-acting basal and fast-acting-prandial insulin combination.

REFERENCES

1. Fazel M. Medical implications of controlled fasting. *J R Soc Med*. 1998;91(5):260-3.
2. Karamat MA, Syed A, Hanif W. Review of diabetes management and guideline during Ramadan. *J R Soc Med*. 2010;103(4):139-47.
3. Benaji B, Mounib N, Roky R, Aadil N, Houti IE, Moussamih S, et al. Diabetes and Ramadan: Review of the literature. *Diabetes Res Clin Pract*. 2006;73(2):117-25.
4. Grajower MM. 24-Hour Fasting with Diabetes: guide to physicians advising patients on medication adjustments prior to religious observances (or outpatient surgical procedures). *Diabetes Metab Res Rev*. 2011;27(5):413-8.
5. Al-Arouj M, Assaad-Khalil S, Buse J, Fahdil I, Fahmy M, Hafez S, et al. Recommendations for management of diabetes during Ramadan. *Diabetes Care*. 2010;33(8):1895-902.
6. Hui E, Devendra D. Diabetes and Fasting During Ramadan. *Diabetes Metab Res Rev*. 2010;26(8):606-10.
7. Ziaee V, Razaei M, Ahmadinejad Z, Shaikh H, Yousefi R, Yarmohammadi L, et al. The changes of metabolic profile and weight during Ramadan fasting. *Singapore Med J*. 2006; 47(5):409-14.
8. Mafauzy M, Mohammed WB, Anum MY, Zulkifli A, Ruhani AH. A study of the fasting diabetic patients during the month of Ramadan. *Med J Malaysia*. 1990;45(1):14-17.
9. Felig P. Starvation. In: De-Groot L, Jameson JL, editors. Endocrinology. New York: Grune & Stratton; 1979. pp. 1927-40.
10. Salti I, Bénard E, Detournay B, Bianchi-Biscay M, Le Brigand C, Voinet C, et al. A population-based study of diabetes and its characteristics during the fasting month of Ramadan in 13 countries: results of the epidemiology of diabetes and Ramadan 1422/2001 (EPIDIAR) Study. *Diabetes Care*. 2004;27(10):2306-11.

11. Cesur M, Corapcioglu D, Gursoy A, Gonen S, Ozduman M, Emral R, et al. A comparison of glycemic effects of glimepiride, repaglinide, and insulin glargine in type 2 diabetes mellitus during Ramadan fasting. *Diabetes Res Clin Pract.* 2007;75(2):141-7.
12. Greenfield M, Kolterman O, Olefsky JM, Reaven GM. The effect of ten days of fasting on various aspects of carbohydrate metabolism in obese diabetic subjects with significant fasting hyperglycemia. *Metabolism.* 1978;27(12 Suppl. 2):1839-52.
13. Horne BD, May HT, Anderson JL, Kfoury AG, Bailey BM, McClure BS, et al. Usefulness of routine periodic fasting to lower risk of coronary artery disease in patients undergoing coronary angiography. *Am J Cardiol.* 2008;102(7):814-9.
14. Al Suwaidi J, Bener A, Suliman A, Hajar R, Salam AM, Numan MT, et al. A population based study of Ramadan fasting and acute coronary syndromes. *Heart.* 2004;90(6):695-6.
15. Driessen SO, Cobelens FG, Ligthelm RJ. Travel-related morbidity in travelers with insulin-dependent diabetes mellitus. *J Travel Med.* 1999;6(1):12-5.
16. Knutsson A. Health disorders of shift workers. *Occup Med (Lond).* 2003;53(2):103-8.
17. Yasushi S, Kouichi S, Yasushi O, et al. Long-term longitudinal study on the relationship between Alternating shift work and the onset of diabetes mellitus in male Japanese workers. *J Occup Environ Med.* 2006;48:455-61.
18. Pan A, Schernhammer E, Sun Q, Hu F. Rotating night shift work and risk of type 2 diabetes: two prospective cohort studies in women. *PLoS Med.* 2011;8(12):e1001141.
19. Kivimäki M, Batty GD, Hublin C. Shift work as a risk factor for future type 2 diabetes: evidence, mechanisms, implications, and future research directions. *PLoS Med.* 2011; 8(12):e1001138.
20. Poole CJ, Wright AD, Nattrass M. Control of diabetes mellitus in shift workers. *Br J Ind Med.* 1992;49(7):513-5.

Index

Please note page numbers with *f* and *t* indicate figure and table, respectively.